PSYCHOLOGICAL MANAGEMENT OF PEDIATRIC PROBLEMS

Volume I
Early Life Conditions and Chronic Diseases

PSYCHOLOGICAL MANAGEMENT OF PEDIATRIC PROBLEMS

Volume I
Early Life Conditions and Chronic Diseases

Edited by

Phyllis R. Magrab, Ph.D.

Associate Professor
Department of Pediatrics
Georgetown University

University Park Press
Baltimore

UNIVERSITY PARK PRESS
International Publishers in Science and Medicine
233 East Redwood Street
Baltimore, Maryland 21202

Typeset by American Graphic Arts Corporation.
Manufactured in the United States of America by
Universal Lithographers, Inc.,
and The Optic Bindery Incorporated.

PSYCHOLOGICAL MANAGEMENT OF PEDIATRIC PROBLEMS
Published in two volumes:
Volume I: **Early Life Conditions and Chronic Diseases**
Volume II: **Sensorineural Conditions and Social Concerns**

Library of Congress Cataloging in Publication Data
Main entry under title:
Psychological management of pediatric problems.

Bibliography: p.
Includes indexes.
CONTENTS: v. 1. Early life conditions and chronic
diseases.—v. 2. Sensorineural conditions and social concerns.
1. Sick children—Psychology. 2. Chronic diseases
in children—Psychological aspects. 3. Child psychiatry.
4. Pediatric neurology. I. Magrab, Phyllis R.
[DNLM: 1. Child psychology. 2. Child development
deviations—Therapy. 3. Pediatrics. WS100.3 P974]
RJ47.5.P78   618.9′2′00019   78-3880

ISBN 0-8391-1218-1 (v. 1)

Contents

vi   Contents

Contents of Volume II

Contributors

Eleanor B. Alter, J. D. (II), Marshall, Bratter, Greene, Allison, and Tucker, Attys, 430 Park Avenue, New York, New York 10022

Ida Sue Baron, Ph.D. (II), Director, Neuropsychology Research Laboratory, Departments of Neurosurgery and Neurology, Children's Hospital National Medical Center; Assistant Professor of Psychiatry and Behavioral Sciences, and of Child Health and Development, George Washington University School of Medicine, Washington, D.C. 20009

Suzanne Pochter Bronheim, M.A. (I), Psychologist, Georgetown University Child Development Center, Washington, D.C. 20007

Philip L. Calcagno, M.D. (I), Professor and Chairman, Department of Pediatrics, Georgetown University, Washington, D.C. 20007

B. Patrick Cox, Ph.D. (II), Assistant Professor of Pediatrics, Georgetown University; Director of Training and Chief Audiologist, Georgetown University Child Development Center, Washington, D.C. 20007

Mary Kate Davitt, M.D. (I), Assistant Professor of Pediatrics, Georgetown University; Director of Neonatology, Georgetown University Hospital, Washington, D.C. 20007

Patricia Edelin, M.A. (II), Assistant Professor of Psychology, Gallaudet College, Washington, D.C. 20002

Ann M. Garner, Ph.D. (I), Professor of Medical Psychology, University of Oregon Health Sciences Center; Training Director of Psychology, Crippled Children's Division, Portland, Oregon 97207

Stephen E. Goldston, Ed.D., M.S.P.H. (I), Coordinator of Primary Prevention, National Institute of Mental Health, Rockville, Maryland 20857

Kathy S. Katz, Ph.D. (I), Instructor of Pediatrics, Georgetown University; Psychologist, Georgetown University Child Development Center, Washington, D.C. 20007

Gerald P. Koocher, Ph.D. (I), Instructor of Psychology, Harvard University Medical School; Chief Psychologist, Sidney Farber Cancer Institute, Boston, Massachusetts 02115

Henry Leland, Ph.D. (II), Professor of Psychology, Ohio State University; Director of Psychology, Nisonger Center for Mental Retardation, Columbus, Ohio 43210

Thomas R. Linscheid, Ph.D. (I), Assistant Professor of Pediatrics, Georgetown University; Director of Psychology, Georgetown University Child Development Center, Washington, D.C. 20007

Phyllis R. Magrab, Ph.D. (I, II), Associate Professor of Pediatrics, Georgetown University; Director, Georgetown University Child Development Center; Chief Pediatric Psychologist, Georgetown University Hospital, Washington, D.C. 20007

John H. Meier, Ph.D. (II), Director, Children's Village USA, Beaumont, California 92223

Zoe L. Papadopoulou, M.D. (I), Assistant Professor of Pediatrics, Georgetown University; Director, Pediatric Hemodialysis Unit, Georgetown University Hospital, Washington, D.C. 20007

Patricia O. Quinn, M.D. (I), Instructor of Pediatrics, Georgetown University; Director of Medicine, Georgetown University Child Development Center, Washington, D.C. 20007

Donald K. Routh, Ph.D. (II), Professor of Psychology, University of Iowa, Iowa City, Iowa 52242

Lee Salk, Ph.D. (I), Professor of Psychology in Psychiatry and Pediatrics, Cornell University Medical College; Pediatric Psychologist, Lenox Hill Hospital; Attending Psychologist, The New York Hospital, Payne Witney Clinic, New York, New York 10028

Stephen E. Sallan, M.D. (I), Assistant Professor of Pediatrics, Harvard University Medical School; Senior Clinical Associate, Sidney Farber Cancer Institute, Boston, Massachusetts 02115

Milton F. Shore, Ph.D. (I), Adjunct Professor of Psychology, Catholic University of America, Washington, D.C.; Associate Chief, Mental Health Study Center, National Institute of Mental Health, Adelphi, Maryland 20783

Anita Miller Sostek, Ph.D. (I), Instructor of Pediatrics, Research Psychologist, Division of Newborn Medicine, Georgetown University, Washington, D.C. 20007

Ellidee D. Thomas, M.D. (II), Professor of Pediatrics, University of Oklahoma Health Sciences Center; Director, Child Study Center, Oklahoma Children's Memorial Hospital, Oklahoma City, Oklahoma 73126

Clare W. Thompson, Ph.D. (I), Emeritus Professor of Psychology, Washington State University, Pullman, Washington; Clinical Psychologist, San Francisco, California

C. Eugene Walker, Ph.D. (I), Associate Professor of Clinical Psychology, Chief, Pediatric Psychologist, University of Oklahoma Health Sciences Center, Oklahoma City, Oklahoma 73190

Gertrude J. Williams, Ph.D. (II), Clinical Psychologist, 11 South Meramer Avenue, St. Louis, Missouri 63105

Diane J. Willis, Ph.D. (II), Associate Professor of Pediatrics, University of Oklahoma Health Sciences Center; Chief of Pediatric Psychological Services, Child Study Center, Oklahoma Children's Memorial Hospital, Oklahoma City, Oklahoma 73117

Preface

Be near
Through life's first mist;
For dark nights' fear
A forehead kissed;

For a family torn,
A sightless son,
A child stillborn;
For a world undone.

Grant Peters

Thousands of children are born each year whose potential for optimal development is challenged by one of the many diseases and chronic conditions of childhood. As we strive to develop new treatments and more effective preventions for childhood illness, we must simultaneously attend to the emotional as well as the medical needs of our affected children. Childhood conditions vary dramatically in their severity and impact on the quality of life of the child and his family. The medical and mental health community is confronted with a complex set of issues in providing adequate care and must respond to the uniqueness of each individual and each condition. Nonetheless, there is a growing body of knowledge and research that can guide us in our management of these patients and families.

It is the purpose of this two-volume series to raise those issues that generally affect the quality of psychological care of pediatric patients and to share the fund of knowledge extant. A variety of prevalent pediatric conditions ranging from mild to severe in their manifestations has been selected to illustrate the needs of pediatric patients. Volume I presents general issues related to mental health aspects of pediatric care as well as specific chapters on early life conditions and chronic diseases, including renal disease, diabetes, oncology, and pulmonary conditions. Volume II focuses on sensorineural conditions such as retardation, hyperactivity, hearing disorders, seizures, and social concerns such as child abuse and divorce. In each chapter a thorough review of current practices in care and intervention and of relevant research is emphasized. Pediatricians, psychologists, psychiatrists, nurses, social workers, and other health-related professionals can benefit from the scholarly review of this information provided by their colleagues in these volumes. Our clinical practice of care must parallel our most advanced knowledge.

My own experiences over the last decade in a pediatric setting have enriched my sensitivity to the needs of children with chronic conditions and to the needs of their families. I am indebted to my many co-workers who have shared their knowledge and human caring and to the many children who have been my mentors in reminding me of the ways of childhood and the special needs of special children. In particular I am grateful to Dr. Philip Calcagno, Chairman, Department of Pediatrics, Georgetown University, whose humanitarian approach to care and readiness to attend to the emotional needs of his patients have served as a model for all our faculty and as a profound source of support to me.

In the preparation of this text, I would like to acknowledge the many members of the Society for Pediatric Psychology who have provided insight and critical review of the material included. I appreciate, as well, the numerous hours of manuscript preparation by my dear friend and able assistant, Sherry Padgett Soliz, and her most competent associates, Donna Ratherdale and Debra Folberg.

Phyllis R. Magrab

Editor's note. Masculine pronouns are used throughout the volumes for the sake of grammatical uniformity and simplicity. They are not meant to be preferential or discriminatory.

To my three smiling, loving, caring children
Ryan
Kylee
Brendan
and my most cherished friend.

PSYCHOLOGICAL MANAGEMENT OF PEDIATRIC PROBLEMS

Volume I
Early Life Conditions and Chronic Diseases

GENERAL ISSUES

General issues in mental health care of pediatric patients include the effects of disease, medical care, and hospitalization on children and their families. Disruptions to the developmental process and socialization are discussed as well as a historical overview of changes in mental health care in hospitals and the community for pediatric medical conditions. The role of the pediatrician and his profound effect on child behavior and child-rearing practices are examined with respect to a variety of situations.

1
Psychological Impact of Chronic Pediatric Conditions

Phyllis R. Magrab and Philip L. Calcagno

The effect of long-term illness and chronic conditions on children and their families is pervasive. It impinges on the normal growth and development of the child, the process and quality of interrelationships, and the total family-life pattern. The duration, the severity, and the nature of the condition are all relevant parameters in determining the psychological effects of any chronic illness, but overriding as a source of extreme stress is the uncertainty that accompanies each day. Whether it be the quality of life, the threat of death, or a combination of the two, planning for the emotional and social well-being of the child and his family is a challenge to all pediatric health care professionals.

We have increased dramatically our ability to save and extend the lives of children as is evidenced in the new treatment and longer survival of renal patients, oncology patients, cystic fibrosis patients, and others. As a result the interrelationship between psychosocial functioning and the disease process has become an important consideration for health planners, who are beginning to document the effect of this interaction as well as the causation of disease by psychosocial stimuli (Kagan and Levi, 1974). In providing medical care, we must be responsive to patient and family needs, apply sound therapeutic techniques, and, importantly, be aware of the intense confrontation that arises with our own feelings of vulnerability. Long-term illness and chronic disease represent significant mental health issues to be studied systematically with the goal of providing optimal care to our children, thus enabling them to achieve their maximal physical, emotional, intellectual, and social potential.

PREVALENCE

The number of families affected by having a child with a chronic condition, defined here as any condition persisting more than three months, is

3

high. Mattson (1972) points to the staggering prevalence of chronic conditions in childhood; Stewart (1967) estimates that more than 30–40% of children up to the age of 18 suffer from one or more disorder, if visual and hearing impairments, mental retardation, speech, learning, and behavior disorders are included. Including only serious chronic illnesses, surveys still indicate that 7–10% of all children are afflicted (Rutter, Tizard, and Whitmore, 1968; Jennison, 1976; Pless, Satterwhite, and Van Vechten, 1976). The most common physical conditions apart from sensory defects are asthma (approximately 2% of the population under 18), epilepsy (1%), cardiac conditions (0.5%), cerebral palsy (0.5%), orthopaedic illnesses (0.5%), and diabetes mellitus (0.1%) (Mattson, 1972). Recent changes in the pattern of childhood morbidity, accompanied by a decline in acute illnesses, have increased the number of chronically ill children both absolutely and relatively, resulting in almost 50% of pediatric practice now being concerned with the chronically disabled child (Holt, 1972). As our health care system responds to the emotional and social needs of these children, the services implied must be developed in concert with the total growth of the child and the changes in survival patterns and treatment techniques.

SOCIALIZATION

In any discussion of child health, seeing the child as a part of a family unit is of pervasive importance. It is in the context of the family that the child develops socially, emotionally, and physically. Confronted with chronic illness and the accompanying stress, separation, and threat of death, families and children need substantial support in the child-rearing tasks essential to the development of the child.

A model of personality development proposed by Kagan (1971) suggests that the active process of socialization of the child is accomplished through four basic mechanisms: 1) the desire for affection and positive regard, 2) the fear of punishment or rejection, 3) the desire to identify with respected and admired persons, and 4) a general tendency to imitate the actions of others. When a chronic condition is superimposed on this process, the threats to the emotional needs of the child and to the family's ability to meet these needs usually distort and inhibit this process. For example, affection may be withheld or overindulged by parents. The pain, the procedures, and/or the separation of child from parents while in the hospital may be interpreted as punishment by the child. Parents, in an effort to compensate for the pain and suffering of the child, may respond with permissive attitudes and fewer delineations of rewards and punishments, thereby inhibiting social learning. The processes of identification and imitation can be subverted by the child's overriding sense of difference because of his illness or condition. The result may be a decreased tendency to socialize actively on the part of the child.

When a chronic illness intervenes, normal socialization is affected by the changes in the child's and family's behaviors and the impact of an altered life space. If one goal is facilitating the socialization process, then understanding responses of the child and family is a primary issue for mental health and health professionals caring for the chronically ill child and planning intervention programs.

IMPACT ON CHILDREN: DEVELOPMENTAL CONSIDERATIONS

The child at all ages is confronted with acquiring new skills through the continuous emergence of language, perceptual-motor, cognitive, and psychosocial functioning. This developmental process is shaped by the texture of the child's environment and its accompanying stresses and supports. The effects of aversive life conditions on a child, such as poor nutrition, inadequate caregiving, and deprivation of stimulation, are well known. Less well known is the impact of a chronic condition on the developmental process.

The normal child moves along the continuum from dependence to independence in psychosocial development, contingent upon simultaneous development of cognitive skills. Opportunities for exploration, peer relationships, and learning are integral aspects of this process. Stubblefield (1974) asserts that mastery of many of the frustrations and disappointments that normally occur in the various developmental periods is dependent upon the hope and expectations of the child that he will be older, stronger, and better able to solve his problems. What happens when a chronic condition inhibits opportunities and gives rise to self-doubts? How is the developmental process affected?

Although the effects of a chronic condition will vary significantly with the age of the child, Hughes (1976) suggests that there are eight basic emotional needs that become challenged: 1) love and affection, 2) security, 3) acceptance as an individual, 4) self-respect, 5) achievement, 6) recognition, 7) independence, and 8) authority and discipline. For the child with a chronic illness, fear of the unknown, of pain, and of death, feelings of weakness and difference, blocked achievement, increased dependence on parents and professionals, diminished discipline—all constitute major threats to these needs. His development may be influenced by feelings of rejection, lack of acceptance, hostility, or lack of affection. Restrictions in day-to-day experiences, interpersonal communication, mobility, self-care, activity level, education, and plans for career and marriage are other factors that will have major effects on the developmental process (Talbot and Howell, 1971).

Behaviorally, children respond to illness along the parameters of activity or passivity, with anxiety and/or depression, with withdrawal and/or anger, depending upon the nature of the condition, the established personality of the child, and the family's response. The age of the child will significantly determine the type of behavior expressed. Stubblefield (1974) points out that, inevitably, chronic illness first produces a depressive reaction including shock, apathy, and detachment, as well as the other regressive processes associated with mourning. A developmental approach to understanding these effects is essential for successful intervention.

Infancy

Consider for a moment the period of infancy in which the development of trust between the mother and child is so important. The classic studies of the attachment process (Harlow and Harlow, 1966) have guided our thinking concerning the psychological well-being of the infant. For the sick infant, the disruptions to this process by frequent separations necessitated by hospitalization, the mother's response to the infant's condition, and the anxiety generated imply significant alterations in the expected mother-infant relationship. Bowlby (1952) documented the need for a warm, intimate, continuous relationship with the mother for the infant to obtain satisfaction, noting that prolonged deprivation of maternal care can have lasting detrimental effects. His work further demonstrated that at approximately six to seven months the infant experiences a form of loss and expresses a kind of mourning, which is precipitated by the separation from the mother. This has special implications for the hospitalized infant. The basis for the need for human attachment develops during infancy, and, to whatever extent possible, health care professionals must maximize the opportunities for affected infants to obtain love, affection, and warmth from a consistent caregiving parent.

Young Children

The young child struggles to develop a sense of autonomy and separateness through initiating activities and ideas in a meaningful way while still maintaining a strong attachment to parenting figures. The behavioral impact of disease affects this struggle in two major ways: 1) families may become overprotective and inhibit opportunity for expression of these feelings and needs, and 2) intrusive prolonged separations as a result of hospitalization may arouse intense anxiety over abandonment.

It has been pointed out repeatedly that separation is the most common manifestation of anxiety in children under four years of age (Prugh et al., 1953; Godfrey, 1955; Robertson, 1958, 1970). Robertson (1958, 1970) described sequencing of protest, despair, and detachment among hospitalized young children as a response to the anxiety aroused by parental separation. Godfrey (1955), in looking at the young child in the hospital, found that stress in response to separation from parents was augmented by a loss of security or confidence in parents and by uncertainty with unfamiliar situations.

For the young child whose cognition is limited in terms of understanding his condition, magical thinking often pervades and feelings of self-blame arise. Children tend to react to treatment procedures as hostile attacks, often viewing them as punishment (Prugh, 1953). Kagan (1971) points out that sensory motives continue to prevail in young children who are concerned with hunger, warmth, stimulation, and physical contact. The impact of pain generated through medical procedures and through the chronic conditions themselves for children of this age thus can have substantial effects on the development of their personality, particularly as they interpret their sensory discomfort as punishment. The guilt that can result may become expressed in unusual ways. Prugh et al. (1953) described hospitalized young children who exhibited temporary inhibitions of unacceptable impulses and who pointed out to doctors or nurses how good they were as a reaction to their guilt.

School Age

The school-age child is dedicated to developing a sense of mastery, a desire to predict and control future events, peer relationships, and a set of moral attitudes and values. A long-term illness or chronic disease can thwart this development substantially. Restrictions and increased dependency may hinder the desire to accomplish and achieve new skills and the ability to maintain meaningful peer relationships. When frequent hospitalizations are required, the effects on this can be dramatic. Jessner (1952) has pointed to other effects, including the fear of loss of control of impulses or of body mastery, compounded particularly by fear of harm of the integrity of body image. The school-age child is unable to develop a firm self-concept and body image without acceptance of his condition.

The practicalities of maintaining sufficient educational input to develop academic skills and a sense of achievement may be inordinately difficult in the face of chronic disease. It is essential in our provisions of health care that opportunities for continued achievement be available. This implies a close working relationship between health professionals and educators, an association not always easy to achieve.

Adolescence

The adolescent is neither child nor adult. Like the child, he is still in a developing stage, but, like the adult, he is coping with issues of vocation, sexuality, and marriage. It is a time of identity formation, characterized by what is affectionately called a period of "storm and stress." It is a difficult time even under the most optimal circumstances. The sense of difference generated by a chronic disease can be excruciating during the adolescent period. At a time when self-concept and body image are being finalized, the intrusion of an illness or of physical changes can produce intense emotional stress. Kagan (1971) defines the desire to control uncertainty as one of the basic characteristics of development. Uncertainty about the future becomes intensified during adolescence for the child with a chronic condition. Depending on his condition, he may have strong doubts around his ability to obtain a job, his sexual potency, and his relationship with peers. The challenge of the future can produce overwhelming anxiety and depression. The normal increased independence from the family is thwarted often, and parents may, in fact, exercise even greater controls than usual if the child becomes overtly ill (Peterson, 1972). Preparation for adulthood may get set aside in the face of a chronic condition. The adolescent may meet his condition with a variety of more adult-like defenses—denial, intellectualization, compensation, anger (Moore, Holton, and Marten, 1969)—but the professional must be careful to remember that he is not yet an adult and habilitation, not rehabilitation, is a guiding concern.

THE FAMILY

For families the diagnosis of a chronic condition in their child implies a shocking loss—a relinquishing of earlier hopes and aspirations, an anticipation of restrictions and reduced potential, a change in routine and habits (Lowit, 1973). The time of diagnosis is a time of crisis for the family. Usual initial responses include disorganization and denial. On the one hand, families may become preoccupied with thoughts of the condition, sometimes unable to function or accomplish their normal activities, and, on the other hand, they may continue with feelings of disbelief and unwillingness to accept the diagnosis. Anger and guilt may follow, often involving displaced anger toward the medical staff or spouse and/or guilt over the child's unmet needs, parenting practices, or genetic heritage. In response to their feelings of loss, a mourning process typically emerges: denial, anger, acceptance. Going through the stages of this process is important because it is through a realistic acceptance by parents of the child's condition that the child himself will have his attitudes confirmed and his adjustment optimized.

Unfortunately the effect of a chronically ill child on a family system is more frequently disintegrative than integrative. It disrupts the established patterns of living and the roles of family members, and often results in divorce (Bruhn, 1977). Anxiety surrounding the health of the ill child may be a common source for the lack of meeting of the psychosocial needs of the child patient, taking the form of overprotectiveness, overcontrol, excessive permissiveness, lack of control, and overindulgence. Talbot and Howell (1971) succinctly summarize the major effects on families, which are elaborated on in the chapters that follow:

Parental disappointment, shame, or guilt
Parental resentment or anger over the burden
Parental anxiety leading to overprotectiveness, overrestrictiveness, over-indulgent care
Overconcentration of attention on the sick child, resulting in underattention to needs of other family members, fatigue, depression, and family impoverishment
Distortion of family life with respect to where to live and what to do
Sibling resentment of the patient as the recipient of special and favored attention and also shame caused by having an abnormal sibling
Sibling vulnerability with respect to parental transference of overprotective attitudes and practices to them, and, if the patient dies, grief and depression in anticipation of outcome

With these issues in mind, it is in the interest of the child that attempts be made to enhance the functioning of the family. Pless, Roghmann, and Haggerty (1972) found that the combined presence of a chronic illness and a low level of family functioning served to increase the probability of a child having deviant behavioral symptoms. A useful clinical pediatric technique for assessing family function was developed related to this study (Pless and Satterwhite, 1973). Providing support to the total family through the medical staff and mental health professionals is essential for all cases of pediatric chronic conditions. Helping the family to understand the condition and their feelings is a major goal. Through the sensitivity of staff and the availability of support services, the disruption and disintegration of family life can be minimized.

THE CONDITION

Perhaps the most significant variable in the adaptation of the child and the family to a chronic condition is the condition itself. A condition varies along a number of significant dimensions: time of onset, duration, severity (life-threatening potential), need for hospitalization, physical manifestations, and mental manifestations. The chapters that follow here and in Volume II attempt to explore various pediatric conditions and their psychological ramifications relevant to these parameters.

The time of onset—early or late in the life of the child—has developmental implications as already noted, as well as an effect on the adaptation of the family. The chapters on genetic conditions and high-risk infants point to the family's feelings of discouragement and guilt and the reevaluation of expectations that accompany early onset of a condition as compared to others that can occur at any time.

The duration and severity of the condition—its chronicity or potential for change—often stand as an unknown, sometimes with the threat of death in sight. The chapters on feeding disorders and enuresis/encopresis reflect generally short-term problems that are responsive to treatment. The chapters on cystic fibrosis, renal disease, oncology, and diabetes present life-threatening conditions with variable potential for control. The very special issues that are raised around the dying child—his anxieties and his fears—are illustrated dramatically in the chapter on oncology. As Spinetta, Rigler, and Karon (1974) and Waechter (1971) point out, for the child there may or may not be overt expression about impending death, but the more subtle fears are equally real and painful.

There are children who are not confronted with fatal illness but with conditions that seriously affect the quality of their lives through physical or mental manifestations. In Volume II the chapters on retardation, seizure disorders, hyperactivity, dyslexia, and hearing problems recount the significant impact that these conditions have on a child's development and family life.

In a society that so values its children, of special concern in pediatric care are the issues of child abuse and the effects of divorce on children. In the case of child abuse, the condition is a parental one, but the effect on the child in terms of physical and psychological harm is far reaching. The parent as the protector and caregiver of the child has the ultimate responsibility for his well-being. When the parent uncontrollably abuses this responsibility, the care of the child becomes a paramount concern to all of society. In the instance of divorce, an increasing phenomenon in our society, the professional support of mental health specialists and pediatricians in developing alternative child-rearing practices is essential for the optimal growth of the child.

MULTIDISCIPLINARY CARE
OF THE CHILD WITH A CHRONIC CONDITION

The care of the chronically ill child will in most cases require the interface of a number of professionals sharing in the medical and psychological management of the child/patient and his family. The pediatrician, through his relationship to the child and his family, plays a key role. He provides medical intervention and such knowledge as is available regarding the etiology of the illness and the predictable variant patterns that may develop during the chronological growth period. The medical specialists provide needed specific expertise around given conditions. By appropriate referral, or through integrated team management, various mental health professionals including pediatric psychologists, social workers, psychiatrists, and nurses make available support around the psychosocial aspects of the condition (see Figure 1).

Consider for example the following four vignettes, each of which illustrates the complicated interaction of the time of onset, the duration, the severity of the condition, and the role of the professionals in working with the child and his family for medical and psychological care. Let us explore the condition of a cataract (noting that the muscles controlling eyeball movements are integrated during the first 12 months of life).

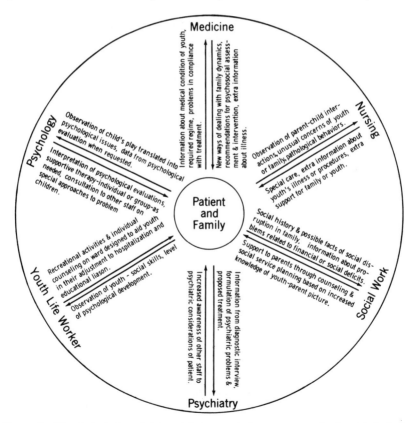

Figure 1.   Visual depiction of integrated teamwork for management of psychological aspects surrounding pediatric problems.

Case 1   An infant is born with an unrecognizable operable cataract and has been treated by the family as a blind child. The family's reactions in the process of acceptance of the circumstances have ranged from rejection and hostility to despair and futility. When the cataract is finally diagnosed, an irreversible psychological impact already has occurred for the infant. Professionals are confronted with reeducating the family members in their approach and attitudes toward the child who is and will continue to be essentially normal.

Case 2   A cataract that is secondary to an intrauterine infectious illness such as rubella is diagnosed at birth. As a result of the infection, other organ systems, e.g., auditory and cardiac, are affected. Feelings of guilt on the part of the parents mingle with concern about the severity of the deficit in relation to overall functioning of the child. Concerns about mental development arise. All of these supersede the effect of the cataract and point to the need for long-term multidisciplinary management with the family and child.

Case 3   A congenital defect in the carbohydrate metabolism, such as enzymatic deficiency of galactose-1-phosphate uridyl transferase activity, exists but allows the infant to appear normal at birth. However, symptoms appear soon after feedings are begun, and cataracts appear. Because the diagnosis was delayed, a significant amount of retardation occurs. The family's expectations of normalcy now must be adapted to fit the limitations imposed by the permanent deficits the child will have. Crisis intervention at the point of diagnosis must occur along with continued psychological support and additional resource access.

Case 4   A preschool child, accidentally traumatized by a foreign body in the eye, subsequently develops a cataract that is treated successfully with surgery. Limited support such as short-term counseling to the child and/or family will be required.

SUMMARY

Chronic conditions affect the fiber of family life and the developmental processes of the child. The basic emotional needs of children become challenged as well as the ability of the family to meet these needs. Time of onset, duration, and severity are the most significant factors in the adjustment of the child and his family to any chronic condition. The ensuing chapters point to the ways in which distortions of normal patterns of living are coped with in various conditions. Although patterns of response and adjustment are often predictable, one must be attuned constantly to the uniqueness of each child and each family unit. In our dedication as professionals to the improvement of the lives of children with problems, we must continue to seek new answers to providing mental health care for children with chronic conditions.

REFERENCES

Bowlby, J. 1952. Maternal Care and Mental Health. World Health Organization. Geneva, Switzerland.

Bruhn, J. 1977. Effects of chronic illness on the family. J. Fam. Pract. 4:1057–1060.

Godfrey, A. 1955. A study of nursing care designed to assist hospitalized children and their parents in their separation. Nurs. Res. 4:52–70.

Harlow, H., and Harlow, M. H. 1966. Learning to love. Am. Sci. 54:244–272.

Holt, K. 1972. The problem in the young. Proc. R. Soc. Med. 65:4–5.

Hughes, J. 1976. The emotional impact of chronic disease: The pediatrician's responsibility. Am J. Dis. Child. 130:1200–1203.

Jennison, M. 1976. The pediatrician and care of chronic illness. Pediatrics 58:5–7.

Jessner, L. 1952. Emotional implications of tonsillectomy and adenectomy on children. Psychoanal. Study Child. 7:126–169.

Kagan, A., and Levi, L. 1974. Health and environment—psychosocial stimulus: A review. Soc. Sci. Med. 8:225–241.

Kagan, J. 1971. Personality development. In N. B. Talbot, J. Kagan, and L. Eisenberg (eds.), Behavioral Science in Pediatric Medicine, pp. 283–350. W. B. Saunders Co., Philadelphia.

Lowit, I. 1973. Social and psychological consequences of chronic illness in children. Dev. Med. Child Neurol. 15:75–90.

Magrab, P., and Bronheim, S. 1976. The child life model and pediatric hospitalization. J. Pediatr. Psychol. 1:7–9.

Mattson, A. 1972. Long-term physical illness in childhood: A challenge to psychosocial adaptation. Pediatrics 50:801–811.

Moore, P., Holton, C., and Marten, G. 1969. Psychological problems in the management of adolescents with malignancy. Clin. Pediatr. 8:464–473.

Peterson, E. 1972. The impact of adolescent illness on parental relationships. J. Health Soc. Behav. 13:429–437.

Pless, I., Roghmann, K., and Haggerty, R. 1972. Chronic illness, family functioning and psychological adjustment: A model for the allocation of preventive mental health services. Int. J. Epidemiol. 1:271.

Pless, I., and Satterwhite, B. 1973. A measure of family functioning and its application. Soc. Sci. Med. 7:613–621.

Pless, I., Satterwhite, B., and Van Vechten, D. 1976. Chronic illness in childhood: A regional survey of care. Pediatrics 58:37–46.

Prugh, D., Staub, E., Sands, H., Kirschbaum, R., and Lenihan, E. 1953. A study of the emotional reactions of children and families to hospitalization and illness. Am. J. Orthopsychiatry 23:70–106.

Robertson, J. 1958. Young children in hospital. Basic Books, New York.

Robertson, J. 1970. Young children in hospital. 2nd Ed. Tavistock Publications, London.

Rutter, M., Tizard, J., and Whitmore, K. 1968. Handicapped children: A total Population Prevalence Study of Education, Physical and Behavioral Disorders. Longmans, London.

Shultz, M. T., McVicar, M. I., and Kemph, J. P. 1974. Treatment of the emotional and cognitive deficits of the child receiving hemodialysis. In N. Levy (ed.), Living or Dying—Adaptation to Hemodialysis, pp. 62–73. Charles C Thomas, Springfield, Ill.

Spinetta, J. J., Rigler, D., and Karon, M. 1974. Personal space as a measure of a dying child's sense of isolation. J. Consult. Clin. Psychol. 42:751–756.

Stewart, W. 1967. The unmet needs of children. Pediatrics 39:157.

Stubblefield, R. 1974. Psychiatric complications of chronic illness in children. In J. A. Downey and N. L. Low (eds.), The Child with Disabling Illness, pp. 509–519. W. B. Saunders Co., Philadelphia.

Talbot, N. B., and Howell, M. C. 1971. Social and behavioral causes and consequences of disease among children. In N. B. Talbot, J. Kagan, and L. Eisenberg (eds.), Behavioral Science in Pediatric Medicine, pp. 1–89. W. B. Saunders Co., Philadelphia.

Waechter, E. H. 1971. Children's awareness of fatal illness. Am. J. Nurs. 71:1168–1172.

2

Mental Health Aspects of Pediatric Care
Historical Review and Current Status

Milton F. Shore and Stephen E. Goldston

"Primum non nocere"
(First do no harm)

Hippocrates

BACKGROUND

Medical care in the United States currently is undergoing a major reevaluation in anticipation of a national health insurance program. As part of that evaluation, the components of high-quality comprehensive medical care are being defined and described in the light of current knowledge. One result has been a rising interest in the mental health elements that should be included in any health service.

The present concern about the mental health aspects of pediatric care can be seen as an outgrowth of three historical forces: the humanist tradition, the increased understanding of the close interweaving of biological and psychological elements, and the growing emphasis on preventing psychological dysfunctions in adult life. This chapter presents an overview of the field rather than an exhaustive review of the literature.

The Humanist Tradition

Aries (1965) has traced the development of the concept of childhood in Western thought. He notes that it is only over the last two centuries that childhood has been identified as a specific stage of development with unique characteristics and needs requiring the special attention of society. The implications of the delineation of childhood as a discrete phase of development have led to major advances in the understanding, as well as in the protection, of the young. Development of the concept of childhood correlates with the rising humanist philosophy that focused on the avoidance and reduction of unnecessary pain or discomfort in both adults and children.

In line with the philosophical changes, there have been major advances in the children's area over the last eight decades. In fact, the twentieth century in the United States has been called by some the Century of the Child. Specialties such as pediatrics arose to give particular recognition to the physical and medical problems of children. In the mid 1800s hospitals exclusively for children were built. The late 1800s saw the establishment of a Section on Pediatrics within the American Medical Association, and in 1930 the American Academy of Pediatrics was founded.

Meanwhile, federal interest in children grew with the establishment of the Children's Bureau in 1912, a national resource and action group concerned with the welfare of the young. The first White House Conference on Children was convened in 1909. State and national child labor laws were passed. Standards of hospital care for children were recommended by professional groups. Special units were established for children in courts, recreational centers, libraries, and even in dentistry (as in the recently developed field of pedodontics). An increasing general concern about developing a national program around parenting through the Federal Office of Child Development, now the Administration for Children, Youth, and Families, has been evident. Recent attention to child abuse has mobilized many of the forces concerned with children's welfare and has resulted in various articles of child abuse legislation.

In addition to the concern with the physical, social, and psychological welfare of children, the recent growth of the children's rights movement and the focus on advocacy have led to a greater desire to bring about major changes in the institutions (schools, hospitals, etc.) that serve children and their families (Berlin, 1975).

The humanist tradition that has played a role in these major changes in child care in the United States may also be seen as playing a role in the selection of pediatrics as a specialty by doctors. It has been noted that the financial rewards in pediatrics are less, but the physical and emotional involvement is often greater than in many other medical specialties (*Medical Economics*, 1975).

Increased Understanding of the
Interrelationship Between Body and Mind

Over the last three decades, knowledge has accumulated about the close interweaving of psychological and physiological processes. Recent studies have led to an improved conceptual understanding of how biological and psychological factors operate in psychosomatic disorders (Reiser, 1975; Wright, 1977). The boundaries of physical and psychological processes in children are even narrower than those in adults. Physical growth and development have been found to be impaired by difficulties in the relationships between infants and their caregivers as, for example, in the case of failure to thrive (Fraiberg, Adelson, and Shapiro, 1975). Not only do psychological conflicts produce physiological disorders, but physiological disorders have marked consequences on the emotional development of children. For example, children who are forced to limit their locomotion during the phase of active exploration may show problems with regard to activity and passivity in later life. Urological investigations because of enuresis have had effects on sexual fantasy development in boys and girls.

**Emphasis on Preventing
Psychological Dysfunction in Later Life**

With the increasing knowledge of developmental psychology and the delineation, acceptance, and utilization of mental health concepts, greater concern has been expressed about the early experiences that can set the stage for later psychological difficulties. Bowlby (1952) has emphasized the negative consequences of breaking early attachments with the mother. In fact, separation experiences in early childhood now have been assumed to adversely affect later development. Broussard and Hartner (1970) have studied the effects of early maternal perception of the neonate as related to later psychological development. They found an association between negative maternal perceptions and later psychological disturbances in the child. Prugh (1975) has noted how a young child, whose development may have been progressing smoothly in a healthy family, after returning from a hospital experience may feel deserted and abandoned, subsequently provoking a pathological family response. This response can result in clear-cut, long-term maladjustments and symptoms.

HISTORICAL HIGHLIGHTS

Before 1952 the subject of the medical hospitalization of children was not studied systematically. However, some publications identified the area as of great concern to child practitioners (Geist, 1965). Despite limited empirical studies, pediatricians, nurses, child development specialists, and other professionals recommended psychological support to children and their families in an effort to reduce the painful effects of the experience of hospitalization.

In 1952, a fortuitous event occurred, which was to be the turning point in the interest in hospitalized children. Prompted by the experiences of young children separated during World War II and the work of Spitz (1946) and others on infant attachments, Bowlby and his associates (1952) became involved in the careful study of the specific aspects of the separation experiences in children that were potentially damaging to later personality development. One of the experiences selected for study was the separation resulting when a young child is placed in a medical setting with limited or no contact with his parents.

In 1952, in Great Britain, using a hand-held camera, Robertson produced the classic movie "A Two-Year-Old Goes to the Hospital" (Robertson, 1952). He followed a two-year-old child separated from her parents through an eight-day hospitalization experience for a minor hernia repair. The film showed vividly how the child (Laura) went through a series of extremely upsetting experiences, later described by Bowlby as the three stages resulting from breaks in attachments in early years: *protest, despair,* and *detachment.* The movie effectively mobilized many professionals, parents, and the general public in a major effort to review the policy of limiting parental involvement and presence in hospital settings where their young children were being treated. A public campaign was launched in Great Britain to bring about major changes in hospital procedures. The need for maintaining an attachment to the parents was reinforced by Robertson's second movie, "Going to Hospital with Mother" (1958a), in which a child, followed in a manner similar to that used with Laura, showed no intense emotional reactions, either in the hospital or upon returning home, when mother was permitted to stay through the hospitalization.

The campaign to change hospital practices in Great Britain led to the establishment of the National Association for the Welfare of Children in Hospitals in 1961. This association's activities are described by Robertson (1966). Meanwhile the British Government established a commission to study the needs of young children in hospitals. The Platt Report (Platt Committee, 1959) recommended major alterations in hospital procedures for young children in Great Britain. Following this report, the Nuffield Foundation (1963) financed an architectural study to show how the physical structure of children's hospitals could be adapted so that parents could stay with their children, thus recognizing formally that the need for maintaining parental attachment was essential for the total care of the child under five years of age.

Concurrent with the increased British interest in the hospitalization of children was the growing involvement of professionals in the United States in the study of the consequences of hospitalization on personality development. Because a theoretical framework had been developed for studying attachment and separation, more systematic research arose (noted by Prugh, 1953). Data on the hospitalization of children, both descriptive and empirical, expanded exponentially in the areas of preparation, parental involvement, staff relations, and physical arrangements.

TWO DECADES OF EXPERIENCE: 1952–1972

In 1960, the American Academy of Pediatrics published "Care of Children in Hospitals." A major addition to the chapters on medical care and administration was material on meeting the emotional needs of hospitalized children and adolescents. Although relatively brief in its treatment of emotional factors, the book recognized that comprehensive care in a hospital includes sensitivity to childhood fears of separation, unfamiliar surroundings, darkness, disfigurement, and exposure.

In 1965, Mason reviewed two decades of research on the emotional needs of the hospitalized child. Citing more than 60 works over that period, he concluded that hospitalization should be viewed as a crisis for a child and his family. This crisis offers an opportunity for significant growth in a child and his family, as well as the possibility of significant maladaptation and dysfunction. He also pointed out the consistency of the research results and the necessity of a community-wide effort to bring about changes in the medical care of children more consonant with mental health principles. He urged greater consideration in medical education of the emotional needs of children, a recommendation that is being implemented very slowly.

In 1966, the National Institute of Mental Health published *Red Is the Color of Hurting: Planning for Children in the Hospital*, a collection of papers originally presented at the annual meeting of the American Orthospsychiatric Association by representatives of such disciplines as pediatrics, psychiatry, nursing, psychoanalysis, social anthropology, and architecture. The purpose of the book was to integrate the current knowledge in the field of hospitalization, especially concerning young children, and to suggest specific recommendations for changes in policy. At that time only 28 out of 5,500 general hospitals in the United States provided facilities for parents to stay overnight with their sick children. The resources needed to develop a positive mental health climate in hospitals for children were delineated from five perspectives: the child, the family, the government, the community, and the physical plant. *Red Is the Color of Hurting* gave impetus to the movement to change hospital practices in pediatric settings. Its concepts have become well known and served as a guide for the physical construction and the program development of the Children's Health Center, Inc., in Minneapolis, Minnesota, in the early 1970s.

EMERGENCE OF PARENT AND PROFESSIONAL ORGANIZATIONS

Even when knowledge increases, large-scale changes in practice and in social policy result only when a constituency has been developed that can bring pressure on those forces that resist change. Robertson (1966) has described how his movie generated discussion in Great Britain, leading to the establishment of the organization "Mother Care for Children in Hospitals," later called the National Association for the Welfare of Children in Hospitals. This organization consisted of both parents and professionals. Through massive publicity, as well as social action, the issue of hospitalization was brought to the attention of the British Government, resulting in a major change in national policy. Although many in Great Britain are still not satisfied with the changes that have occurred, we in the United States remain far behind our British colleagues.

A number of organizations have sprung up in the United States to bring to the attention of policy makers the need to view hospitalization of children from a psychosocial and mental health perspective. In 1965, an interdisciplinary group of child care workers, pediatricians, nurses, and mental health professionals established the Association for the Care of Children in Hospitals (ACCH). This group has become the primary resource for information for all disciplines interested in the hospitalization of children—social work, psychology, psychiatry, pediatrics, child life, nursing, etc. Through the publication of bibliographies, guidebooks, and a journal, it has attempted to encourage professionals involved in the medical care of children to bring about more humane and empirically proven changes in pediatric care.

The National Association of Children's Hospitals and Related Institutions (NACHRI) was founded in 1968 primarily for administrators of children's facilities who were interested in playing a role in establishing and fostering those settings believed best able to meet the specific needs of children. If specific structures for children are not built recognizing the unique needs of children and youth (which have taken many decades to identify, describe, and accept), children will continue to be cared for as miniature adults. Accordingly, this organization has as a major objective the construction of autonomous administrative and physical structures for children's services.

Special groups in specific disciplines have also arisen. In 1968, psychologists established the Society for Pediatric Psychology. The society has attempted to identify specific training needs for psychologists who work in nonpsychiatric medical settings. The group has stressed the contribution of psychologists not only to the traditional activities of mental health evaluation and treatment, but also to establishing a positive mental health climate in the total hospital setting. The issue of the *Journal of Pediatric Psychology* (1976) entitled "Children, Families and the Hospitalization" has brought up to date some of the theoretical, programmatic, and research knowledge that has emerged since *Red Is the Color of Hurting.*

All of the above organizations were initiated primarily for administrators and professionals. Unlike the course of development in Great Britain, parents in the United States have found it necessary to establish their own separate associations aimed at making the lay public aware of the problems of hospitalization of children and at recommending to parents how they can act to promote changes in hospital settings consonant with the needs of children and their families. Two of the most well-known organizations for parents are Children in Hospitals (established in 1971) and Parents Concerned for Hospitalized Children (established in 1972).

As Prugh (1976) pointed out in a recent article, despite all these organizations and the efforts of many dedicated people, changes in pediatric hospital practices in the United States have been slow. Hopefully the recent interest in child advocacy, which recognizes the need for institutional change and legitimizes efforts to bring about such change, will accelerate the pace of development of high-quality mental-health-oriented medical programs for children.

IMPACT OF HOSPITALIZATION

Certain assumptions and concepts have guided the concerns about the impact of hospitalization on children, concerns that are not only of theoretical interest but that, as in Britain, have become a major movement aimed at improving children's medical care:

1. *The recognition over the last three decades that behavior such as attachment is a significant area of study and can be subjected to vigorous and careful investigation.* Harlow and his associates (McKinney, Suomi, and Harlow, 1975) have shown that precipitous separation in monkeys leads to severe disturbances in relationships when they grow into maturity. Their work with monkeys has given legitimacy to the concept of attachment by creating bridges between laboratory scientists and the clinicians whose observations of the effects of separation in humans have been described vividly for a number of years. Bowlby (1975) has tied the separation experience to an ethological framework, hypothesizing that attachment behaviors in humans are based on biological evolutionary principles associated with innate releaser mechanisms needed for the survival of the human species.
2. *The realization that psychic pain can have an effect as profound as or even greater than physical pain, especially in children.* Experiences

of isolation, abandonment, loneliness, neglect, and emotional deprivation produced by hospital settings are often so painful that they not only impair the convalescent process but appear to produce an iatrogenic emotional disease. A. Freud and D. T. Burlingham (1944) graphically described how children in Britain during wartime experienced the separation from their parents as more frightening and painful than the realistic dangers of the bombings.

3. *The effect of hospitalization must be viewed within a developmental framework.* Mastery of the hospital experience is dependent upon the resources, cognitive and affective, that a child has available to him as a result both of personal experiences and of maturational level, biologically and psychologically. Prugh (1966) has described vividly the various anxieties children have at different ages and how hospitalization can stimulate and exacerbate those fears, resulting in severe distress. For instance, annihilation anxiety appears in the very young child. Later, children have strong fears of separation. Three- to five-year-olds show concern about body damage. Older children fear regression. Among adolescents, privacy, sexuality, and loss of identity are major concerns. Because needs of adolescents differ markedly from those of young children, hospitals must have different facilities and total care programs for children of different ages. It has now become axiomatic that the attachment of a child under five to his family should not be broken if he is hospitalized and that facilities should be available in the hospital for family members to be with the child through the hospital stay.

4. *The child within the context of his family.* Unfortunately, in approaching the hospitalization experience, the focus has been only on the child and his specific needs within the hospital. The family, as well as the child, is in crisis and needs support. Richmond (1958) has outlined the stages parents and families go through in dealing with a severely ill child. After the initial phase of denial and disbelief used to deal with the immediate crisis, fear and frustration set in as the illness continues. If the guilt and depression associated with the second phase are dealt with, a third phase of intelligent inquiry and planning can follow in which family members (parents) can learn to handle the ill child more appropriately. Each family will deal with the situation in the members' characteristic way of handling stress. But as these stages progress, and with the assistance and understanding of the hospital staff, the efficiency of the family in caring for the ill child should increase.

Over the years families have been discouraged from participating in the care of the child. Instead, parent substitutes and professional personnel have aggressively taken over all control.

Recently there has been increased recognition that the professionals must work with the family, assisting family members in supporting the child in the hospital and after returning home. Even siblings, who often regress during the crisis, can be helped in dealing with the ill child. When families care for their children in the hospital using medical personnel only on a consultative basis (Kennedy, 1966), the results indicate that children respond better and hospital costs are reduced.

5. *"Anticipatory guidance" techniques to help a child master the potentially traumatic experience of hospitalization.* Early research stressed the negative effects of hospitalization. Current work focuses on what can be done to alleviate the traumatic aspects of the experience. Preparation for hospitalization (such as visits before admission, story books, and movies) has been found to be very helpful. Robertson (1958b) has shown how the presence of mother or mother substitute is essential for the young child to cope with the experience. Playrooms, puppet shows, group sessions, dance, and television are some of the techniques used to assist young children in the hospital. Although the experience of hospitalization can be physically painful, techniques are available to alleviate or reduce the emotional consequences.

6. *An interdisciplinary approach toward dealing with the hospitalization of children.* Knowledge from a number of different disciplines is needed to look at the child from different points of view and to integrate the material into a treatment plan useful for the total care of the child. A unique discipline that has arisen within hospital settings involves the child life worker. These personnel are trained child development specialists whose knowledge of normal growth and development and of children's emotional reactions to stress qualify them to handle children in hospital settings. Also, within this discipline are teachers to assist in the learning area. Specialized mental health services need to be available for consultation and treatment when specific psychopathological disturbances occur. Architects are needed to adapt the physical structures to more humane care. Comprehensiveness of care is the most important element in assisting the child and his family through the experience.

7. *Hospital settings must be responsive to new knowledge about health care.* Major changes in medical care have made it possible to reduce the need for hospitalization, with greater use of outpatient and ambulatory care facilities. Hospitals must constantly evaluate what some have called the "myths of medical care." Many activities in an institutional setting are based more on tradition than on effectiveness. For example, some settings still require lengthy hospitalization

for surgical procedures that are currently being done on outpatient or overnight bases in other settings. Some settings continue to have limited visiting hours or to restrict sibling visits to over ages 12 to 16, ages which are determined arbitrarily, ostensibly for medical reasons. Hospitals must have an evaluative program aimed at studying procedures and feeding back into the system ways of implementing changes that are in line with changing needs and the constantly expanding knowledge of physical and emotional growth.

SOME MENTAL HEALTH PRINCIPLES FOR DEVELOPING EFFECTIVE INPATIENT HOSPITAL PROGRAMS FOR CHILDREN

During the past two decades, general mental health principles have been integrated slowly into pediatric settings. Hospitals have incorporated some of the essential elements; however, few have planned, organized, and implemented a total, integrated program of medical and emotional care. There are five major principles to be considered: 1) the avoidance of hospitalization, 2) preparation if hospitalization is inevitable, 3) brief hospitalization as a goal, 4) adequate resources to assist the child in coping with the experience, and 5) follow-up work with the child and the family.

1. *Hospitalization should be avoided if possible.* Recent advances in medical care permit more opportunities for outpatient treatment for conditions previously requiring inpatient hospitalization. Constant evaluation should be fostered to accelerate the trend of moving away from the hospitalization of children. Alternatives such as home care should be encouraged, with financial incentives offered by third-party payers to programs that reduce the use of hospital facilities.

2. *Whenever possible, children should be prepared for hospitalization.* Such preparation should take place when inpatient status is imminent and also should be part of a child's total educational program. Visits to hospitals by school classes and greater activity on the part of hospital personnel in the community (including visits of hospital personnel to schools) are components of a total community-based helping service, of which the hospital is one part.

3. *When hospitalization must occur, it should be as brief as possible.* Support services should be present within the community in order to permit a child to leave the hospital as early as possible. Family members should be trained to provide for the total care of the child at home.

4. *During hospitalization the following provisions and resources should be available to assist the child in dealing with the experience:*

a. Facilities for parents to stay overnight with young children. This means the planning of rooms not only for children but also for parents to talk to one another and not be isolated from adult company.

b. Ways of maintaining contacts with the family as much as possible during the administration of medical and surgical procedures, including unrestricted visiting for parents and siblings.

c. Staff trained to explain to children and their families what is happening in a constructive, understandable manner.

d. An educational program that can continue the child's formal learning while in the hospital.

e. Opportunities to translate passivity into activity. This means the expression of fantasy, as well as opportunities to move about, use play objects, and actively master the situation by continued learning, despite the restricted environment. Hyperactive and counterphobic children merit special consideration because their normal coping patterns may be misinterpreted as active adjustment to hospitalization, when in reality they are as fearful as the withdrawn, depressed child.

f. Playrooms that permit free play so that the fantasies and fears related to hospitalization can be expressed and worked out in an accepting environment.

g. The opportunity to bring objects from home to which a child is attached, and to have them available whenever needed.

Prugh (1975) has also recommended, *as a standard practice, visits by hospital staff to the child's home shortly after hospitalization to assist the family in dealing with the child when he returns.* Through such visits, any possible pathological interpersonal processes resulting from the hospitalization experience can be identified early and hopefully reversed. This recommendation suggests the possibility that a single staff member be charged with the responsibility of continuity of care for the child and his family beginning with preadmission and continuing through posthospitalization home visits.

THE PRESENT

In 1975, the Children's Health Center, Inc. of Minneapolis, Minnesota was built. Unlike other children's hospitals, which have well-established traditions that need to be changed in order to implement mental health principles, this new center set its own traditions from the beginning. Mental health services are available at the hospital as a specialized service. In addition, mental health principles are used throughout the hospital in an effort to set up a total evironment that recognizes the emotional needs of children and youth. To foster a positive environment, a psychologist was appointed Vice President for Ecology. All organizational levels at the hospital are encouraged to adapt mental health principles to their operation. The success of this hospital program has shown that the incorporation of mental health concepts into hospital settings is neither expensive nor a romantic dream incapable of implementation. Many hospitals currently are renovating, expanding, or building new facilities. These new settings offer an opportunity to rethink the ways health care has been delivered to children and their families and to alter current practices so that they are more in line with the new comprehensive ecological thinking.

THE FUTURE

Although interest in the mental health aspects of the health care of children originated with concerns over hospitalization in line with research of maternal deprivation, attachment behavior, and separation from mother, the field has now broadened to encompass all health care for the young. The following areas, in addition to hospitalization, need consideration and exploration in the near future.

Psychological Aspects of Medical Care for Adolescents

The medical needs of adolescents differ from those of young children and adults, thereby necessitating settings different both in structure and form. Just as the Nuffield Foundation in Great Britain (1963) developed architectural plans for how children under age five and their parents could best be accommodated in hospital facilities, architectural plans are needed for medical wards for teenagers. Hospitals usually have improvised teenage programs by adding juke boxes and/or game rooms to wards. Certainly there are better ways to utilize space so as to give adolescents greater opportunities to cope with the hospitalization experience without impairing their psychological and social growth.

In addition to space, the specific developmental aspects of illness in adolescence need to be addressed. Sider and Kreider (1977) have described the specific aspects of adolescent development in body image, independence, relatedness, and identity formation that must be understood in trying to deliver medical care to the adolescent. Schowalter (1977) has discussed the impact of bodily illness on the adolescent that puts him at high risk for psychological disorders. Both articles imply that within adolescent medicine, a relatively new field, more attention needs to be paid to the psychological factors that seriously affect adolescent health care. New techniques in self-care, in the sharing of physical concerns in group settings, and in the involvement of adolescents in the care of peers or younger children need to be explored.

Psychological Aspects of Outpatient Care

As the focus on inpatient care decreases and that on outpatient care increases, we are faced with questions as to what preparation is necessary for children and their families in outpatient settings. The long wait in outpatient pediatric settings without adequate play activities fosters boredom, anger, and fear. Waiting rooms can become health education centers where parents and young adults can learn about preventive health through television or other techniques. The waiting room can also be used for diagnostic purposes to understand and assist families if problems are manifested. In addition, many hospital waiting rooms are natural settings for fostering the development of social contacts between families, many of whom have been isolated in their everyday life. The self-help movement has brought to our attention how nonprofessionals can assist one another successfully in times of personal physical and psychological crises. Hospitals should be aware of these groups and encourage such contacts when appropriate.

Mental Health Intervention in the Emergency Room

The use of mental health principles in crisis settings such as the emergency room needs to be explored (see Axelrod, 1976). Emergency work necessitates quick action with minimal time for preparation or exploration. Innovative and creative ideas are needed to assist children and their families in the emergency rooms. For example, it may be necessary that special attention be given to follow-up of patients and their families over a longer period of time. Training in the mental health aspects of crisis intervention should be provided to medical staff.

Mental Health Aspects of Long-Term Care

We have not yet adequately dealt with the mental health effects of long-term chronic medical problems. How does one maintain close association with a family over an extended hospitalization? What should be done with families having children requiring chronic care? While some work has been done in this area, especially by social workers, further research is needed.

Some Specific Aspects of Health Care Not Yet Studied

Aspects yet to be studied include, for example, the effects of many specific medical conditions on psychological functioning which are not clearly understood. Techniques for handling specific illness need to be devised. Each disease has its own psychological as well as physiological component. In addition to general mental health issues, the intimate interweaving of the medical requirements and mental health issues needs to be explored carefully for each disease entity. This volume addresses some of these issues.

The Hospital as a Community Facility

The hospital setting provides a unique opportunity for total socio-psychological assessment of family functioning. As a result the hospital can serve as an information and referral center for all services within the community that can best meet the needs of specific families.

The Need to Address Major Constraints on Change in Pediatric Settings

Despite the urgings of many concerned people, hospital standards specifically for the care of children have not been written. Accreditation standards for children's medical settings should be a separate section in the general accreditation standards in order to incorporate the latest information in the field of comprehensive child health care. (The 1976 Manual of the Joint Commission on Accreditation of Hospitals does not even list "children" in its index.)

Insurance coverage needs to be related more to current medical and mental health knowledge. In the children's area such factors as reimbursement to parents staying with the young child would be included (as in Great Britain), because the presence of parents can be seen as necessary for the total care of the child. Insurance companies need to foster greater use of outpatient care, rather than inpatient hospitalization as they do at present. In addition, more emphasis should be placed on preventive care with financial incentives available for all procedures that avoid the expensive and possibly traumatic procedures of hospitalization.

Although some mention has been made of the cost effectiveness of pediatric care that includes mental health (Kennedy, 1966), a large number of carefully planned studies done over an extended period of time need to be undertaken to obtain a true understanding of costs, both immediate costs and costs in terms of later personal adjustment. Although short-term costs may be high in working with children, a reduction in the length of hospital stay or the reduced use of expensive services later in life need to be used as criteria of effectiveness.

Further research needs to be done on the positive effect of constructive programs aimed at alleviating the potential traumatic effects of pediatric services. For example, although preparation for hospitalization in general has been found to be useful, the effects of different kinds of preparation for hospitalization have not been studied. Siegel (1976) has outlined a number of areas for further research such as the optimal preparation time for children of various ages, and the relationship between past experiences and the ability to profit from a specific type of preparation.

There is a great need for total comprehensive health services delivered to children and families in an integrated fashion by a multidisciplinary staff. Changes in training and better staff communication are essential. As medical care for children is being extended to reach those who currently do not have adequate access to it (such as the financially disadvantaged), there will be a number of new challenges. New outreach services need to be developed. Paraprofessional training programs need to be fostered. Different levels of specialized care need to be identified. Utilization of current manpower in more constructive and efficient ways is necessary. The organization of services with greater focus on continuity and coordination is imperative.

Hospitals have important primary prevention functions. Broussard and Hartner's (1970) research on maternal perceptions of the infant and Klaus and Kennell's (1976) work on the establishment of appropriate affective bonding in the early days of life while mother and infant are still in the hospital have both shown how hospitals can play a major part in setting a constructive pattern for future psychological development.

The current trend in health care is to view health within the total context of life ("well-being"), not as a state of the absence of disease. Within this view, hospital settings should not be seen as only a place for physical healing or an institution for marking time during recuperation. Instead, hospitals can be settings that foster growth and development and contribute to the quality of life. Humanizing health care in line with our growing knowledge of physical and mental health can contribute to more constructive personal and interpersonal functioning in children who happen to be ill and in their families. Such benefits are in society's best interests, both socially and economically.

REFERENCES

American Academy of Pediatrics. 1960. Care of Children in Hospitals. Evanston, Ill.

Aries, P. 1965. Centuries of Childhood: A Social History of Family Life. Random House, New York.

Axelrod, B. H. 1976. Mental health considerations in the pediatric emergency room. In M. F. Shore and S. E. Goldston (eds.), Families, children and hospitalization, J. Pediatr. Psychol. 1(4):14–17.

Berlin, I. N. (ed.). 1975. Advocacy for Child Mental Health. Brunner/Mazel, New York.

Bowlby, J. 1952. Maternal Care and Mental Health. 2nd Ed. World Health Organization Monograph #2. Geneva, Switzerland.

Bowlby, J. 1975. Attachment theory: Separation anxiety and mourning. In S. Arieti (ed.), American Handbook of Psychiatry, 2nd Ed., Vol. VI, pp. 292–309. Basic Books, New York.

Broussard, E., and Hartner, M. 1970. Maternal perception of the neonate as related to development. Child Psychiatry Hum. Dev. 1(1):16–25.

Earnings on the six biggest medical specialties. 1975. Med. Econ. 53(122):154.

Fraiberg, S., Adelson, E., and Shapiro, V. 1975. Ghosts in the nursery: A psychoanalytic approach to the problems of impaired infant-mother relationships. J. Am. Acad. Child Psychiatry 14(3):387–421.

Freud, A., and Burlingham, D. T. 1944. War and Children. International Universities Press, New York.

Geist, H. 1965. A Child Goes to the Hospital: The Psychological Aspects of a Child Going to the Hospital. Charles C Thomas, Springfield, Ill.

Kennedy, D. A. 1966. Planning a new children's hospital. In M. F. Shore (ed.), Red Is the Color of Hurting: Planning for Children in the Hospital, pp. 63–73. Superintendent of Documents, Government Printing Office, Washington, D.C.

Klaus, M. H., and Kennell, J. H. 1976. Maternal Infant Bonding: The Impact of Early Separation or Loss on Family Development. The C. V. Mosby Company, St. Louis, Mo.

McKinney, W. T., Suomi, S. J., and Harlow, H. F. 1975. Experimental psychopathology in non-human primates. In S. Arieti (ed.), American Handbook of Psychiatry, 2nd Ed., vol. VI, pp. 310–334. Basic Books, New York.

Mason, E. 1965. The hospitalized child: His emotional needs. N. Engl. J. Med. 272:406–415.

Nuffield Foundation. 1963. Children in Hospital: Studies in Planning. Oxford University Press, New York.

Platt Committee, Great Britain. 1959. The Welfare of Children in Hospitals. Her Majesty's Stationery Office, London.

Prugh, D. G., Staub, E. M., Sands, H. H., Kirschbaum, R. M., and Lenihan, E. A. 1953. A study of the emotional reactions of children and families to hospitalization and illness. Am. J. Orthopsychiatry 23:70–106.

Prugh, D. G. 1966. Emotional aspects of the hospitalization of children. In M. F. Shore (ed.), Red Is the Color of Hurting: Planning for Children in the Hospital, pp. 17–37. Superintendent of Documents, Government Printing Office, Washington, D.C.

Prugh, D. G., and Jordan, K. 1975. Physical illness or injury: The hospital as source of emotional disturbances in child and family. In I. N. Berlin (ed.), Advocacy for Child Mental Health, pp. 208–248. Brunner/Mazel, New York.

Reiser, M. F. 1975. Changing theoretical concepts in psychosomatic medicine. In S. Arieti (ed.), American Handbook of Psychiatry, 2nd Ed., Vol. VI, pp. 477–500. Basic Books, New York.

Richmond, J. 1958. The pediatric patient in illness. In. M. H. Hollender (ed.), The Psychology of Medical Practice, pp. 195–211. W. B. Saunders Co., Philadelphia.

Robertson, J. 1952. A two-year-old goes to hospital. (Film). New York University Film Library, New York.

Robertson, J. 1958a. Going to hospital with mother. (Film). New York University Film Library, New York.

Robertson, J. 1958b. Young Children in Hospitals. Basic Books, New York.

Robertson, J. 1966. Effecting change in the hospitalization of children. In M. F. Shore (ed.), Red Is the Color of Hurting: Planning for Children in the Hospital, pp. 47–63. Superintendent of Documents, Government Printing Office, Washington, D.C.

Schowalter, J. E. 1977. Psychological reactions to physical illness and hospitalization in adolescence. J. Am. Acad. Child Psychiatry 16(3):500–516.

Shore, M. F. (ed.). 1966. Red Is the Color of Hurting: Planning for Children in the Hospital. Superintendent of Documents, Government Printing Office, Washington, D.C.

Shore, M. F., and Goldston, S. E. (eds.). 1976. Families, children and hospitalization. J. Pediatr. Psychol. 1(4):14–17.

Sider, R. C., and Kreider, S. D. 1977. Coping with adolescent patients, Med. Clin. North Am. LXI(4):839–854.

Siegel, L. J. 1976. Preparation of children for hospitalization: A selected review of the research literature. In M. F. Shore and S. E. Goldston (eds.), Families, children and hospitalization, J. Pediatr. Psychol. 1(4):14–17. 26–29.

Spitz, R. 1946. Hospitalism: Inquiry into the genesis of psychiatric conditions in early childhood. In K. Eissler et al. (eds.), Psychoanalytic Study of the Child, Vol. 1, pp. 53–74. International Universities Press, New York.

Wright, L. 1977. Conceptualizing and defining psychosomatic disorders. Am. Psychol. 32(8):625–629.

3

Emotional Factors in Pediatric Practice
An Overview

Lee Salk

The need to examine emotional factors in pediatric practice requires little justification; one must simply look back to one's own early experiences in the medical scene. It doesn't matter whether it was a routine visit to the pediatrician, a minor surgical procedure, or perhaps a prolonged illness or chronic disease. Memories of how one was treated are indelible and in all likelihood have shaped subsequent attitudes toward health professionals. Trust or distrust of health professionals greatly influences whether or not one seeks medical care when necessary.

MENTAL HEALTH ROLE OF THE PEDIATRICIAN

The pediatrician clearly holds a very influential role for the mental health of future generations. Recently it has become widely known how profound the effects of early experience on later behavior can be. We know that newborn infants are selective in many of their reactions, habituate to various stimuli, and can show conditioned responses. The pediatrician, as a major purveyor of information to parents, can make this kind of knowledge available. When parents understand how profound their impact is on their newborn infants, they are more responsive to them and feel more important in their role as parents.

Sociologists, anthropologists, biologists, and educators, along with psychologists, have shown how early environmental conditions can help shape personality, learning ability, and capacity to tolerate stress and can effect structural and biochemical alterations of the body. These effects during early development are not only very profound but are often extremely difficult to change.

The pediatrician sees more human beings during their most critical phases of development than any other professional. He can detect developmental and psychological problems and is in a position to recommend further study of the problem and methods for dealing with it, or he is able to refer the patient to another professional for treatment. However, although the pediatrician, logistically, is in a position for early detection of psychological and development disorders, he is often unable to do so because of a lack of training in the skills and methods of detecting these disorders. Moreover, the pediatrician may be overwhelmed by medical problems to the extent that little time is available for training to develop skills necessary for the early diagnosis of psychological problems. All too often, the patient's problem is well developed and of long standing by the time it comes to the pediatrician's attention; by then, intensive psychotherapy may be required, or the problem may not be treatable at all.

The pediatrician's potential for determining early developmental and psychological problems represents one important aspect of his mental health role. Perhaps more important is the pediatrician's vast influence on the attitudes of many parents toward child-rearing practices. Usually it is the pediatrician who tells a parent that, when the child cries, he should "pick him up" or "let him cry it out" or "ignore it." Such contradictory advice is not uncommon among pediatricians and is often based only on their personal preference and not on any logical theory or body of scientific data.

This is not meant to be derogatory in any way of the pediatrician's practice but merely to provide a focus on the dilemma of the pediatrician, who is looked upon as an expert in child-rearing practices but more often than not lacks the knowledge and training for such a role. Part of the reason for the gap in pediatric training lies in the fact that medical centers rely solely on psychiatry for training in human behavior rather than on the broader behavioral sciences that focus more on psychological theory and social organization (Brown, 1969). Traditionally, it has been the psychiatrist whom the pediatrician consults for knowledge about human behavior; yet, the problems pediatricians face do not require the traditional psychiatric approach. Their problems generally require a broader knowledge of psychological theory as well as a familiarity with current research findings, usually found in the psychological journals.

These issues are emphasized because the human infant is highly susceptible to early experiences, and the pediatrician plays a heavily influential role with regard to the nature of these early experiences, which in turn can have a profound effect on later behavior and adjustment. The pediatrician therefore has a very important role in the mental health of future generations. Impressive as it is for the pediatrician to hold such an important mental health role, it is somewhat paradoxical to find that this same individual receives little preparation for it.

Clearly pediatricians must receive more and intensive training in the behavioral sciences, particularly in personality dynamics and development. Furthermore, the pediatrician should have a consultant available who is trained in the behavioral sciences and equipped to screen, diagnose, and advise on problems pertaining to development, learning, behavior disorders, nervous system dysfunction, and patient management, and also on child-rearing practices. The specialist currently described as a pediatric psychologist has arisen from the need of the pediatricians for such a consultant. Basically the pediatrician can continue to assume responsibility for his patient without loss of continuity, and in this way can become more sensitized to psychological factors and become more adept in "feeling out" potential problems. By working closely with such a consultant the pediatrician is able to deal with patients medically and at the same time offer a good mental health service.

Significance of Early Feeding
Practices: An Example of Pediatric Influence

The pediatrician's impact during the infancy period is very broad. New parents are appropriately interested in doing what is best for their newborn infant, and they have a multitude of questions about the physical and psychological care of their children. Parents generally accept a pediatrician's opinions as "gospel."

One of the most important influences the pediatrician has is on the parents' feeding relationship with the newborn. Feeding in infancy is much more than providing nutrition for the infant. It involves a relationship between mother and child. During the early months of life, much of the interaction that takes place between mother and child centers around the feeding process. This relationship should be gratifying and lead to satisfaction, reduction of tension, and good nutrition.

Parents need to know that the newborn has a very strong need for sucking satisfaction. The need for sucking is congruent with the need for food. A series of fascinating reflexes and impulses seem to be triggered by hunger pangs. Hunger pangs lead to a more intense need for sucking gratification and to a cry of pain and discomfort. A cry usually motivates a mother to pick up her baby and satisfy it. When the baby is hungry, there is increased sensitivity around the mouth and the rooting response is intensified so that a gentle touch by any object near the baby's mouth causes the baby to open its mouth and grasp the object with a vigorous sucking action.

The newborn's sucking needs are not always fulfilled during the feeding process. Some babies fed by bottle may show what appears to be an enormous appetite. In my experience these babies have been sucking from a nipple with a large hole in it. In satisfying his sucking need, such a child must consume more food than is nutritionally necessary. A nipple hole must be small enough so that the baby has to work hard to get its nutrients but large enough so that he does not become exhausted in the process.

Breast-fed babies rarely have this problem because they acquire most of their milk in the early minutes of feeding, and, although allowing them to suck for long periods does give them more milk than they need, it also offers them sucking satisfaction without the ingestion of large quantities of food in the process. On occasion a mother may be a "prolific" milk producer and may find it helpful to give the baby one breast per feeding to ensure that there is enough sucking satisfaction but not too much food.

Parents should be discouraged from using pacifiers to meet the sucking need. It is important that an association be made between the baby's sucking need and the intake of food. Careful regulation of the amount of food in conjunction with satisfaction of the sucking need generally prevents the baby from having to seek other means for gratification. From a psychological point of view it is far better to provide stimulation by picking up, carrying about, and playing with the baby than by using a pacifier. Parents who use pacifiers frequently are, in a sense, "plugging up" rather than "picking up" their babies.

Intense frustration in the feeding relationship and lack of gratification of the sucking need may cause problems in relation to food later in life. Some people have a tendency to gorge themselves or to turn to food when they feel insecure or frightened because food is associated in their subconscious with love and security. Eating as a substitute for other emotional satisfaction can lead to many behavioral problems.

The controversy over breast feeding versus bottle feeding has been addressed by many psychologists from the viewpoint of behavioral development. In this author's view, breast feeding provides many built-in satisfactions that make it more advisable than bottle feeding. It gives the greatest opportunity for contact between mother and child. It gives the baby a feeling of security by being held and supported during feeding, and there are tactile stimulation and movement during the holding.

It is important to note that breast feeding is not the only essential element in the development of a healthy feeding relationship. Whether the baby's need for sucking is met, whether the baby is held during feeding, and whether he is fed within a reasonably short time after hunger sets in are also important factors. A self-demand kind of schedule to eliminate undue frustration in the early feeding process is crucially important so that the mother can feed her baby in a way that is pleasant to herself and her baby, and so that they are free to enjoy each other's company.

It is the pediatrician's role to counsel new parents on other problems they may face with the newborn, such as sleep problems, irritability, and when not to leave a child with others. Pediatricians should also be sensitive to how new parents deal with their frustration, anger, and emotional impulses in order to help prevent overwrought parents from abusing their infants.

THE PEDIATRICIAN AND BEHAVIOR PROBLEMS

Various classification systems are available for the classification of behavior problems, but these have little practical value for the pediatrician who is faced with many complaints from parents about the behavior of their children. While these complaints focus on a behavior problem *for* the parent, they do not necessarily reflect a behavior problem *in* the child.

It is important for the psychologist or other mental health professionals working with pediatricians to distinguish between children with problems and problem children. For example, a child whose family is in a state of disruption because of divorce is a child with a problem. His disturbed behavior is most likely appropriate to his life situation at that moment and transitory in nature. A child with a history of destructive behavior, who becomes sullen and threatens suicide, is a problem child. Although the distinction is not always easy to make, basically a "child with a problem" is reacting to problem circumstances whereas "a problem child" is one with intrapsychic problems.

When attempting to establish the causes of problem behavior, it is important to give very serious and careful consideration to organic factors. It is always possible to find something that has gone wrong in someone's life or some stress factor that is easily implicated with a behavior problem. For this reason, some metabolic disorders, neurological diseases, and malignancies can go unnoticed. All possible physiological explanations for mood changes, feelings of weakness, aggressive outbursts, hyperactive behavior, "day dreaming," etc. should be considered when establishing a diagnosis and preparing a plan for treatment.

Genetics and Behavior

Genetic factors in an individual are linked invariably with physical or physiological effects. Genetic factors are rarely considered to have any significance in the individual's behavior. However, there are unquestionable genetic influences on behavior. At least, genetic factors contribute to the individual's potential in certain areas of behavior. Intellect and temperament are merely two of the many possible behavioral variables that may be considered to be connected to the individual's forebearers.

It is easy to understand why the genetic origins of behavior are neglected except when dealing with behavioral extremes such as intellectual giftedness, retardation, schizophrenia, or manic-depressive states. To determine which aspects of human behavior are genetic and which are largely caused by environmental influences is extremely difficult, if not impossible at this point. It is far easier to "ferret out" the genetic influences on behavior in animals because the parentage and the environment can be controlled.

While it is easier to recognize genetic influences and disorders at the physical and physiological level since they lend themselves to clear, observable factors, consideration also must be given to the possibility that some behavioral patterns may be inherited. For example, after years of recording detailed developmental histories from parents, I have observed family patterns occurring over a series of generations for such traits as lateness in walking, enuresis, difficulty in learning to read, and a tendency toward temper outbursts. It is undeniable that these patterns also might have resulted from environmental factors. However, when there are warm, loving, "well-balanced" parents in a relaxed home environment with two children who have enuresis until the age of eight but who are otherwise healthy, and whose father, grandfather, and paternal uncles also had enuresis until approximately the same age, the possibility of a strong genetic predisposition is substantial. The same kind of family pattern is seen in some children who begin walking alone at approximately 17 months of age and in others who do not begin to put words together until about two years of age.

Parents suffer a great deal of guilt about a child's disturbed behavior because of our tendency to attribute everything to environmental influences, particularly parental influences. For this reason, it is extremely important for the pediatrician, psychologist, and psychiatrist to take very careful and detailed family histories of developmental patterns, with special emphasis on the presenting problem. In fact, if more emphasis were placed on history, perhaps going back two or three generations, professionals might uncover more evidence of genetic behavior patterns. In this way, it might be possible through follow-up and genetic counseling to prevent the transmission of some genetic disorders.

I have evaluated numerous adopted children, in many instances two or three in the same family, all of whom were adopted within days after delivery. The differences among these children's emotional makeup and temperaments are impressive. What are particularly striking are the differences between the children and their adoptive parents. Many of these children were brought to me because of behavior disorders or parent-child conflict. In every instance, the parent had been told by some other professional, or had assumed, as is generally the case, that the child's problems resulted from being adopted and the feeling of rejection by their biological parents. While this may be the case in some instances, it cannot be the diagnosis for all adopted children. I have been impressed by the warmth, sincerity, and great skill many of these parents have shown in raising their children and cannot help but conclude that some of their problems are based on incompatibility caused by temperamental or constitutional differences that perhaps are genetic in origin. At the same time, one cannot rule out the possibility of congenital influences. Elimination of the guilt factor made it much easier for the parents to understand the problems and to work out successful methods for dealing with them.

Many professionals take a prejudicial view of the issue of genetic versus environmental factors. Some recognize behavior as being entirely genetic in origin, while others believe it is influenced totally by environmental factors. A prejudice of this sort can be detrimental to good patient care and careful diagnosis, because it may lead to the categorical referral of children with certain genetically determined character traits in psychotherapy. It may also cause the professional to neglect making a recommendation for psychotherapy when disturbed behavior is in fact attributable to intrapsychic factors.

An experienced, sensitive clinician who respects a careful analysis can generally make a proper diagnosis of the etiology of a behavioral problem.

Role of the Pediatrician

In viewing the problem of behavior disorders from the vantage point of the pediatric practitioner, it is important to recognize certain facts. The most important one concerns the question of prevention versus treatment. It is undeniable that psychotherapy should be given when behavior problems are evident. However, the number of trained professionals available to do the job is seriously limited. Even if every physician, psychiatrist, psychologist, social worker, and nurse were put to the task of dealing with emotional problems, they could not handle the existing need effectively. Moreover, the techniques available for treatment are extremely time consuming. Even when success is achieved, it is oftentimes after damage to the individual, to the family, and to society has occurred already. Today at least one-half of the hospital beds available in this country are occupied by patients suffering from a significant behavior disorder. This fact alone points to the need for early identification and prevention/elimination of the conditions that lead to behavior disorders.

Despite the many controversies in the mental health field, it is known that many emotional disorders are the result of conditions that are present very early in a child's development, and that aberrant patterns of behavior that develop at that time are extremely difficult, if not impossible, to reverse in adulthood. This is not meant to imply that treatment of emotional disorders is impossible. In most instances psychotherapeutic treatment produces varying degrees of success. However, the view that psychotherapy can "cure" any emotional disorder is incorrect; in fact, there are very few dramatic "cures" comparable to those for physical disorders.

Clearly, if an individual's personality is influenced by early experiences, preventive efforts must be concentrated on the very young. It is astonishing that, while most mental health professionals have recognized the tremendous effect of early experience on later behavior, little has been done to assist those people who are clearly responsible for behavioral development of infants and children, namely, parents and pediatricians. As a general rule, most parents have been left to their own devices when faced with questions and concerns about minor emotional problems. At best, they have been given conflicting information, recipes on handling problems, or assurances that the child will "outgrow it." It is precisely these minor emotional problems that can lead to serious problems if poorly handled. More help seems to be available for major emotional disorders than for minor problems or "normal" problems that require some guidance and understanding.

Most often, parents turn to the pediatrician for help with these problems. While some pediatricians are receptive to these requests, most are so pressed for time in handling emergencies that these requests are treated superficially. Because the pediatrician is the focus of these requests and placed in this very important role, it is essential that more emphasis be given to training pediatricians in behavioral development. Parents' requests for information on child rearing, normal everyday emotional confrontations, and diagnosis of serious emotional problems must be met by the pediatrician in a systematic manner.

The time has come for the pediatrician to focus his attention more on well-baby *psychological* care; postgraduate courses, workshops, and conferences should be geared to this need. In addition, pediatricians should establish closer working relationships with psychologists who are trained and experienced in this task. Currently available services are for the most part either intensive psychotherapy or nonexistent.

More training in the responsibilities of parenthood *before* people become parents also is needed. The content of such training is extremely important. Parents are highly vulnerable to *any* ideas and frequently follow information that is detrimental to their child's healthy emotional development. For example, parents are sometimes encouraged to be unresponsive to their infants' need to be held and cuddled to "avoid spoiling them." This notion is not only incorrect but it can be upsetting to a warm, loving, parent-child relationship. Parents, who are indeed the first line of emotional care, are equally as misinformed as they are well intentioned. Generally they tend to follow the advice of others. Parents frequently feel that others are better informed than they are when, in fact, others may be equally misinformed. The recognition of this need has led to improving the availability to parents and pediatricians of information concerning child raising that is understandable and incorporates accepted psychological theory.

CHILDHOOD ACCIDENTS AND EMOTIONAL FACTORS

The pediatrician is logically the one whom parents seek when a child has an accident. For this reason it is essential for pediatricians to understand the psychological significance of accidents and be alert to children who are accident prone.

Accidents are commonly regarded as events that have occurred by chance, bad luck, or misfortune but that, in all cases, were not the result of a plan perpetrated by any person. A great majority of so-called accidents are not accidents at all but result from impulses on the part of the victim of which he lacks conscious awareness. Many people who have a substantial propensity for accidents are considered accident prone. Considerable psychological research has shown that the frequent sufferer from accidents usually has some active role in their causation. As far back as 1926, Marbe (1926) demonstrated that a person who has had an accident is much more prone to have another accident than the person who has never had an accident is likely to have his first accident.

Fuller (1948), in a study of nursery school children, found that 50% of the accidental injuries among girls occurred in 14% of the girls. She noted that the accident-prone child tended to be impulsive, high strung, overactive, obstinate, aggressive, and insolent. Similar personality profiles of accident-prone children were reported by Birnbach (1948), Fuller and Baune (1951), Krall (1953), Fitt (1956), Longford (1953), and Burton (1968).

Accident-prone children tend to be concerned with immediate satisfaction and to be unwilling to put off gratification. They seem to want excitement and adventure, and want it in the present. Planning ahead or preparing for the future is usually absent in their behavior. Perhaps the most interesting feature of the accident-prone person is his unusual resentment of people in authority. He is extremely rebellious against any restrictions, and he is even intolerant of self-discipline. In a sense, he is rebelling against his own good judgment and self-control.

Another element in the psychodynamics of accident proneness is guilt. An accident can represent a destructive act, in this case, a rebellion against authority. The destructive act is an unconscious attempt to destroy the authority person. For the child, and for most adults as well, the authority is the equivalent of the authoritative parent. Hence, the destructive impulse or wish is directed against the parent, which leads to unconscious guilt feelings. Guilt is a most unpleasant feeling to bear, and suffering is an effective way of expiating guilt. The accident or self-inflicted punishment then serves to express a destructive impulse and at the same time alleviate the guilt for doing so. The child, free of guilt and not having expressed open hostility to the parental authority, can feel that parental love has not been lost or threatened.

Accident-prone children are almost always the product of a strict upbringing or are children who lack affection and have developed a very strong degree of resentment against people in authority. They harbor deep-rooted feelings of aggression and have not learned ways of channeling these feelings in a socially useful manner.

Studies of the development of aggression in children have shown that maximal aggression occurs when there is permissiveness in conjunction with parental rejection, hostility, and periodic but unpredictable episodes of severe parental punishment. The child is left feeling unprotected in a context in which there are no adequate controls and from which he is unable to identify with his parents.

A study by Baumrind, made in 1967, provides clear evidence that parental strictness combined with punitive and rejecting attitudes fosters dissatisfaction and displaced aggression in the child. It is precisely this tendency toward the displacement of aggression that provokes accident proneness and self-inflicted destructive actions. While the dynamics of the suicidal person are generally different, there are many individuals who have terminated their own lives through accidents that were unconscious expressions of impulses, which, although destructive, were not meant to be suicidal.

When accident proneness is recognized in children, psychotherapeutic intervention should seriously be considered. Treatment must not only focus on the child but definitely should involve the parents as well. While this kind of family therapy represents the ideal arrangement, it is often very difficult to establish simply because of the nature of the problem itself. As we have seen, the parental attitudes toward the child combine permissiveness with periodic strictness, rejection, hostility, and occasional severe punishment. Such parents are hardly amenable to the idea of psychotherapy and often simply reject any suggestion that there is a psychogenic basis to their child's accidents.

More often than not, the accident-prone person does not receive adequate psychological help until he has reached adulthood, when he can make the choice himself and is not at the mercy of hostile, punitive, and rejecting parents.

I have observed, over the years, a number of children who were marginally accident-prone, that is, they tended to have episodes when accidents were more frequent. Investigation disclosed that these children were not receiving sufficient positive parental attention and had quickly learned they could invariably gain their parents' recognition when they were hurt. Often these were the "busy" parents who had little time available except for crises. Their children, picking this up very quickly, understandably made accommodations for the situation the parents created. For the child it is far better to gain negative attention than it is to be ignored.

Accident-proneness is a complex problem with serious consequences, but these tendencies can be prevented. The question of permissiveness versus restrictiveness is not the primary issue; rather, it is the question of warmth and nurturance. These elements have been the major deficit in the growing child's parental experience. The child who experiences a strict regimen, occasional hostility, and severe punishment once in a while need not resort to accident-prone behavior to discharge his pent-up emotions, provided he feels genuine warmth in a context in which his parents can meet his physical needs and respect his struggle for self-esteem.

PSYCHOLOGICAL EFFECTS
OF DISEASE AND THE PEDIATRICIAN

Pain, discomfort, disease, any disruption of the physiology of the human body brings about psychological reactions. Among the many reactions are anxiety, depression, fatigue, anger, agitation, and changes in body image. These effects can sometimes trigger underlying emotional problems and can also alter personal relationships. Chronic diseases frequently require alteration in a person's life-style while degenerative diseases generally cause a gradual but profound change in one's relationships. For example, an independent and self-sufficient person may have to adjust to being passive and dependent upon those who previously were dependent upon him.

For examples of what the psychological effects of disease, as discussed in Chapter 1 and elaborated throughout this book, can be, let us examine the categories of blood disease and cardiac problems.

Emotional Factors in Blood Disease

Blood diseases in children present varied complications to the pediatrician. These depend on the nature of the disease, its severity, and the method of treatment required.

In my work with pediatricians, parents, and children, I have become most familiar with the impact of hemophilia, sickle cell anemia, thalassemia, and leukemia on the patient, the family, and the physician. While each of these diseases differs, certain problems are more or less common to all of them. All of these diseases have tragic implications, not only because of the direct outcome on the patient's life, but also because of the broad impact of the disease on all aspects of development.

The only appropriate psychological adjustment patients with these diseases can make is an inadequate one. The emotional reactions of these patients are often regarded as emotional disturbances, but they represent understandable reactions, given the circumstances. Their emotional health is usually more impressive than their emotional pathology.

A visit to a clinic where children with thalassemia are receiving periodic blood transfusions dramatizes this point. As painful as the procedure is, they accept it willingly and their regular visits simply become a part of life for them. The depression and concomitant aggressive reaction demonstrated by the patient with sickle cell anemia or hemophilia during a crisis exemplify an appropriate and restitutive emotional reaction that is motivated by the patient's desire to be well. His anger results from being dependent upon others for treatment.

The stresses on the patient with a hematologic disorder are related directly to a real fear of death. Most of these children learn sooner or later that their disorder can contribute to a shortened life-span, and they understandably become preoccupied with this fear. In addition, treatment is often painful and forces children to leave the mainstream of their lives. They often miss school and other activities, and other children ask what is wrong. Children with hematologic disorders have to work harder to keep up with others, and this creates a stress. They have periods of diminished strength, and their activities are limited. Many times they are unable to compete with their peers in normal physical activities.

In regard to performance in school, children with hematologic disorders usually have difficulties. They miss school and have trouble keeping up. Generally speaking, many of them show a drop in grades and a decrease in motivation toward the end of grammar school. As they grow older, many show increased depression, agitation, lack of motivation, and quietness or withdrawn behavior.

These children feel different from other children and often ask, "Why do I have to have this illness?" or "Will I ever get over it?" They begin to behave differently, partly because their disorder makes them different. Their problems with siblings are also affected; sibling rivalry can become intensified. These children usually show some repressed resentment toward their parents for "having caused their sickness." This resentment is real and harder to handle, particularly in cases in which the blood disease has a hereditary basis.

During adolescence even the unafflicted child has problems. For the child with a blood disease, the problems multiply. In patients with thalassemia, for example, the absence of secondary sexual development creates particular problems that undermine the child's sense of self-esteem. These adolescents are frequently left out of normal, healthy social situations. The facial and skin changes that occur with this disease also add to these children's problems.

Most children are asked by some well-meaning adult, "What do you want to be when you grow up?" Children who suffer from hematologic diseases are rarely asked that question because of the general expectation that many of them will die before adulthood. These children sense that grown-ups do not discuss their future with the same enthusiasm and detail as they do with other children.

Many afflicted children who do reach adulthood have difficulty getting jobs and have a difficult time making a vocational adjustment. Most employers would rather hire "healthy" people than people who require periodic treatment, who look different from others, or who show periodic diminution of energy.

Parents of children with hematologic problems undergo a great deal of stress upon all of their defense mechanisms. Generally speaking, they demonstrate shock and guilt when the diagnosis is made. Initially they feel they cannot adjust, and they go through a period of depression, agitation, and turmoil before accepting reality. They tend to indulge these children and give them everything because of their underlying feelings of guilt as well as their sincere interest in providing happiness and satisfaction to their children. Parents have trouble establishing discipline and generally apply double standards when dealing with the afflicted child in comparison with a healthy sibling. The ensuing inconsistency causes anxiety in the child and often reliance on somatic complaints to gain control over the parents.

In offering necessary care to the afflicted child, parents often have to neglect their other children. Simply getting a hemophiliac or thalassemia patient to a hospital for a transfusion requires quite an "engineering" feat with regard to transportation, care of the other children, and all the other necessary particulars in the everyday life of the average parent. It is hard for these parents to take vacations or to have babysitters. They must always be aware of the child's physical problem and the need for emergency care from time to time. The major concern of these parents, needless to say, is the constant fear of complications and possible death of the child.

Hematologic conditions cause parents a great deal of grief, anguish, and stress. It is understandable for them to harbor periodic fantasies of "I wish it were all over," or "I can't stand these problems any longer and feel like running away." The tremendous responsibility brought to bear on the parents often creates stresses on a marriage or mobilizes the strengths within each person.

It is essential for these patients and their familes to maintain a feeling of trust in their pediatrician and hematologist. Every effort should be made through the physician-family relationship to enhance independence in the patient and to offer practical help to the family in the everyday management of the problem. The physician who recognizes the complications will find a grateful patient whose trust and respect will go a long way toward the successful management of the child's illness.

Hemophilia: A Study of Adjustment Factors   Salk, Hilgartner, and Granich (1972) conducted a study of 34 families of hemophiliacs. The goals of the study were to determine the needs and the adjustment problems of the hemophiliacs and their families, to specify some of the psychosocial factors affecting the course of the disease, and to develop recommendations for new approaches for hemophiliacs and their families.

Two questionnaires, one for parents and one for patients, were used by trained interviewers in the study. Some questions dealt with socioeconomic and educational data, but most of the questions were open-ended. From these data it was established that there was a great deal of emotional turmoil within the family regarding the initial diagnosis. "We felt that our world had come to an end," "Grieved," "Overwhelmed," "A devastating experience." These were some of the not surprising reactions and expressions used by the parents. In spite of the basic shock the parents experienced when learning the diagnosis and extensive effects of the disease upon their lives, 83% of the families stated that they learned to take the disease in stride and developed a realistic attitude toward it. They claimed they learned to manage and live with the disease, and an overwhelming majority of them described their children as outgoing and friendly, not only within the family, but also outside the family.

When the patients themselves were asked to evaluate the impact of the disease on their lives, they reported that the greatest area of effect was in physical functioning, largely because of the physical consequences of hemophilia itself. Because of physical consequences, they had to be absent from school more frequently and had more difficulty with maintaining a consistent social life. In the area of family relations, almost all of the patients saw the effects of the disease as negative. A few stated that the effects brought the family closer together.

The overall impression gained from these interviews indicated that, while the families and patients recognized that hemophilia had negative effects on their lives, they made a reasonably good adjustment to the handicap.

For the parents of hemophiliacs, the major adjustment problem reported was in the area of family relationships, financial stress, and mobility. They found it difficult to make any plans in advance and they showed a need to remain close to a major medical facility when going away on vacations. In spite of these inconveniences, very few expressed disappointment or resentment of this factor.

At the completion of the study, a series of recommendations based upon the problems identified was made. First, when families are initially informed of the diagnosis, a great need exists for helping them deal with the emotional upset that occurs. There is shock, guilt, and self-blame from the inevitable feeling that the parents are responsible for causing the disorder. A great deal of fear also exists as to what the consequences of hemophilia will be. Not only is it important to help the family through this upset, but it is also necessary for treatment purposes in the long run. It was felt that, until the emotional problems were handled, it was very likely that therapeutic efforts would be hampered. Guidance and counseling services should be provided to deal with the immediate psychological upset, and group meetings with other parents of hemophiliacs would tend to reduce the sense of isolation these families might feel and help them learn about the realities of hemophilia itself.

In general it was found that the positive adjustment made by both the patient and the family showed no significant difference between the family life of hemophiliacs and that of the population at large. Whatever weaknesses existed in the family were further stressed by the disease; whatever strengths these families had were mobilized to cope with the problems. This study clarified the need for close follow-up of the patient's and the families' emotional reactions to the sequelae of a chronic illness. Clearly, the outcome of treatment depends to a great extent upon the capacity of physicians to deal with the emotional aspects of the physical problems.

Emotional Sequelae and Pediatric Cardiology

In the field of pediatric cardiology, perhaps even more than in some of the other pediatric subspecialties, dealing with the emotional sequelae of the organic pathology is of the utmost importance. Anxiety in the patient and family is clearly understandable and can have a very significant impact on the patient's organic pathology. Intense anxiety can directly exacerbate the patient's symptoms and confound the diagnostic picture.

The pediatric cardiologist may have difficulty separating symptoms that are caused by the patient's anxiety from those that are attributable to the cardiac condition itself. Cardiac conditions can result in severe anxiety because of the great symbolic importance of the heart. Everyone knows that a functioning heart is synonymous with life. Symbolically in literature, poetry, and song, various emotions are expressed using the heart as the symbol of feeling, for example, "I am brokenhearted," "My heart skipped a beat," and "My heart longs for you." The pediatric cardiologist must have a relationship with the patient and the family that is characterized by trust and in which openness and communication prevail. Psychologically, the greatest adjunct to successful treatment is this mutual trust and understanding.

One must regard many of the behavioral patterns seen in the pediatric cardiac patient and the family as normal and appropriate to the medical situation. The anxiety and concern of the parents as well as increased dependency of the child on his parents are understandable. Weakness, fatigue, and avoidance of competitive situations also are to be expected if the child's heart condition is severe.

However, there are hazards based on the fact that the child suffering from a cardiac condition may learn to use symptoms for secondary gain. Problem areas could include avoidance of family responsibilities, withdrawal from facing educational challenges in school, and attempts to gain more attention in situations in which sibling rivalry is a problem.

These problems are extremely perplexing to the physician and the family, because attributing a patient's cardiac symptoms to emotional factors can be extremely hazardous if this information proves to be incorrect. Understandably, this puts the physician and the family in a real "bind." There is a definite tendency to give the child the benefit of the doubt to avert a possible tragedy. Children can pick this up quickly and, when necessary, use it effectively.

The cardiac patient who feels unloved can use cardiac symptoms to gain the needed attention or to cause anguish in those from whom he feels a sense of deprivation. To achieve the greatest potential health with minimal emotional disturbance, closeness with the family and careful follow-up of the patient by the physician are of the utmost importance. Here, the pediatric cardiologist's greatest tool is patience.

Most children learn to adapt effectively. Eventually, this adjustment leads to a certain character formation, which is clearly related to behavioral responses to the cardiac illness. With the major strides made in cardiac surgery, many of these children have a unique and ironic problem. That is, after successful surgical repair they can engage in normal activities and can lead a normal life. A number of children who have great difficulty in adjusting to a normal life after successful cardiac surgery are hesitant, anxious, and tend to cling to their old patterns of behavior, which have involved self-preoccupation, cautiousness concerning activity, and an avoidance of stressful situations. However, this is indeed a happy state of affairs when the psychological problem becomes one of helping a child to adjust to good health. It is essential that the physician take a very understanding and supportive attitude in encouraging the patient to adjust to the new-found health. It is too easy to regard the patient as a malingerer and to criticize him for clinging to old symptoms. The patient is simply reacting in a way consistent with his character structure that has grown out of an adjustment to an illness.

In view of all of these problem areas, it is apparent that the trust and understanding that are essential to pediatric practice are of particular significance in the field of pediatric cardiology.

THE PEDIATRICIAN AND ADOLESCENT PROBLEMS

As adolescence emerges, it is quite common for a parent to think that something is seriously wrong with a child, and the parent may entertain questions about the need for seeking professional help. It is often said that the "normal" adolescent appears to be an "abnormal" human being; that is, behavior that seems to indicate some form of mental imbalance in a person much younger or older is a somewhat routine phenomenon around the age of puberty and for some time thereafter. This behavior does not necessarily reflect a serious emotional disorder, particularly in a youngster whose early experiences have been positive and who seems to have made a good adaptation to various developmental stages.

This is a very trying time in life. The youth is not full grown yet is no longer a child. Physically the adolescent has undergone changes unparalleled in rate, except for those in the first year.

The problems of adolescence brought to the pediatrician, adolescent medicine specialist, and pediatric psychologist are, more often than not, problems of parents who have to cope with adolescents. If being an adolescent is extremely difficult, being the parent of one can be equally overwhelming. Parents are perplexed that some hostile, belligerent "stranger" seems to have taken the place of the loving child that once inhabited their home. All of a sudden, he seems to have no regard for parents and has contemptuous feelings toward the basic values of their life and any rules, regulations, or customs that exist within the family.

When working with adolescents and their parents, it is important to recognize that the conflict between them can be a useful one. The adolescent is concerned about his individuality, is struggling for independence, and is trying to achieve the skills necessary for dealing with the situations of adult life. Many of these issues come forth in the struggle between parent and adolescent. While they may not be resolved, they at least can be brought out into the open for the adolescent to become more aware of the issues involved.

In our culture, it seems as if some conflict between generations must take place to enable a young person to take his own turn in life as an adult. Having something to struggle against is very helpful to young people trying to establish an identity. It is not only important for them to find out what they are but also what they are not.

Most adolescents try to find out what their parents' ideas, values, and wishes are so that they can turn around and do the opposite. Their purpose is not so much to be negativistic as it is to assert their own views. For this reason, it is extremely upsetting to parents to try to reason with their adolescents and convey ideas heavily weighted in experience and good judgment.

Most parents try desperately to convince their adolescents of their own wisdom and attempt to get the adolescent to accept their values. This represents the greatest problem parents experience with their adolescents. It would be far more effective for these parents to express their views directly and openly while not trying to enforce them on their adolescents. In fact, they should encourage their adolescents to express their feelings on various subjects even though they may be diametrically opposed to the parents' own views.

Some parents claim, "What's the use of telling my adolescents how I feel? They only do what they want anyway." Parents who decide not to express views and values to "their emerging adult" will find that their child has to go through much greater difficulty to assert individuality because the parents' positions are either not expressed or are somewhat vague. "How," said one adolescent in a frustrating moment, "can I do the opposite of what my parents want unless I know what it is they want?"

Stone and Church (1968) state that most writers on adolescence

have been struck by the adolescent's agonies of self-consciousness, his preoccupation with who he is and where he belongs. They have noted his proneness to idealism, religious conversion, moodiness and changes of mood, to feelings that life is futile, and to rebellion and inconoclasm. Adolescence has come to be known as a time of inner turmoil, as a period of Sturm and Drang, of "storm and stress." This inner turmoil finds external expression, and the adults who have to deal with adolescents come in for their share of turmoil, too.

It is interesting to note that in many primitive societies the transition from childhood to adulthood takes place simply and smoothly, generally in the form of some ceremony called puberty rites or initiation ceremonies. In some societies the child decides when he is ready to assume the rights of adulthood and then undertakes the particular initiation ritual of that culture.

Some initiation rites are simple and some are more complicated, but in few instances do they last more than a few weeks. In our culture, in marked contrast to primitive societies, the transition from childhood to adulthood takes approximately seven years.

It seems that adolescent turmoil as it exists in our culture represents a period of great turmoil and struggle for both the adolescent and parents. The fact that this is not a universal phenomenon suggests that society plays an important role in this struggle. This is important to recognize for those of us who work with adolescents and their parents. The point to be stressed most for professionals dealing with adolescent problems is the need to work with parents—to help them understand the adolescent's struggle and accept his erratic behavior, marked fluctuation in mood, and disparity in expressed values. And parents need to recognize that a normal adolescent in our culture has some of the characteristics of an emotionally disturbed person during other stages in life. One may venture to say that in our culture an adolescent who dresses precisely the way parents want, who "parrots" their values and ideas, who will do all things they request, and who accepts their values in preference to those of peers, is more than likely emotionally disturbed.

Clearly, the pediatrician must understand the psychodynamics of adolescents in order to assist parents in dealing with the problems that surround this stage in life.

Drug Abuse

The adolescent who has learned to solve everyday problems on his own with parental support generally finds gratification in being able to overcome such problems, thereby getting a sense of accomplishment. It is possible for a youth to learn that oftentimes one can gain greater satisfaction in the long run by putting off immediate gratification. Psychoanalysts call this dealing with the "reality principle" rather than the "pleasure principle." Adolescents who abuse drugs are usually unable to function according to the reality principle. They have little tolerance for frustration and have to dissipate their anxieties quickly. They are unable to channel their anxiety into constructive use. If a youth cannot gain a sense of self-esteem through achievement, accomplishment, and putting off immediate gratification, he may discover that many drugs offer an immediate sense of well-being or self-esteem "internally." That is, the person's sense of self-esteem or "high" comes about through manipulation of the body's internal mechanisms rather than through environmental factors. It would seem, therefore, that the best way of preventing youngsters from abusing drugs would be to help them learn to use their own resources to get a sense of self-esteem or a "high."

I have found individuals who live in a socioeconomic environment that provides them with little opportunity for achievement and expression highly susceptible to drug abuse. This is exemplified by the drug problem in poverty and ghetto areas where individuals have either lacked the opportunity to develop their skills or have been unable to find expression for the skills that they do have because of discrimination. I have also found that many teenagers from affluent areas are highly susceptible to drug use. They are victims of intense peer pressure and oftentimes live in families where the parents have been relatively weak figures in the child's life with respect to the development of social and ethical values. This is not limited to the affluent who live in suburbs. But many suburban fathers spend considerably less time with their children. Peer pressure in suburban areas is often greater than peer pressure among the affluent who live within urban communities. Many fathers and mothers are self-made people who use themselves as examples to their children. They hold themselves high in their children's eyes, giving the children little opportunity for self-expression. The parental role does not include helping the children find their individuality. These children often claim that "whatever we do, our parents never seem to be satisfied." For this reason they are inclined to turn to their peer culture for recognition, and away from parental authority and values.

The best means for helping prevent drug abuse lies in the child's early relationship with the family. Recent programs have been adopted that are geared toward the education of youngsters about the effects of drugs. In this author's opinion, this is not the ideal way of dealing with the problem. Dr. Richard B. Stuart (1972) at the University of Michigan demonstrated that drug education may lead to drug experimentation. He used 600 junior high school students exposed to drug education programs and compared them with a control group of 350 students at the same public school system who were not given drug education. He found that the educated group demonstrated a sharp increase in experimentation. Other surveys conducted in California and Texas produced similar evidence showing that drug education programs have some harmful effects, but the Michigan study has rather conclusively supported this point.

By providing youngsters with a sense of self-esteem during early development and by helping them gain greater confidence through being able to engage in sustained activity that provides gratification, they will be far less inclined to experiment with drugs.

SUMMARY

This chapter highlights some of the many psychological issues that cross the path of the pediatrician. The focus has been on providing greater understanding for the pediatrician, pediatric psychologist, and other mental health professionals to help them see their role better and be able to work in concert with each other toward more effective methods of diagnosis, treatment, and prevention of serious emotional problems.

REFERENCES

Baumrind, D. 1967. Child care practices anteceding three patterns of preschool behavior. Genet. Psychol. Monogr. 75:43–88.

Birnbach, S. 1948. A comparative study of accident repeater and accident free children. New York University Press, New York.

Brown, J. H. 1969. Behavioral sciences and the medical school. Science 163:964–967.

Burton, L. 1968. Vulnerable children. Schocken Books, New York.

Fitt, A. 1955. An analysis of road accidents to children in Great Britain. Aust. N.Z. J. Psychol. 7:129–134.

Fuller, E. 1948. Injury prone children. Amer. J. Orthopsychiatry 18:708–723.

Fuller, E., and Baune, H. 1951. Injury proneness and adjustment in a second grade. Sociometry 14:210–225.

Krall, V. 1953. Personality characteristics of accident repeating children. J. Abnorm. Soc. Psychol. 48:99.

Langford, W. 1953. Pilot study of childhood accidents. Pediatrics 11:405–415.

Marbe, K. 1926. Praktische Psychologue der unfalle und Betriebsschaden. Oldenbourg Muchen, Berlin.

Salk, L., Hilgartner, M., and Granich, B. 1972. The psychosocial impact of hemophilia on the patient and his family. Soc. Sci. Med. 6:491–505.

Stone, I. J., and Church, J. 1968. Childhood and adolescence—a psychology of the growing person. Random House, New York.

Stuart, R. December 3, 1972. The New York Times.

EARLY LIFE CONDITIONS

The early life years are especially significant in the growth and development of the child. For the normal infant and young child, feeding practices and toilet training are major areas in which the expression of problems can occur, and the influence of parental practices can be substantial. For the high-risk infant or infant with an inherited disorder, the perinatal-neonatal period is a time of adjustment for all family members when the many medical and psychosocial issues begin to be raised. The impact of the early years is explored in the chapters that follow.

4

The High-Risk Infant and His Family

Patricia O. Quinn,
Anita Miller Sostek, and Mary Kate Davitt

It is generally felt that problems in the perinatal-neonatal period are responsible for a large proportion of developmental and neurological handicaps seen in children. To minimize these handicaps it is essential to be able to identify as precisely as possible which infants are at risk. Even more importantly, good identification of the infant at risk can concentrate attention on the areas of greatest need, thereby reducing the incidence of potential problems. This chapter addresses such identification and techniques for early intervention.

MEDICAL CONDITIONS CONTRIBUTING TO RISK STATUS

The infant at risk comes from a population made up of approximately 30% of pregnancies broadly defined as high risk because of maternal disease affecting the fetus, problems during labor and delivery, or complications of a previous pregnancy. The vast majority of infants resulting from these pregnancies do well in the neonatal period as a result of careful prenatal monitoring and anticipatory care of the mother and infant during the perinatal period. In spite of this, however, a small group of high-risk infants will be subject to one or more life-threatening conditions. If the infant survives, he may remain at risk for later physical and psychological handicaps. To fully appreciate this risk, an understanding of the nature and frequency of the more common neonatal problems is necessary.

The most important factors determining outcome, both for survival and risk of later handicap, are *birth weight* and *gestational age*. Prematurity alone is not as important as the fact that with increasing prematurity the number of other complications increases dramatically. The actual incidence of prematurity varies with the population group being considered. In their extensive review, Abramowicz and Kass (1966) listed socioeconomic status, lack of prenatal care, multiple gestation, extremes of maternal age, low maternal weight, and complications of pregnancy, specifically anemia, bacteria, and toxemia, as being the more important factors.

Prematurity

The incidence of prematurity in the United States, as determined by Chase and Byrnes (1970) is summarized in Table 1 below. Infants comprising the largest group of prematures, those of 37 weeks gestation and over, have a morbidity and mortality not significantly different from term infants. Survival and outcome of infants less than 37 weeks vary with gestational age; mortality ranges from a reported 2% in infants of 36 weeks to as high as 8% in those born at 31 weeks. Infants of less than 32 weeks gestation comprise the most vulnerable group. Representing less than 2% of live births, they account for nearly half of the neonatal deaths. Again in this group, increasing gestational age carries an increased survival rate. Overall survival approaches 70% in most intensive care nurseries. Factors adversely affecting survival include respiratory distress, asphyxia, intracranial hemorrhage, sepsis, hyperbilirubinemia, metabolic derangements, and nutritional inadequacies. Each of these factors is discussed later in greater detail.

The most significant factor determining survival and outcome of the preterm infant is the occurrence and severity of *respiratory distress*, or *hyaline membrane disease.* Hyaline membrane disease (HMD) is a state of pulmonary immaturity that seriously hinders the infant's ability to obtain adequate oxygen. In a survey by Miller and Futrakul (1968), HMD occurred in 16% of preterm infants with birth weights less than 2,500 g. The incidence varied from 4% in the infants of greater than 36 weeks gestation to as high as 76% in infants less than 28 weeks. Usher, Allen, and McLean (1971) reported similar rates. Although severity and mortality tend to increase with decreasing gestational age, reported survival rates vary widely, depending on the modality of therapy and the occurrence of complications. Newer types of therapy, especially the use of continuous distending airway pressure and greater experience with

Table 1.   Incidence of prematurity in the United States

Gestational age (weeks)	Live births (%)
37–39	17.5
<37 (total)	6.7
36	2.9
32–35	2.5
28–31	0.8
<28	0.6

ventilatory assistance, coupled with advanced methods for providing other supportive care such as improved nutrition, have significantly reduced mortality. Those infants who do survive, however, have frequently suffered such insults as birth asphyxia, periods of hypoxia, varying degrees of nutritional deprivation, hyperbilirubinemia, and metabolic abnormalities. In addition, they are often subject to such potentially devastating complications as intraventricular hemorrhage, necrotizing enterocolitis (a serious condition of intestinal inflammation and necrosis), and sepsis (systemic blood-borne infection). The smaller or more premature the infant, the greater the risk for such complications.

One of the serious complications of the treatment of respiratory distress in the preterm infant is oxygen damage to the retina of the eye known as *retrolental fibroplasia*. Caused by an excessive oxygen concentration in the blood that supplies the retina, the condition may range from mild visual impairment to complete blindness. Awareness of the pathophysiology and better techniques for measuring the blood oxygen level during oxygen administration have helped to reduce the incidence of this disorder significantly, but it has not yet been eliminated completely. It is now seen primarily in very small infants who require supplemental oxygen for protracted periods.

Intraventricular hemorrhage (hemorrhage occurring within the ventricles of the brain) is a particularly devastating event for the preterm infant. It is, after hyaline membrane disease, one of the leading causes of death in this group (Valdes-Dapena and Arey, 1970). Until recently, it has been thought to leave survivors with an almost certain prospect of serious neurological injury, because the hemorrhage occurs first in the germinal matrix (the area in the brain containing rapidly dividing cells destined to become cerebral cortex) and then ruptures into the ventricles. However, with the development of technology to diagnose more subtle forms, it may be found that smaller degrees of hemorrhage are associated with a better prognosis.

Hyperbilirubinemia and *kernicterus* were once causes of considerable morbidity and mortality in the newborn period, primarily associated with red blood cell breakdown caused by maternal-fetal blood group incompatibility. Bilirubin, a normal breakdown product of disintegrating red blood cells, tends to accumulate in the blood of many newborns because of liver immaturity, which delays clearance of the material. Kernicterus, bilirubin deposition in the brain, occurs when fat soluble bilirubin is present in the blood in concentrations exceeding the ability of blood albumin to bind it. This allows bilirubin to diffuse into the central nervous system where it causes cellular damage and death. The basal ganglia of the brain are especially susceptible, but other areas of the brain can also be affected. With the popularization of the techniques of exchange transfusion by Diamond, Allen, and Thomas (1951), followed by widespread use of phototherapy, kernicterus is fortunately rarely seen in term infants. However, the threat still remains for the preterm infant, especially the small, critically ill infant. Studies have described pathological lesions of kernicterus in the brains of preterm infants dying from other causes whose bilirubin levels were well below those considered dangerous even for sick preterm infants (Gartner et al., 1970). Newer techniques are being developed to help in assessing the risk for such infants so that exchange transfusion can be done before bilirubin levels pose a threat. However, until they are more widely available, kernicterus remains a risk for the small, sick premature.

Small for Gestational Age

It recently has been appreciated that not all low-birth-weight infants (those weighing less than 2,500 g) are actually premature. Approximately one-third of such infants are actually mature (over 38 weeks gestational age). Various authors have reported that from 2 to 10% of term infants have birth weights less than 2,500 g (Coleman and Rienzo, 1962; Greenwald, 1964). These infants who are *small for gestational age* (SGA) represent a very different group from true prematures. The clinical problems that complicate their neonatal period are different, as are their survival rates and outcomes. The SGA infant has a mortality rate (3.4%) significantly lower than that for the preterm infant less than 36 weeks, but higher than that for term, normally grown infants (Coleman and Rienzo, 1962). Because these differences were not appreciated before the 1960s, earlier studies concerning survival and long-term outcome of low-birth-weight infants usually included both premature and small-for-dates infants in varying proportions, depending on the population studied. Thus, the conclusions drawn from these studies are of questionable validity.

The causes for low birth weight in the term infants can best be categorized in three major groups: infectious, genetic, and nutritional (Warkany, Monroe, and Sutherland, 1961). First, infants with *chronic intrauterine infections* are often small-for-dates. The usual infections encountered are cytomegalic inclusion virus, rubella, toxoplasmosis, and syphilis. Other agents such as varicella (chicken pox) are also thought to occasionally cause intrauterine infection with possible teratogenic (causing malformation) effects. These infections have a potentially widespread effect on the developing fetus, causing malformation of many organ systems: cardiovascular, skeletomuscular, genitourinary, hematopoietic, and the central nervous system. The combined frequency of these infections in the fetus is estimated at 6-16 per 1,000 live births (Alford, Reynolds, and Stango, 1974).

The second group, *genetic causes,* includes major chromosomal abnormalities, such as trisomy 18, and many syndromes associated with severe malformations (e.g., Cornelia de Lange syndrome). These are relatively rare, and make up only a small proportion of the total group of SGA infants.

The third group of SGA infants represents the majority of cases. In this group, the decrease in birth weight is associated with *maternal-* and/or placental abnormalities that affect the supply of nutrition to the developing fetus. These include such conditions as toxemia of pregnancy, multiple gestation near term, maternal hypertensive or renal disease, sickle cell anemia, and infarctions and premature separation of the placenta. In addition, other maternal factors, specifically low socioeconomic status, multiparity, extremes of maternal age, use of narcotics, heavy cigarette smoking, maternal stature, low pre-pregnancy weight and chronic maternal malnutrition, play a role in retarding intrauterine growth.

The consequence of these conditions for the fetus is chronic malnutrition of varying severity and duration during the time of rapid fetal growth, the third trimester. This results in a fetus deprived of normal adipose tissue and carbohydrate stores, and with impaired linear and, in severe cases, head (brain) growth. Such infants are likely to suffer from birth asphyxia and from profound prolonged hypoglycemia in the immediate postpartum period. As a group, they are less susceptible to hyaline membrane disease, because chronic intrauterine stress serves to accelerate lung maturity. However, because of asphyxia during labor and delivery, aspiration of amniotic fluid and meconium is a significant cause of respiratory distress.

In addition to difficulties in physiological adaptation, infants suffering from intrauterine malnutrition have a significantly higher incidence of congenital malformations of all kinds: 5.4% of live births in one report, contrasted with 1.5% in the appropriate weight premature (Coleman and Rienzo, 1962; Warkany, Monroe, and Sutherland 1961). Although improvements in intra- and postpartum monitoring and advances in corrective surgical techniques have improved survival of SGA infants, they remain at risk for long-term handicap.

Birth Asphyxia, Sepsis, Congenital Malformations, Metabolic Disorders

There are a number of problems affecting infants of all weights and gestational ages that must be mentioned. *Birth asphyxia* has commonly been held to be responsible for a significant proportion of the neurological handicap seen in infants. More recent information would seem to modify that assumption. Low Apgar scores (score given at one and five minutes after birth to assess cardiorespiratory adaptation) alone are not predictive. The duration of asphyxia, the general condition of the infant before the asphyxial insult occurs, and problems after resuscitation all play a significant role in determining outcome. For example, the chronically malnourished SGA infant who is intermittently asphyxiated throughout labor and requires prolonged resuscitation at birth has a much poorer prognosis than the well-nourished infant who suffers a brief asphyxial insult just before delivery and is easily resuscitated, even though the Apgar scores of the two infants may be identical.

Sepsis (systemic bacterial infection) is another important problem. Because of the inability of the newborn to limit infection, meningitis is a frequent occurrence with sepsis, with the highest incidence and mortality seen in low-birth-weight infants. Other associated factors are complications of labor and delivery, especially if associated with fetal distress, prolonged rupture of membranes, and amnionitis (Overall, 1970). The high mortality continues in spite of newer antibiotics partly because of the difficulty in diagnosing neonatal sepsis. For the same reason, neurological sequelae are also high. Horn et al. (1974) reported 33% with handicaps in their small series of patients.

Congenital malformations have already been mentioned in the discussion of the small-for-dates infant. Their general frequency is estimated to be two major malformations per 100 live births. Many are now surgically correctable and have minimal sequelae (some obstructions of the gastrointestinal tract, for example), but others are not so readily eliminated. The infant having cyanotic congenital heart disease or meningomyelocele, for example, remains at high medical and neurological risk throughout most of his life.

Finally, the infant with *metabolic disorder*, such as hypothyroidism, galactosemia, or phenylketonuria, even with early diagnosis and good medical management remains at risk, especially when treatment requires strict limitation of essential nutrients, as in phenylketonuria. The long-term management and outcome are still unclear for such patients.

DEVELOPMENTAL OUTCOME

Increased survival has been demonstrated with the advent of regionalization and neonatal intensive care. With the existing concern for the quality of life, these recent increases in survival rates for high-risk infants are being viewed in relation to the long-term developmental outcome of survivors. The growing technology responsible for the survival of the seriously ill neonate is one factor contributing to the spiraling cost of medical care. Justification of such expenditures is necessary.

Initial reports dealing with these infants were discouraging. Serious neurological sequelae and mental retardation were reported in as high as 60 to 80% of low-birth-weight (LBW) populations. Lubchenco et al.'s (1963) 10-year follow-up of LBW infants born between 1947–1950 found 68% (43/63) to have CNS and/or visual handicaps, and 25% had IQs of less than 80. Growth retardation, social and/or emotional problems, or school failure were reported in 30% of this population.

Studies of infants born earlier, in 1946 only, were not as bleak, and showed incidences of physical, mental, or behavioral difficulties similar to a control group at the age of 18 years (Douglas and Gear, 1976). It must be kept in mind, however, that these infants were neither as small nor as seriously ill, and no ventilatory assistance was provided.

Advanced perinatal care with attention to metabolic disturbances, improved early nutrition, better temperature regulation as well as ventilatory assistance, has made a marked impact on the outcome of infants with these problems. For example, Drillien's (1964, 1967) initial prospective studies found that approximately 60% of LBW infants were abnormal. These findings were discouraging indeed, with her prediction of greater handicaps with increasing numbers of survivors. Improved prognosis with advanced technology was demonstrated in her later studies (Drillien, 1972a, 1972b), however. Following 283 LBW infants born between 1966 and 1971, she found 22% neurologically abnormal at one year, with only 6% rated as severe. Furthermore, only 27 (9%) of the children were found to be severely handicapped at three years of age. Similarly, in another group of 72 infants born between 1966 and 1969, only 7.4% had abnormal mental or physical development (Rawlings et al., 1971).

The literature on LBW infants who also required ventilatory assistance reports mixed results. Marriage and Davies (1977) found that 15% of such infants born between 1966 and 1973 had neurological abnormalities. However, the proportion of abnormals for the last four years of the study (1970–1973) was almost double (16%) that for the first four years (9%) (1966–1969). In another study, 27 infants weighing less than 1,000 g and born between 1966 and 1974 were followed by Stewart et al. (1977). Only 7% were considered to have major handicaps, and 15% were reported to have minor handicaps. IQs for 13 of the 14 younger children (ages between 15 months and three years) were considered normal (greater than 80).

A two-year follow-up study of 73 infants born from 1970 to 1973 was done by Fitzhardinge et al. (1976), who found neurological abnormalities in 39% of the males and 18% of the females and that 16 of the infants were severely handicapped. Although mean Bayley scores at one year were 93.5 (mental) and 81.3 (motor), 41% of the abnormal group scored less than 80 on the Bayley Scales of Infant Development (Bayley, 1969). Significantly, 48% of the sample were either neurologically abnormal or scored below 80 on the Bayley tests.

In trying to determine the risk for an individual infant, it has been traditional practice to utilize what is known about outcome and adapt that information to the infant in question. Birth weight, gestational age, perinatal and postnatal complications and their severity, and the condition of the infant at discharge are considered. In the nursery at Georgetown University Hospital, follow-up is planned for infants who have any one or a combination of the factors listed in Table 2. Of a sample of 102 infants assessed at birth, 90 were available for follow-up and 45 (50%) actually returned for further testing. Data were generally similar to those reported above. Of the infants born prematurely, 30% (10/31) were found to be neurologically abnormal at follow-up, and 52% scored less than 80 on the Bayley Scales of Infant Development (uncorrected for age).

Bayley mental scores correlated with birth weight (see Figure 1) ($r = 0.48$, $n = 37$, $p < 0.01$), whereas motor scores appeared to be a function of neurological abnormalities rather than birth weight ($r = 0.40$, $n = 37$, $p < 0.05$) (see Figure 2). Overall mean Bayley scores at six months were 81.1 ± 21.9 on the mental development index (MDI) and 87.9 ± 20.0 on the psychomotor development index (PDI) (uncorrected for gestational age). Scores were 100.1 ± 23.0 MDI, 98.7 ± 22.8 PDI, and 74.1 ± 17.1 MDI, 83.8 ± 17.8 PDI for terms and prematures (uncor-

Table 2.   Criteria for inclusion in Georgetown follow-up program[a]

Birth weight less than 1,800 g
Gestational age less than 34 weeks
Respiratory distress requiring oxygen for longer than 48 hr, or assisted ventilation
Major congenital malformation
Asphyxia requiring resuscitation longer than 5 min, or with complications
Documented sepsis
Meningitis
Necrotizing entercolitis
Congenital infection
Chromosomal abnormality or dysmorphic syndrome
Birth weight less than 2,250 g (5 lb) at term
Any significant persistent neurological abnormality noted in the nursery (e.g., seizures, spasticity)
Hyperbilirubinemia exceeding albumin-binding capacity or requiring exchange transfusion

[a] Occurrence of any one of the criteria is sufficient to warrant inclusion in the program.

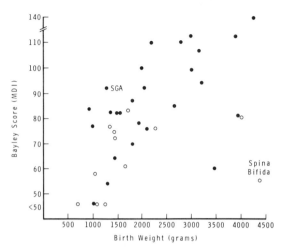

Figure 1.   Performance on the Bayley mental scale at six months by birth weight. (O = abnormal neurological examination.)

rected), respectively. In the group weighing less than 1,500 g, 50% were neurologically abnormal or suspect, and 78% scored less than 80 on the Bayley mental tests (uncorrected). Because these results are from early first-year data and it is important to follow the sample longitudinally, assessment through at least two years of age is planned.

Small-for-dates infants or those suffering from intrauterine growth retardation have approximately the same rate of neurological abnormalities as appropriate for dates infants (Drillien, 1967; Lubchenco et al., 1974). In a study of intrauterine growth retardation and neonatal hypoglycemia, Lubchenco (unpublished data) found a high incidence of developmental retardation and soft neurological signs (32%). Fitzhardinge and Steven's (1972) study of the small-for-dates infant showed a similar incidence of minimal dysfunction (25%). IQs were all reported within the normal range, but 50% of the boys and 36% of the girls had poor school performance. Degree of growth retardation did not relate to outcome, and major neurological sequelae were strikingly low in this sample (1%).

Language delays are also being reported in at-risk populations. A recent study of two-year-olds by Zarin-Ackerman, Lewis, and Driscoll (1977) found risk groups performing significantly lower than matched controls on the language tests administered.

Some mention also should be made of the group of infants born preterm weighing more than 2,500 g. Lubchenco et al. (1974) found this group to have a high incidence of neurological handicaps, and the Fisch et al. (1975) follow-up of respiratory distress syndrome (RDS) survivors

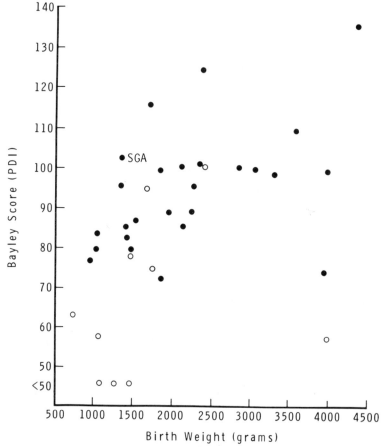

Figure 2.   Performance on the Bayley motor scale at six months by birth weight. (O = abnormal neurological examination.)

showed significantly more neurological abnormalities in the infants of this higher-birth-weight category.

FACTORS INFLUENCING OUTCOME

Even with the establishment of increased risk, prediction of outcome cannot be based simply on the data presented. Studies of risk factors and subsequent development rarely demonstrate a cause and effect relationship. It is therefore important to determine the other factors affecting the developing infant and to determine the possibility of manipulation or intervention in these areas to improve outcome.

The 10-year study by Werner, Bierman, and French (1971) of infants born on the island of Kauai in 1955 is a good example of varying longitudinal influences. Tests done at 20 months of age showed that infants with higher perinatal stress ratings scored lower than those with no stress recorded. At 10 years, the correlation between perinatal difficulties and IQ was no longer present, but outcome was related to parent education level, previous IQ scores, and socioeconomic status (SES). These results from the older sample indicate that, in the long run, perinatal influences were less important and that environmental factors became significant. The work of Pasamanick and Lilienfeld (1955), which initially postulated a continuum of reproductive casualty, later demonstrated the influence of SES on outcome (Pasamanick, Knobloch, and Lilienfeld, 1956; Pasamanick and Knobloch, 1960).

It would seem then that SES has a strong influence on development. It was the importance of environment that led Sameroff to the postulate of a *"continuum of caretaking casualty"* (Sameroff and Chandler, 1975) based on an organismic model of development. In this model, "Transactions between child and his caretaking environment seem to break or maintain the linkage between earlier trauma and later disorder." It is this caregiving environment that must be taken into consideration if successful predictions of outcome are to be made.

However, we all know children subjected to many early traumas and poor environments whose outcomes are much above expectation. It appears that it is not environment or risk alone that determines outcome. The infant himself, with all his individual characteristics and traits, can influence his own environment. Studies by Thomas, Chess, and Birch (1968) delineated the temperamental characteristics that provide each infant with his individuality. Using parent interviews to identify nine categories of infant reactivity, they described "difficult" and "easy" babies. It is these "difficult" infants who are at greatest risk for developmental problems.

Carey (1970), using these same categories, developed a parental questionnaire for use in his pediatric practice. His later reports (1972) demonstrated a relationship between difficult temperaments and clinical conditions such as colic, night waking, and accident proneness.

The infant, therefore, is not a passive participant in the process of caregiving and elicits particular responses from those around him. So we see the interaction betweeen caregiving environment and individual temperament playing a role in the behavior and outcome of each newborn.

ASSESSING THE BEHAVIORS OF THE HIGH-RISK NEWBORN

With increasing knowledge of the sensory and motor abilities of the newborn over the past 15 to 20 years, psychologists and pediatricians have developed methods for assessing neonatal behavior. The importance of such assessments is twofold. First, it may be possible to identify early neurological or behavioral precursors of later developmental disorders. Second, careful evaluation of the newborn may enable the hospital staff to prepare parents for what to expect of their high-risk infant's behavior.

Graham Scale

One of the earliest neonatal assessments was the Graham (1956) scale, which consists of five subscales and ratings. The maturation scale includes motor strength and tactile adaptive responses (the newborn's reactions to stimuli obstructing breathing). Visual and auditory responses comprise the sensory scales, and pain thresholds, irritability, and muscle tone are rated. The Graham scale scores the infant's characteristic performance. Rosenblith (1961) modified the Graham scale by scoring the newborn's best, rather than characteristic, performance and by eliminating the pain threshold scale for technical reasons.

Brazelton Scale

In an effort to examine behaviors with social significance, Brazelton (1973) and his collaborators developed a newborn behavioral assessment scale, which is currently the most widely used instrument in both clinical and research settings. The Brazelton scale consists of a series of reflexes, and begins with four habituation items using a light, rattle, bell, and pin prick. The response decrements are followed by the neonatal reflexes, motor-tone evaluations, uncovering, undressing, and responses to aversive stimuli. Each item is administered during the appropriate behavioral state, initial and predominant states are determined, and state changes are counted during the exam. During the course of the assessment, note is made of skin color, motor maturity, hand-mouth coordination, startles, irritability, consolability, cuddliness, and self-quieting. Finally, the newborn's ability to orient to animate and inanimate sensory stimuli is measured during the period of maximal alertness. The Brazelton items can be scored according to empirically derived factors of irritability, alertness, and motor tone (Bakow et al., 1973; Strauss and Rourke, in press), or according to the a priori scoring dimensions of social interactive processes, motoric processes, state modulation, and responses to stress (Adamson, Tronick, and Brazelton, 1975). Additionally, some investigators compare groups of infants on an item-by-item basis.

Although the Brazelton was developed for assessment of normal, term infants, use of the scale for high-risk newborns has recently increased sharply. DiVitto and Goldberg (in press) assessed full-terms, healthy prematures, sick prematures, and infants of diabetic mothers. Brazelton scoring dimensions yielded significantly more worrisome ratings for social interactive and motoric processes for the high-risk newborns, and the sicker babies cried less. Similarly, both postmature and small-for-dates newborns have poorer social interactive and motoric process scores than normal full-term controls (Als et al., 1976; Field et al., 1977, in press).

Studying the influence of high-risk factors on Brazelton performance in normal infants, Lester et al. (1976) found that birth weight, maternal age, and the infant's sex and race related to an empirically derived attention-orientation factor, and five-minute Apgar scores related to temperament-arousal. The a priori scoring dimensions were differentially sensitive to high-risk factors (Sepkowski, Coll, and Lester, 1977), and each dimension was best predicted by a different combination of variables. Birth weight or gestational age contributed substantially to all four dimensions and the summary score, and motoric processes were most closely related to the high-risk factors.

High-risk newborns in the nurseries at Georgetown University Hospital are evaluated using the Brazelton Neonatal Assessment Scale at the time of discharge. Preliminary data have been collected on a sample of 102 high-risk newborns, which consisted of 70 prematures and 32 full-terms. The criteria for risk included the conditions listed in Table 2 with the exception of chromosomal abnormalities, which were excluded. An additional 36 infants were included as a full-term normal control group. The prematures (less than 37 weeks) are divided into three groups: 1) healthy preterms (transient respiratory distress (RDS) only), 2) a respiratory distress, ill group without central nervous system (CNS) involvement, and 3) ill preterms with CNS involvement (seizures, meningitis, intracranial hemorrhage, hydrocephaly). The term infants were similarly divided into 1) healthy (low-risk controls), 2) ill without CNS involvement (aspiration pneumonia, erythroblastosis fetalis, cardiac complications, etc.), and 3) ill with CNS involvement. Table 3 presents descriptive

Table 3. Mean descriptive values for newborn sample

	Healthy	Ill (no CNS)	CNS illness	Total group
Preterm				
n	25	36	9	70
Gestational age	32.74	33.03	32.50	32.86
Birth weight (g)	1,690.32	1,834.72	1,707.22	1,766.76
Age at testing (days)	28.20	28.58	46.67	30.77
Full-term				
n	36	20	12	68
Gestational age	40.00	38.83	40.00	39.66
Birth weight (g)	3,319.89	3,116.50	3,409.58	3,275.90
Age at testing (days)	2.94	12.35	15.75	7.97

information about each group including the number (*n*), gestational age, birth weight, and age at testing. Age at testing reflects length of stay, because the Brazelton was administered within a week before discharge.

The Brazelton was scored according to the five-point adaptation of Adamson et al.'s (1975) a priori dimension system described by Sostek and Anders (1977). A score of 1 is optimal and a score of 5 is worrisome. The data were analyzed for gestational age and diagnosis, and the means are presented in Table 4. The social interactive cluster, which includes orientation, alertness, cuddliness, and consolability, did not differ among groups. These data contrast with Field et al. (1977, in press) and DiVitto and Goldberg (in press) who found social interactive processes less optimal in high-risk newborns. The discrepancy may be accounted for by the high frequency and extent of parent-infant and caregiver contact in our nurseries, including as much social and sensory stimulation as possible.

Motoric processes include reflexes, activity, muscle tone, motor maturity, hand-mouth coordination, and defensive movements. They were poorer for prematures than full-terms and differed according to diagnosis. Motoric processes were poorest for the CNS ill group, intermediate for the ill babies without CNS involvement, and best for the healthy newborns (see Figure 3). Similar findings on Brazelton performance in high-risk newborns were reported by Field et al. (1977, in press) and DiVitto and Goldberg (in press). Additionally, in normals, motoric processes were also most extensively explained by high-risk factors

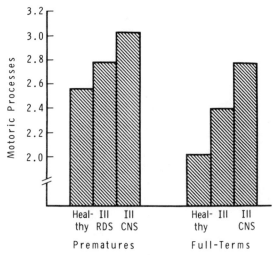

Figure 3.   A priori dimension score for motoric processes for prematures and full-terms varying in medical condition.

Table 4. Brazelton scoring dimensions: Means for gestational age and diagnosis

| | Gestational age | | | Diagnosis | | | |
Dimension	Preterm	Full-term	p	Healthy	III (no CNS)	CNS illness	p
Social interactive processes	2.82	2.46	N.S.	2.59	2.70	2.67	N.S.
Motoric processes	2.77	2.32	<0.05	2.31	2.66	2.95	<0.05
State modulation	2.60	2.34	<0.10	2.46	2.31	2.91	N.S.
Response to stress	0.43	0.28	N.S.	0.26	0.45	0.38	N.S.
Total	8.62	7.40	=0.02	7.62	8.12	8.91	N.S.

(Sepkowski, Coll, and Lester, 1977). In a related report on a different neurological examination, prematures' reflexes were weaker and had longer latencies than those of term newborns (Howard et al., 1976).

State modulation, which includes the response decrement, state lability, and irritability items, tended to be poorer for the preterms. When the poorly modulated infants (scores of 4 or 5) were examined, preterms were more likely to be flat, depressed (10/16), and full-terms were more likely to be labile (changeable) (11/13) (Fishers exact probability = 0.01). These data are comparable to many recent observations that high-risk newborns cry less frequently and less robustly (Zeskind, Lester, and Eitzman, 1977; Field et al., in press; DiVitto and Goldberg, in press).

Gestational age interacted with diagnosis for physiological response to stress, which consists of excessive startles, tremors, and skin color changes. Prematures had more marked responses than all full-terms except the ill group without CNS involvement (see Figure 4). This interaction may have been because of poor skin color regulation in the full-term cardiac patients. The total Brazelton cluster score also differed between gestational age groups. Prematures again responded more poorly than full-terms.

To control for the extrauterine experience of the premature group (tested at a mean age of 36 days), the full-term healthy group was retested at a mean age of 39 days. On all clusters, however, the control group responded more optimally on repeated testing than any of the original groups. The Brazelton Neonatal Assessment Scale, therefore, distinguished between high-risk groups, in the expected direction. Later

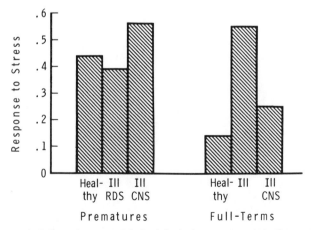

Figure 4.   A priori dimension scores of physiological response to stress for prematures and full-terms varying in medical condition.

analysis in this chapter examines relationships between birth weight and newborn behavior as well as the Brazelton and infant outcome.

In addition to neonatal assessment indices, specific features of newborn behavior are also affected by risk status. Miranda (1976) found that preterm infants at 40 weeks gestational age, with 8 weeks postnatal experience, preferred more complex visual patterns than newborn term infants. Additionally, infants' cry behaviors differ relative to risk status (Zeskind, Lester, and Eitzman, 1977). High-risk newborns cried less to painful stimuli, and both their initial cry sound and overall cry length were shorter. Furthermore, the cry of high-risk newborns had a higher pitch.

PREDICTION OF OUTCOME

For purposes of early identification and intervention, it is clearly desirable to be able to predict outcome as soon as possible. Any effective screening instrument must be able to predict later problems accurately and minimize false positives, i.e., individuals identified as abnormal who are not. Currently, very few measures of infant functioning have well-established long-term predictive value.

Neonatal Tests

Several measures of neonatal condition have been related to infant outcome. In the Collaborative Perinatal Project of the National Institute of Neurological Diseases and Stroke, one-minute Apgar ratings of 350 newborns correlated with eight-month Bayley mental and motor performance (Serunian and Broman, 1975). The Bayley scores of infants with extreme Apgar ratings (0–3 and 7–9) differed significantly, as did the Apgars of eight-month-olds classified as normal or abnormal. Similarly, Hunt (1975) reported significant correlations between five-minute Apgar ratings and six-month developmental quotients. Other medical variables, such as neurological suspect judgments based on birth records (Honzik, Hutchings, and Burnip, 1965) and abnormal neurological findings during the first year (Drillien, 1972b), also have been shown to have prognostic significance for infant development.

There is evidence as well that neonatal behavioral status in normals relates to later development. Five-point a priori dimension scores derived from the Brazelton neonatal assessment scale correlated with Bayley mental performance at 10 weeks (Sostek and Anders, 1977). Furthermore, those infants with worrisome Brazelton clusters had significantly lower Bayley scores than the more optimal newborns. Rosenblith (1974) examined newborns participating in the Collaborative Study with the Graham/Rosenblith scale and found that muscle tone and general matu-

ration related to eight-month Bayley scores, four-year motor performance, and overall condition. Newborns with hypersensitivity to light and/
or discrepancies in muscle tone between upper and lower limbs had
particularly poor outcomes (Anderson and Rosenblith, 1964; Rosenblith
and Anderson, 1968; Rosenblith, Anderson, and Denhoff, 1970). In a
retrospective study, Anderson and Rosenblith (1971) found some evidence that victims of sudden death had poorer tactile adaptive responses
in the newborn period.

Abnormal classification based on the Brazelton scale predicted
seven-year abnormalities as accurately as a newborn neurological exam
and yielded fewer false positives (Tronick and Brazelton, 1975). Using
the visual preference test to categorize neonates as normal, suspect, or
abnormal, Miranda's (1976) predictions of outcome between 15 and 60
months of life also compared favorably with neurological assessments.

Infant Tests

Although some prediction to later development is clearly possible from
neonatal assessments, for the most part the outcome ages are well within
the infant period. Similarly, early infant tests have been found to relate
to later infant performance. Looking at Bayley and Cattell Infant
Intelligence scores, Hunt (1975), for example, found significant correlations between 6, 12, and 24 months.

Attempts to relate infant development to intelligence beyond infancy
have met with less success; however, correlations between infant and childhood or adult assessments have indicated little or no developmental
stability (Honzik, McFarlane, and Allan, 1948; Bayley, 1949; King and
Seegmiller, 1971; Lewis and McGurk, 1972; McCall, Hogarty, and
Hurlburt, 1972). Lewis (1973) concluded that infant tests do not predict
later intelligence because they only evaluate particular abilities at particular times.

Reviewing a large body of literature, Honzik (1975) noted that the
strength of predictions from infant to child intelligence varied in relation
to the interest interval, age of the infant at testing (predictions improve
between one and three years), and the nature of the sample. Predictions
were better for girls than boys (McCall, Hogarty, and Hurlburt 1972),
and socioeconomic status seemed to influence the stability of test scores
(Willerman, Broman, and Fiedler, 1970). Finally, Drillien's (1961) findings suggest that poor prediction may be a function of limitation of most
samples to normal, healthy infants. Correlations between infant performance and later outcome increased with the inclusion of retarded groups.

The relatively poor predictive value of single neonatal or infant
assessment scores has led to investigations of multiple predictors.
Pasamanick and Knobloch (1960) emphasized the importance of taking
medical factors into account in predicting infants' intellectual poten-

tial. In retrospective analyses of the Collaborative Perinatal Project, preschool intelligence and seven-year outcome were best predicted by multiple prenatal, perinatal, and postnatal measures including medical and psychological variables (Smith et al., 1972; Broman, Nichols, and Kennedy, 1975). In terms of seven-year IQ, the accuracy of prediction increased substantially through one year of age, but improved only minimally by adding assessments of development between one and four.

Cumulative Risk Indices

Retrospective analyses, however, cannot provide information useful for determining any individual's prognosis. To this end, the cumulative risk score has been developed to take into account information gathered at all examinations prior to and including the present. Prediction from the perinatal period alone is difficult because many problems are transient, disappearing after the perinatal period. Furthermore, some disabilities do not manifest themselves until complex behaviors such as independent locomotion or language emerge (Drillien, 1972b), and some home environments are more conducive for compensation than others.

Parmelee and his colleagues (Parmelee, Kopp, and Sigman, 1976) developed a cumulative risk index that includes neonatal, three-and four-month, and eight- and nine-month assessments. At each age, the cumulative risk index consists of standardized scores for every assessment performed, up to and including the present. They include the following items.

Neonatal
    1. Obstetric complications
    2. Postnatal events
    3. Newborn neurological examination
    4. Visual attention
    5. Sleep polygraph
Three- and four-months
    1. Pediatric events and examination
    2. Gesell test
    3. Visual attention
    4. Sleep polygraph
Eight- and nine-months
    1. Pediatric events and examination
    2. Gesell test
    3. Cognitive test
    4. Hand precision/sensorimotor schemes
    5. Exploratory behavior

(See Parmelee et al., 1976, for more detailed descriptions.)

Each evaluation is standardized with a mean of 100 and a standard deviation of 20, and the cumulative risk score consists of the mean of the standardized scores to date. The cumulative risk index was developed on a premature sample, and the assessments were administered at adjusted conceptual ages (40 weeks = newborn, etc.). Typically, the risk score classifies fewer infants as high risk at each successive age, and the prognostic value of the procedure for two-year outcome is currently under investigation.

Another approach to the cumulative risk concept was developed recently by Field et al. (in press). In contrast to Parmelee et al. (1976), who studied only prematures, Field and her collaborators based the cumulative scoring on three groups of newborns varying in status: 1) prematures with respiratory distress, 2) normal full-terms, and 3) postterm, postmatures. Assessments were made during the newborn period and at four, eight, and 12 months. The types of evaluations are similar to Parmelee's although some of the specific assessments differ (e.g., Brazelton Neonatal Assessment Scale, Bayley Scales of Infant Development, Carey difficult temperament rating). The Field procedure differs most substantially from Parmelee's in the use of weighted rather than standardized scores. On the basis of empirically derived analyses, beta weights were calculated for each variable, and their relative contribution to 12-month outcome was determined. The accuracy of the cumulative individual classifications was 83% at newborn and four months and 88% at eight months.

As predictors of infants' outcome, cumulative risk indices have greater promise than single or multiple risk variables measured at any one time. The cumulative index has a built-in allowance for the influence of ongoing infant-environment interactions. Particular problem areas can be identified and taken into account in recommending interventions. Furthermore, a developmental perspective can be maintained, and infants with disabilities that are regressing can be treated differently than those whose problems are increasing or newly emergent.

MODIFICATION IN THE HOSPITAL
EXPERIENCE: STIMULATION AND PARENT INVOLVEMENT

In general, interventions to improve the newborn's condition may occur at any of three points: prenatal, perinatal, or neonatal. The first two areas focus mainly on the pregnant woman, and therefore lie in the realm of obstetrics and social services. Neonatal intervention begins at the time of birth and consists of the quality of care, opportunities for parent-child interaction, and the amount of sensorimotor input (stimulation) available to the infant.

Many of the studies presented earlier have found that the infant at risk has an increased incidence of later physical, behavioral, and intellectual handicaps. These ill infants, besides suffering from prenatal and perinatal insults, are also subject to much less stimulation and maternal contact in their early neonatal environment. For this reason, stimulation programs have been instituted in many special care nurseries. Several recent studies provided extra stimulation for premature and/or low-birth-weight infants and compared them with control groups receiving routine care.

In one of these studies, premature infants given extra vestibular stimulation gained more weight and were found to be superior in both motor and adaptive development (Neal, 1968). Solkoff et al. (1969) increased handling of premature infants and found greater initial weight gain, but no differences in Bayley scores at seven to eight months. During six weeks in the nursery, Scarr-Salapatek and Williams (1973) provided visual, tactile, and kinesthetic stimulation to low-birth-weight infants who were premature and/or socioeconomically deprived. Weekly home visits were made through 12 months of age in an effort to improve maternal care. At one year, the experimental group had Cattell IQ scores 10 points above the control groups' (95.3 versus 85.7).

Studying prematures, Powell (1974) increased stimulation and maternal involvement. Bayley scores (mental and motor) were higher at six months corrected age, but the mothers' behaviors toward the infants at home were not influenced by the extra handling in the nursery. Brown and Hepler (1976), however, maintain that stimulation programs succeed best with parental involvement.

These studies indicate that cognitive and motor skills can be improved by early multimodal sensorimotor stimulation. This is consistent with the view, developed from studies of normal infants, that intellectual development depends on sensorimotor interactions with the environment. Because it is likely that the same principles apply to ill neonates, sensorimotor interactions providing stimulation to an infant with CNS dysfunction may significantly affect his outcome.

In terms of socioemotional development, the literature suggests that parent-infant relationships differ between high-risk and normal full-term infants. Most of the studies focused on the first year of life, and noted that prematures' mothers engaged in more caregiving behaviors and less play (Campbell, 1977; Crawford, 1977), smiled less frequently, and maintained less ventral body contact (Leifer et al., 1972; DiVitto and Goldberg, in press). During the hospital period, the prematures' mothers persisted more in feeding efforts, and, at a nine-month home visit, they were less emotionally and verbally responsive (Brown and Bakeman, 1977).

More important than these relatively subtle differences, there is extensive evidence that low-birth-weight infants are more likely to be battered, abused, and neglected (Klein and Stern, 1971; Powell, 1974; Schmidt and Kempe, 1975). This overrepresentation of high-risk infant in parenting disorder samples did not occur in Black populations, however, suggesting that prematurity may be less disruptive for Black parents (Elmer and Gregg, 1967).

The causes of interactional differences probably lie in a variety of special problems. The premature or ill infant is likely to be unresponsive to parental stimulation, especially early during the hospitalization. Additionally, the parents' attachment may be limited by their process of mourning for a full-term normal newborn, and they may be unwilling to invest themselves emotionally for fear of losing the infant. More information about problems and ways in which parents can be helped is presented in the following section.

These social and emotional difficulties encountered by the parents of high-risk infants are often exacerbated by hospital-visiting policies in the intensive care nursery. Even under the most liberal conditions, parents and high-risk newborns experience far more separation than parents and full-term normal newborns. Furthermore, intensive care nurseries, until very recently, routinely deprived the parents of visitation privileges and caregiving involvement.

Barnett et al. (1970) established the feasibility of permitting physical contact between parents and premature infants, including caregiving activities during the first 20 days of hospitalization. A primary concern in excluding parents from the nursery had been the fear of increased infection, but it actually occurred less frequently following parental visitation. Parents, in fact, were observed to scrub more extensively than either nurses or house staff.

Comparisons between physical contact and separated (visual contact only) groups demonstrated that contact increased maternal confidence prior to discharge for primiparas (Seashore et al., 1973), improved family adjustment (Leifer et al., 1972), and hastened weight gain in the newborn (Leiderman et al., 1973). Mothers of separated infants positioned their babies less appropriately and were less skillful in feeding and burping (Klaus and Kennell, 1970; Seashore et al., 1973; Field, 1977). Furthermore, Klaus and Kennell (1976) found higher 42-month IQ scores in the early contact group.

There are indications that individual variables such as birth order, sex of the infant, and the family's socioeconomic status can influence the degree to which increased contact is efficacious (Leiderman and

Seashore, 1974; Field, 1977). The body of findings on increased contact in the intensive care nursery suggests that separation plays a large part in altering the parent-child interaction pattern both during and following a high-risk infancy. Support for this premise comes from these data demonstrating that low frequency of maternal visiting was predictive of serious parenting disorders including battering, failure-to-thrive, and abandonment (Fanaroff, Kennell, and Klaus, 1972).

In addition to allowing as much parent-infant contact as possible, increasing parental participation in the care of the infant can be beneficial. It has been suggested, for instance, that allowing mothers to store breast milk permits them to serve a unique function and assume an important responsibility (Klaus and Kennell, 1976). Institution of a stimulation program that the parents could administer increased the frequency of parental visiting (Rosenfield et al., 1977). Parents seem to benefit from a feeling of responsibility for some part of their infant's care, and such involvement is probably even more helpful than increased contact alone. Additionally, there is some suggestion that infants benefit most from parent-administered stimulation and care. Several stimulation programs have already been established, and a growing body of literature is now available. Texts such as *Intervention Strategies for High Risk Infants and Young Children,* edited by Tjossem (1976), and *Developmental Programming for Infants and Young Children,* edited by Schafer and Maersh (1977), provide more information and review current research on this topic.

THE FAMILY: COUNSELING AND COPING

The parents of the sick newborn have several important and difficult emotional tasks to accomplish during their infant's illness and after his recovery. Although they are described in sequence, in actuality the chronology may be artificial. First, the parents, after being confronted with the reality of their ill newborn, must grieve the anticipated normal baby of their hopes. This grief can be just as deep and painful as if that normal baby had actually lived and then died. The parents must come to accept the existing infant as their own, and then cope with the emotional stress that comes with having a loved one critically ill. Finally, if the infant survives, they must still face the uncertainty of the future.

Drotor et al. (1975) have described the adaptation of parents whose infant has a congenital malformation as divided into five stages: shock, denial, sadness and anger, equilibrium, and reorganization. It has been our experience that parents of a very premature or ill infant experience much the same feelings, although some stages may be of differing intensity, depending on whether the infant's problem has serious life-long implications or whether there is hope for survival with complete recovery.

It is essential that the physician and other health professionals be sensitive to the emotional needs of the parents because parenting and the future well-being of the infant will be affected by how these needs are met. A closer look at the stages mentioned above gives some insight into these needs.

Shock or disbelief is the first apparent reaction, frequently leaving a feeling of numbness or immobility. For the mother of the premature, it may begin when she realizes that she is going to deliver prematurely, or it may not occur until after the fact. It is quickly followed by denial or disbelief. This is the stage of "I don't believe this has happened to me." The urge to flee, to run away, is often reported, and avoidance of the infant is often a manifestation of this feeling. Very soon, the feelings of sadness, and often anger, begin to be paramount. There is a sadness over the loss of the dreamed of, anticipated, perfect child. There is anger on the part of each parent at themselves and at each other. The anger is actually a reaction to guilt. For example, the mother of the premature feels as though she was unable to nurture her developing fetus adequately, that she is biologically unable to bear a normal baby. Parents with infants with genetic problems feel that they are unfit persons. The question of medications taken, physician's advice not followed, or similar concerns may arise to augment this guilt. There is anger toward the infant as well, as the cause of the parent's ordeal. The religious convictions of parents frequently enter into the picture and the affected infant may be seen as punishment. During this time, it is difficult for the parents to become attached to their infant. This can be intensified by the fear that the child may die.

During the period of time that the parents are working through these first three stages, there are a number of things that hospital staff can do to facilitate the parents' work. First, it is important that the feelings of the parents be recognized as normal and that an attitude of permissiveness about these feelings be maintained. Parents should not be judged to be unfeeling or bad because for a time they find it difficult to accept and love their infant. Second, as soon as possible, the parents should be encouraged to see and touch their infant. What the parents imagine their child to be like is often far worse than the reality.

In addition to explaining what is wrong with the infant, at this time, what is normal, healthy, and appealing can also be pointed out. This is not an attempt to minimize problems or have the parents deny their grief but to help reassure them that their infant is indeed one that they can grow to love. During this time, parents are frequently not ready to cope with a great deal of factual information. When possible, it is better to wait in presenting complicated medical data. The physician should be as optimistic as he *honestly* can be, even though the infant's situation may be grave. If the infant does die, the parents' attachment does not make mourning more difficult; in fact, it may even facilitate the parents' grieving (Kennell, Slyter, and Klaus, 1970).

During this time, it is important that the parents be allowed to express their feelings. The nursing, medical, and other personnel should spend time with the parents, helping them explore their feelings. While the mother is still in the hospital, restrictions should be relaxed to allow extended visiting by the father with the mother. It is important to encourage the parents to communicate their feelings with each other. Frequently, in a desire to protect and help, one parent may try to conceal his true feelings and put forward a brave front. This only serves to hinder their mutual adjustment. Encouraging the parents to share their sadness, guilt, and fears will help them become more aware of their own feelings. In so sharing they will be able, in many cases, to draw mutual strength and feel more able to cope with their situation.

Once these processes are underway, the parents will soon be able to move into the final stages of equilibrium and then reorganization. This does not mean that feelings of fear and sadness do not reappear. A new crisis in the premature infant may rekindle many of the old feelings. When a child is permanently handicapped, sadness may never completely be gone, but will resurface periodically or remain low key, but chronic. During this time of equilibrium, the parents begin to cope with their infant's problem. They are more able to accept and process information. They can start to assume responsibility for the physical care of their infant. It is important for the staff to encourage the parents to visit, touch, hold, feed, and care for the infant as soon as possible. The parents will benefit greatly from being assured that their presence is important for their infant as well as for them. The nursery should allow parents free access for visiting their infant, and, when the baby's condition permits, they should be allowed privacy with their infant so that bonding can proceed optimally.

In planning for discharge, the parents should feel comfortable in their ability to care for their infant. They should be given the opportunity to ask questions and voice whatever fears or anxieties they may have about their child's health. As much as possible, they should be given an accurate idea of what to expect and clear instructions on how to proceed should a problem arise. It is frequently helpful for the parents to know they can contact the nursery—at any time of the day—should a worrisome question arise. After discharge the process of reorganization continues as the parents get to know their infant better. However, should developmental problems arise, the feeling of disbelief and sadness may recur and need to be dealt with again.

Prognosis raises serious questions and there is considerable disagreement about the usefulness of discussing the possibility of retardation or brain damage with parents before it is evident to them. If there is strong medical certainty that this has occurred (as in Down Syndrome or severe intraventricular hemorrhage), it is generally agreed that the parents need to know—and have every right to know—what the future holds for them and their baby. When, however, there is uncertainty, care must be exercised. It is probably best in these circumstances to be as optimistic as honesty permits. Parents frequently will seek a great deal of information independently, from textbooks, friends, and magazines. Thus the question of retardation frequently comes from them. It is important that they be made aware of the poor predictability of most available measures of newborn behavior and of the variety of factors that contribute to outcome. Unless strong evidence points to the contrary, reassurance that, as far as can be determined, the baby's future looks optimistic is helpful for them and for parent-infant bonding.

Finally, in families where the adaptation does not seem to be proceeding well, the professional help (from psychiatric, social work, or other mental health professionals) should be offered and encouraged. There is a higher incidence of marital dissolution in families with a retarded or chronically ill child, and, as noted before, parenting disorders occur more often when parents and newborn infants have been separated for prolonged periods. Furthermore, the handicapped child can only cope with the world if he has a family within which he is loved and accepted.

SUMMARY

The infant at risk currently being treated in intensive care nurseries provides a population that requires intensive intervention and follow-up by professionals for many years.

Initial reports dealing with the developmental outcome of these children were discouraging, but recent techniques have improved prognosis. Recent studies providing increased stimulation and parental involvement have also indicated that cognitive and motor skills can be improved by early multimodal sensorimotor stimulation. Increasing parent-infant contact and parental participation in counseling sessions facilitates the long-term adjustment process for the infant and his family.

ACKNOWLEDGMENTS

We would like to acknowledge and thank the staff and consultants of the Developmental Clinic of the Georgetown University Hospital University

Affiliated Program of Child Development. For the newborn aspects, special thanks go to Dr. K. Sivasubramanian, Patricia Peters, the nursery staff, and Dr. John Scanlon. We also acknowledge the generous help of Wendy Burgette and the patient manuscript preparation of Jamie White.

REFERENCES

Abramowicz, M., and Kass, E. 1966. Pathogenesis and prognosis of prematurity. N. Eng. J. Med. 275:878–885, 938–943, 1001–1006, 1053–1059.

Adamson, L., Als, H., Tronick, E., and Brazelton, T. B. 1975. A priori profiles for the Brazelton Neonatal Assessment. (Unpublished).

Alford, C. A., Reynolds, D. W., and Stango, S. 1974. Current concepts of chronic perinatal infections. In L. Gluck (ed.), Modern Perinatal Medicine, pp. 285–306. Year Book Medical Publishers, Chicago.

Als, H., Tronick, E., Adamson, L., and Brazelton, T. B. 1976. The behavior of the full-term yet underweight newborn infant. Dev. Med. Child Neurol. 18:590–602.

Anderson, R. B., and Rosenblith, J. F. 1964. Light sensitivity in the neonate, a preliminary report. Biol. Neonat. 7:83–94.

Anderson, R. B., and Rosenblith, J. F. 1971. Sudden unexpected death syndrome. Biol. Neonat. 18:395–406.

Bakow, H., Sameroff, A., Kelly, P., and Zax, M. 1973. Relation between newborn behavior and mother-child interaction at 4 months. Presented at the Biennial Meeting of the Society for Research in Child Development, March, Philadelphia.

Barnett, C. R., Leiderman, P. H., Grobstein, R., and Klaus, M. H. 1970. Neonatal separation: The maternal side of interactional deprivation. Pediatrics 45:197–205.

Bayley, N. 1949. Consistency and variability in the growth of intelligence from birth to eighteen years. J. Gen. Psychol. 75:165–196.

Bayley, N. 1969. The Bayley Scales of Infant Development. Psychological Corporation, New York.

Brazelton, T. B. 1973. Neonatal Behavioral Assessment Scale. Spastics International Medical Publishers, London.

Broman, S., Nichols, P. L., and Kennedy, W. A. 1975. Preschool IQ: Prenatal and early developmental correlates. Lawrence Erlbaum Associates, Hillsdale, N.J.

Brown, J., and Hepler, R. 1976. Stimulation—a corollary to physical care. Am. J. Nurs. 76:578–581.

Brown, J. V., and Bakeman, R. 1977. Antecedents of emotional involvement in mothers of premature and full-term infants. Presented at the Biennial Meeting of the Society for Research in Child Development, March, New Orleans.

Campbell, S. B. 1977. Maternal and infant behavior in normal, high-risk, and "difficult" infants. Presented at the Biennial Meeting of the Society for Research in Child Development, March, New Orleans.

Carey, W. B. 1970. A simplified method for measuring infant temperament. J. Pediatr. 77:188–194.

Carey, W. B. 1972. Measuring infant temperament. J. Pediatr. 81:414.

Chase, H. C., and Byrnes, M. E. 1970. Trends in prematurity: United States, 1950–1967. Am. J. Pub. Health Nat. Health 60:1967–1983.

Coleman, H. I., and Rienzo, J. 1962. The small term baby. Obstet. Gynecol. 19:87–91.

Crawford, J. W. 1977. The premature infant and mother-infant interaction: A preliminary report. Presented at the Biennial Meeting of the Society for Research in Child Development, March, New Orleans.

Diamond, Z. K., Allen, F. H., and Thomas, W. D., Jr. 1951. Erythroblastosis fetalis VII: Treatment and exchange transfusion. N. Engl. J. Med. 244:39–49.

DiVitto, B., and Goldberg, S. The development of parent-infant interaction in full-term and premature infants over the first four months of life. In T. Field, A. Sostek, S. Goldberg, and H. H. Shuman (eds.), Infants Born at Risk. Spectrum, Jamaica, N.Y. In press.

Douglas, J. W. B., and Gear, R. 1976. Children of low birthweight in the 1946 cohort: Behavior and educational achievement in adolescence. Arch. Dis. Child. 51:820–826.

Drillien, C. M. 1961. The incidence of mental and physical handicaps in school age children of very low birthweight. Pediatrics 27:452–464.

Drillien, C. M. 1964. The growth and development of the prematurely born infant. Livingstone, Edinburgh.

Drillien, C. M. 1967. The incidence of mental and physical handicaps in school age children of very low birthweight. Pediatrics 39:238–247.

Drillien, C. M. 1972a. Aetiology and outcome in low birth weight infants. Dev. Med. Child Neurol. 14:563–574.

Drillien, C. M. 1972b. Abnormal neurologic signs in the first year of life in low-birthweight infants: Possible prognostic significance. Dev. Med. Child Neurol. 14:575–584.

Drotor, D., Baskieivicz, A., Irwin, N., Kennell, J., and Klaus, M. 1975. The adaptation of parents to the birth of an infant with a congenital malformation: A hypothetical model. Pediatrics 56:710–721.

Elmer, E., and Gregg, G. S. 1967. Developmental characteristics of abused children. Pediatrics 40:596–602.

Fanaroff, A. A., Kennell, J. H., and Klaus, M. H. 1972. Follow-up of low birth weight infants—the predictive value of maternal visiting patterns. Pediatrics 49:287–290.

Field, T. M. 1977. Maternal stimulation during infant feeding. Dev. Psychol. 13:539–540.

Field, T. M., Dabiri, C., Hallock, N., and Shuman, H. H. 1977. Developmental effects of prolonged pregnancy and the postmaturity syndrome. J. Pediatr. 90:836–839.

Field, T., Hallock, N., Ting, G., and Dempsey, J. A first year follow-up of high risk infants: Formulating a cumulative risk index. Child Dev. In press.

Fisch, R. O., Bilek, M. K., Miller, L. D., and Engel, R. R. 1975. Physical and mental status at 4 years of age of survivors of the respiratory distress syndrome. J. Pediatr. 86:497–503.

Fitzhardinge, P. M., and Steven, E. M. 1972. The small-for-date infant: Neurologic and intellectual sequelae. Pediatrics 50:50–57.

Fitzhardinge, P. M., Page, K., Arstikaitis, M., Boyle, M., Ashby, S., Rawley, A., Netley, C., and Sawyer, P. R. 1976. Mechanical ventilation of infants of less than 1501 grams birth weight: Health, growth and neurologic sequelae. J. Pediatr. 88:531–541.

Gartner, L. M., Snyder, R. N., Chabon, R. S., and Bernstein, J. 1970.

Kernicterus: High incidence of premature infants with low serum bilirubin concentrations. Pediatrics 45:906–917.

Graham, F. K. 1956. Behavioral differences between normal and traumatized newborns: I. The test procedures. Psychol. Monogr. 70(20):Whole No. 427.

Greenwald, P. 1964. Infants of low birth weight among 5,000 deliveries. Pediatrics 34:157–162.

Honzik, M. P., 1975. Value and limitations of infant tests: An overview. In M. Lewis (ed.), Origins of Intelligence: Infancy and Early Childhood, pp. 59–93. Plenum Press, New York.

Honzik, M. P., Hutchings, J. H., and Burnip, S. R. 1965. Birth record assessments and test performance at 8 months. Am. J. Dis. Child. 109:416–426.

Honzik, M. P., McFarlane, J. W., and Allan, L. 1948. Stability of mental test performance between 2 and 18 years. J. Exp. Educ. 17:309.

Horn, K. A., Zimmerman, R. A., Krostman, J. D., and Meyer, W. T. 1974. Neurological sequelae of group B streptococcal neonatal infections. Pediatrics 53:501–504.

Howard, J., Parmelee, A. H., Jr., Kopp, C. B., and Littman, B. 1976. A neurological comparison of pre-term and full-term infants at term conceptional age. J. Pediatr. 88: 995–1002.

Hunt, J. V. 1975. Environmental risk in fetal and neonatal life and measured infant intelligence. In M. Lewis (ed.), Origins of Intelligence: Infancy and Early Childhood, pp. 223–258. Plenum Press, New York.

Kennell, J. H., Slyter, H., and Klaus, M. H. 1970. The mourning response of parents to the death of a newborn infant. N. Engl. J. Med. 283:344–349.

King, W., and Seegmiller, B. 1971. Cognitive development from 14 to 22 months of age in black, male, first-born infants assessed by the Bayley and Hunt-Uzgiris scales. Presented at the Biennial Meeting of the Society for Research in Child Development, March, Minneapolis.

Klaus, M. H., and Kennell, J. K. 1970. Mothers separated from their newborn infants. Pediatr. Clin. North Am. 17:1015–1037.

Klaus, M. H., and Kennell, J. K. 1976. Maternal-infant bonding. The C. V. Mosby Company, St. Louis, Mo.

Klein, M., and Stern, L. 1971. Low birth weight and the battered child syndrome. Am. J. Dis. Child. 122:15–18.

Leiderman, P. H., Leifer, A. D., Seashore, M. J., Barnett, C. R., and Grobstein, R. 1973. Mother-infant interaction: Effects of early deprivation, prior experience and sex of infant. Early Dev. 51:154–172.

Leiderman, P. H., and Seashore, M. J. 1974. Mother-infant neonatal separation: Some delayed consequences. Presented at the CIBA Foundation Conference on Parent-Infant Relationships, November 4–8, London, England.

Leifer, A. D., Leiderman, P. H., Barnett, C. R., and Williams, J. A. 1972. Effects of mother-infant separation on maternal attachment behavior. Child Dev. 43:1203–1218.

Lester, B. M., Emory, E. K., Hoffman, S. L., and Eitzman, D. V. 1976. A multivariate study of the effects of high risk factors on performance on the Brazelton neonatal assessment scale. Child Dev. 47:515–517.

Lewis, M. 1973. Infant intelligence tests: Their use and misuse. Hum. Dev. 16:108–118.

Lewis, M., and McGurk, H. 1972. The evaluation of infant intelligence. Science 78:1174–1177.

Lubchenco, L. O., Bard, H., Goldman, A. L., Coyer, W. E., McIntyre, C., and Smith, D. M. 1974. Newborn intensive care and long-term prognosis. Dev. Med. Child Neurol. 16:421–431.

Lubchenco, L. O., Grueter, B., and McIntyre, C. A. Intrauterine growth retardation, neonatal hypoglycemia and neurologic sequelae. (Unpublished).

Lubchenco, L. O., Horner, F. A., Reed, L. H., Hix, I. E., Metcalf, D., Cohen, R., Elliott, H. C., and Bourg, M. 1963. Sequelae of premature birth. Am. J. Dis. Child. 106:101–115.

McCall, R. B., Hogarty, P. S., and Hurlburt, N. 1972. Transitions in infant sensorimotor development and the prediction of childhood IQ. Am. Psychol. 27:728–748.

Marriage, K. J., and Davies, D. A. 1977. Neurological sequelae in children surviving mechanical ventilation in the neonatal period. Arch. Dis. Child. 52:176–182.

Miller, H. C., and Futrakul, P. 1968. Birth weight, gestational age and sex as determining factors in the incidence of respiratory distress syndrome of prematurely born infant. J. Pediatr. 72:628–635.

Miranda, S. B. 1976. Visual attention in defective and high risk infants. Merrill-Palmer Q. Behav. Dev. 22:201–228.

Neal, M. V. 1968. Vestibular stimulation and developmental behavior of the small premature infant. Nurs. Res. Rep. 3:1–5.

Overall, J. C., Jr. 1970. Neonatal bacterial meningitis. J. Pediatr. 76:499–511.

Parmelee, A. H., Kopp, C. B., and Sigman, M. 1976. Selection of developmental assessment technique for infants at risk. Merrill-Palmer Q. 22:177–199.

Pasamanick, B., and Knobloch, H. 1960. Brain damage and reproductive casualty. Am. J. Orthopsychiatry 30:298–305.

Pasamanick, B., Knobloch, H., and Lilienfeld, A. M. 1956. Socioeconomic status and some precursors of neuropsychiatric disorders. Am. J. Orthopsychiatry 26:594–601.

Pasamanick, B., and Lilienfeld, A. M. 1955. Association of maternal and fetal factors with the development of mental deficiency: I. Abnormalities in the prenatal and paranatal periods. J. Am. Med. Assoc. 159:155–160.

Powell, L. 1974. The effect of extra stimulation and maternal involvement on the development of low-birth-weight infants and on maternal behavior. Child Dev. 45:106–113.

Rawlings, G., Stewart, A., Reynolds, E. O. R., and Straug, L. B. 1971. Changing prognosis for infants of very low birth weight. Lancet March 13:516–519.

Rosenblith, J. F. 1961. The modified Graham Behavior Test for Neonates: Test-retest reliability, normative data and hypotheses for future work. Biol. Neonat. 3:174–192.

Rosenblith, J. F., and Anderson, R. B. 1968. Prognostic significance in discrepancies of muscle tension between upper and lower limbs. Dev. Med. Child Neurol. 10:322–330.

Rosenblith, J. F., Anderson, R. B., and Denhoff, E. 1970. Hypersensitivity to light, muscle tones discrepancies. Biol. Neonat. 15:217–228.

Rosenblith, J. F. 1974. Relations between neonatal behaviors and those at eight months. Dev. Psychol. 10:779–792.

Rosenfield, A. G., Vohr, B. R., Cowett, R. W., and Oh, W. 1977. The effects of an intervention program on parental visiting in a special care nursery. Presented at the meeting of the Society for Research on Child Development, March, New Orleans.

Sameroff, A. J., and Chandler, M. J. 1975. Reproductive risk and continuum of caretaking casualty. In F. Horowitz, E. Hetherington, S. Scarr-Salapatek, and G. Siegel (eds.), Review of Child Development Research, Vol. 4. University of Chicago, Chicago.

Scarr-Salapatek, S., and Williams, M. L. 1973. The effects of early stimulation on low birth weight infants. Child Dev. 44:94–101.

Schafer, D. S., and Maersh, M. S. (eds.). 1977. Developmental Programming for Infants and Young Children, Vols. I–II. University of Michigan Press, Ann Arbor.

Schmidt, B. D., and Kempe, H. C. 1975. Neglect and abuse of children. In V. C. Vaughan and R. J. McKay (eds.), Nelson Textbook of Pediatrics, pp. 107–111. W. B. Saunders, Philadelphia.

Seashore, M. J., Leifer, A. D., Barnett, C. R., and Leiderman, P. H. 1973. The effects of denial of early mother-infant interaction on maternal self-confidence. J. Personal. Soc. Psychol. 26:369–378.

Sepkowski, C., Coll, C. G., and Lester, B. M. 1977. The effects of high-risk factors on neonatal behavior as measured by the Brazelton Scale. Presented at the Biennial Meeting of the Society for Research in Child Development, March, New Orleans.

Serunian, S. A., and Broman, S. H. 1975. Relationships of Apgar scores and Bayley mental and motor scores. Child Dev. 46:696–700.

Smith, A. C., Flick, G. L., Ferriss, G. S., and Sellman, A. H. 1972. Prediction of developmental outcome at seven years from prenatal, perinatal and postnatal events. Child Dev. 43:495–507.

Solkoff, N., Yaffe, S., Weintraub, D., and Blaste, B. 1969. Effects of handling in the subsequent development of premature infants. Dev. Psychol. 1:765–768.

Sostek, A. M., and Anders, T. F. 1977. Relationships among the Brazelton neonatal scale, Bayley infant scales and early temperament. Child Dev. 48:320–323.

Stewart, A. E., Turcan, D. M., Rawlings, G., and Reynolds, E. O. R. 1977. Prognosis for infant weighing 1000 grams or less at birth. Arch. Dis. Child. 52:97–104.

Strauss, M. E., and Rourke, D. L. Multivariate analysis of the Brazelton scale in several samples. In A. J. Sameroff (ed.), Assessing an assessment: The Brazelton Neonatal Behavioral Assessment Scale. Monogr. Soc. Res. Child Dev. In press.

Thomas, A., Chess, S., and Birch, H. G. 1968. Temperament and behavior disorders in children. New York University Press, New York.

Tjossem, T. D. (ed.). 1976. Intervention strategies for high risk infants and young children. University Park Press, Baltimore.

Tronick, E., and Brazelton, T. B. 1975. Clinical uses of the Brazelton neonatal behavioral assessment. In B. Z. Friedlander, G. M. Sterritt, and G. E. Kirk (eds.), Exceptional Infant, 3:137–156, Brunner/Mazel, New York.

Usher, R. H., Allen, A. C., and McLean, F. H. 1971. Risk of respiratory distress syndrome related to gestational age, route of delivery and maternal diabetes. Am. J. Obstet. Gynecol. 111:826–832.

Valdes-Dapena, M. A., and Arey, J. 1970. The causes of neonatal mortality: An analysis of 501 autopsies on newborn infants. J. Pediatr. 77: 366–375.

Warkany, J., Monroe, B., and Sutherland, B. 1961. Intrauterine growth retardation. Am. J. Dis. Child. 102:127–279.

Werner, E. E., Bierman, J. M., and French, F. E. 1971. The Children of Kauai. University of Hawaii Press, Honolulu.

Willerman, L., Broman, S. H., and Fiedler, M. 1970. Infant development, preschool IQ and social class. Child Dev. 41:69–77.

Zarin-Ackerman, J., Lewis, M., and Driscoll, J. M. 1977. Language development in 2 year old normal and risk infants. Pediatrics 59:982–986.

Zeskind, P. S., Lester, B. M., and Eitzman, D. V. 1977. Cry behaviors of low and high risk infants. Presented at the Biennial Meeting of the Society for Research in Child Development, March, New Orleans.

5
Inherited Disorders
Down Syndrome and Phenylketonuria

Kathy S. Katz

Our knowledge of the mechanism of inheritance of genetic disorders has expanded greatly in the past 20 years. We can now predict the incidence of occurrence and reoccurrence for many of the inherited disorders. It is also now possible to identify in utero a child that will be affected by one of a number of genetic disorders.

Our increasing knowledge has brought with it the necessity for families, with the help of health-related professionals, to make difficult decisions regarding affected children and possible future children.

The birth of a child with a genetic disorder has an enormous impact on the family. Often from the outset, the disorder will have far-reaching implications for both the child and his parents. The disease itself in many instances is a handicapping condition with which the child and his family must learn to cope. Parents often experience a debilitating degree of guilt at having passed on a defect to their child. They must often then make painful decisions regarding having additional children when there is a risk that these children will be affected as well.

The need for support from a variety of health-related professionals is great for the families of a child with an inherited disorder. The decisions that must be made for the child and for the benefit of other members of the family require experience and a thorough understanding of the particular implications of the disorder. These decisions require help and expertise from a professional in the field.

Decisions often must be made at times when the family is under great emotional stress. The members of the family need help in these times to sort out and come to grips with their feelings so that realistic decisions can be made. Here, too, professional counseling can help relieve the burden of the family's trying to work out these problems alone.

There are a number of genetic disorders in which the chromosomal defect is well understood and the constellation of characteristics particular to the disorder are well recognized. Among these are the chromosomal defects resulting from sex chromosome irregularities. In Turner Syndrome the individual has an XO complement rather than the normal

89

XX chromosome pattern. Although having female physical characteristics, these girls do not normally develop sexually at puberty, and they are infertile. Other congenital physical anomalies may be present and a characteristic pattern of cognitive deficits is common.

Klinefelter Syndrome is another sex chromosome disorder in which the male-appearing individual has an XXY chromosomal pattern instead of the XY pattern of normal males. Like Turner Syndrome, Klinefelter Syndrome also has a constellation of specific characteristics of physical and cognitive growth. Both of these sex chromosome disorders have significant emotional implications at puberty and thereafter. Counseling can be helpful in helping the child and his family understand and adjust to the conditions.

There are several other well-recognized inherited disorders each having specific physical characteristics and each having significant emotional implications for the affected individual and other family members. A discussion of each individual disorder is not possible within the scope of this chapter. For the purpose of providing guidance to the health-related professional in counseling families of children with an inherited disorder, two exemplary disorders are discussed in detail. One of these, Down Syndrome (mongolism), is a relatively commonly occurring disorder, and, for this reason, many pediatric professionals may be called upon to provide services to a Down Syndrome child. The other disorder that is discussed here is phenylketonuria (PKU), less common than Down Syndrome but of particular interest, because, with careful management, mental retardation, which was formerly an inevitable characteristic of the disease, can be avoided.

Both disorders require the support of a variety of health professionals in helping the family cope with the problem. Down Syndrome on the one hand is a disorder in which the child bears a life-long handicap of mental retardation. He and his family will need guidance at various times throughout his life. The PKU child, on the other hand, has the potential for fully normal functioning, but the treatment of the disease itself may represent a management problem that is a serious burden for the child and his family, one for which professional help is needed.

Family counseling is an important aspect of the management of inherited disorders. The critical issues with which families must deal have no easy solutions. The guidance of the health professional can do much in helping families handle these stresses.

DOWN SYNDROME

Down Syndrome, formerly called mongolism, occurs in 0.1% of all births. It is the most common specific cause of mental retardation, with more than 3,000 children with Down Syndrome born every year (Antley and Hartlage, 1976). Because the condition is usually recognized at birth, from the outset the child and his family must face a problem with widespread social and emotional implications. The health professional, in informing parents of the condition and providing follow-up counseling and information, may play a critical part in the family's adjustment to the child and his handicap.

History of Down Syndrome

In 1866, a London physician named Langdon Down described a condition which he called "mongolian idiocy." Down felt that the physical characteristics he observed were similar to those of Mongol peoples and that the mental defect was caused by degeneration of racial type. Also in 1866, Seguin described a group of patients demonstrating what he called "Furfuraceous cretinism." From Seguin's descriptions, these individuals apparently showed the same disorder described by Down; thus, Down and Seguin are credited as the discoverers of the syndrome.

Down's description of the syndrome showed him to be a good clinical observer, and, while certain of the characteristics he described are not present in all individuals with Down Syndrome, he did include most major features: flat, broad face, eyes obliquely placed with small palpebral fissures, small nose, and thick tongue (Down, 1866). Down also noted certain personality characteristics including humor and mimicking that have remained as a stereotype for the personality of the Down Syndrome individual.

Early theories about causation of Down Syndrome ranged from Down's assumption of racial degeneration caused by familial tuberculosis to suspected thyroid deficiency. Some early theorists were aware that mongolism occurred in births to mothers of advanced age. In more recent years, the search for the etiology of Down Syndrome has focused on genetic factors. The finding by Tijo and Levan in 1956 that the normal diploid chromosomal number was 46 and the subsequent finding by Ford and Hamerton, also in 1956, that the haploid number was 23 in human spermatocytes have had important repercussions in the understanding of human chromosomal disorders. In 1959, Lejeune, Gautier, and Turpin proved that Down Syndrome persons had a total diploid number of 47 rather than the normal 46. This extra chromosome, appearing in every cell of the individual's body, was found to be responsible for the constellation of physical and mental characteristics that appears in Down Syndrome (Penrose and Smith, 1966).

Chromosomes in Down Syndrome

The 46 chromosomes in the normal human cell are assigned numbers by pairs; thus, there are pairs numbered 1 through 23 with the pair number

23 assigned to the sex chromosomes. In the great majority of Down Syndrome individuals, an extra chromosome appears along with the number 21 pair, making three chromosomes in that group. This occurrence is called trisomy 21, and this term is frequently used synonymously with Down Syndrome.

Trisomy 21   Trisomy 21 occurs through a failure of proper cell division during meiosis. This failure to separate is called nondisjunction and results in both members of a chromosome pair being retained, making the gametric chromosome number 24 rather than 23.

Nondisjunction is a sporadic occurrence and is not inherited. The reason for its occurrence appears to be related to advanced maternal age (Lillienfeld and Benesch, 1969). It is theorized that, because ova are present at birth in the female, the older she is at the time of fertilization of the ova, the greater the chance for chromosome damage or misdivision. This may be a consequence of the many years the ova have been exposed to environmental stresses such as viruses and irradiation.

Trisomy 21/Normal Mosaicism   This type of Down Syndrome occurs when the chromosome misdivision takes place after a number of normal cell divisions have already occurred. The normal cells continue to divide into more normal cells, but the misdivided cells continue to produce those with the extra chromosome; thus, the individual then has some cells that are normal and some that are trisomy 21. The later the misdivision, the greater the number of normal cells, and these individuals may have fewer of the Down Syndrome features and higher intellectual functioning (Fishler, Koch, and Donnell, 1976). Mosaicism is nonhereditary because the misdivision occurs spontaneously after normal cell division has already begun.

Translocation   This chromosomal error results in producing a Down Syndrome child who presents the same physical characteristics as the child with trisomy 21. Through chromosomal analysis, however, it is found that a fusion or translocation has occurred between one chromosome number 21 and another chromosome, usually number 14. This translocation error is found in about 4% of those children diagnosed as Down Syndrome. About one-third of children with the translocation error have acquired it from a parent carrier. This, then, is the one form of Down Syndrome that may be inherited. While its occurrence is fairly rare, translocation is found more frequently among the Down Syndrome children born to young parents. In about 2% of these cases the parent is found to be a translocation carrier, although the parent himself or herself is normal in both appearance and intellect. Either parent can be a translocation carrier and produce Down Syndrome children, but the risk of passing on the chromosomal error appears greater for the mother than for the father. The translocation error also can appear sporadically with neither parent found to be carriers.

Mosaicism also occurs among Down Syndrome children with the translocation error. This happens when the translocation occurs after normal cell division has already begun. The child then has a complement of cells of which some are normal and some contain the translocation. As with trisomy 21 mosaicism, some of the mosaic translocation children may show fewer of the physical characteristics of Down Syndrome and may have higher intellectual functioning.

Incidence of Down Syndrome

The general risk of Down Syndrome must be considered relative to maternal age. With increasing maternal age the chance for an error in chromosome division increases. Among women under age 30 the incidence of having a child with Down Syndrome is about 1:1,500. This incidence increases dramatically with age to 1:750 for women 30–34 years, 1:280 for women 35–39, and 1:130 for women 40–44. For women over 45, a Down Syndrome child occurs in one of every 65 births (Smith and Wilson, 1973).

The chances of a family having another Down Syndrome child after a first has been born depend on the age of the parent and whether the child is found to have trisomy 21 or translocation error. If the mother of a trisomy 21 child is under 30, she runs about a 1% risk of having another Down Syndrome child. If she is over 30, the risk is about the same as for other mothers her age.

The risk for the parent of the child with translocation depends on whether or not one of the parents carries the translocation gene. If the mother is a carrier, the chance is 10% or higher that she will bear another Down Syndrome child. If the father is the carrier the risk is only about 2%. If both parents have normal chromosomes themselves, the risk is the same as for other mothers of the same age (Smith and Wilson, 1973).

Prenatal Diagnosis

It is possible through amniocentesis to analyze the chromosomes of a developing fetus. This procedure involves withdrawing a small amount of amniotic fluid by inserting a needle through the mother's abdominal wall and into the uterus. Amniocentesis can be performed during the 13th and 14th weeks of pregnancy. If the fetus is found to be abnormal, the parents may then decide to terminate the pregnancy. Amniocentesis is recommended in cases in which a pregnant woman belongs to one of the older age groups or in cases in which either of the parents is a known translocation carrier.

Physical Characteristics of the Child with Down Syndrome

A number of physical characteristics are typical of the person with Down Syndrome, but not all characteristics are seen in every Down Syndrome person. Changes also occur over time so that certain features may be present at birth but disappear or diminish with age. Additionally, some features that are characteristic of Down Syndrome also may be found in normal individuals.

Head and Face   The head is usually small, round, and flattened in the occiput area. The fontanels, or soft spots, are larger than usual and late in closing. Ears are relatively small and often the helix is folded over. Ear lobes are small or adherent.

The eye openings, called the palpebral fissures, tend to slant upward. At the inside corner of the eyes are small folds of skin known as epicanthal folds. Because the eyes are slightly reminiscent of oriental features, the term mongolism sometimes is attributed to Down Syndrome. Epicanthal folds are in fact found in about 30% of normal infants but tend to disappear with age (Penrose and Smith, 1966). Epicanthal folds also disappear among Down Syndrome individuals but at a slower rate. Eye abnormalities such as strabismus, nystagmus, and cataracts occur frequently in Down Syndrome.

The nose is small and the bridge low, contributing to the flat facial profile.

The oral cavity is relatively small so that, although the tongue is of normal size, it tends to protrude from the mouth. This is also a consequence of the poor muscle tone that is characteristic of Down Syndrome children, causing the lower jaw to frequently hang slack.

The skin tends toward dryness and develops wrinkles at an earlier time than does skin among normal individuals. Thus, the Down Syndrome adult often appears older than one would expect for his age.

Voice   The voice of most Down Syndrome individuals has a rather husky hoarse quality. Speech onset is delayed relative to other skills, and articulation is usually poor.

Hands and Feet   Hands and feet appear small with short fingers and toes. The fifth finger, especially, is short and may have only a single flexion crease. Incurving of the fifth finger, or clinodactyly, is also common. The palmar creases are distinctive in that there is usually a single transverse crease called a *simian line*. On the feet there is a wide space between the first and second toes. There is also a deep vertical crease on the sole running between the first two toes.

Muscle Tone   One of the most distinctive features in early childhood is the hypotonia common to most Down Syndrome children. While muscle tone improves with age, it initially contributes significantly to delays in motor milestones. In a study by Jackson, North, and Thomas (1976), 10 signs were found to be most discriminating in diagnosing Down Syndrome in a group of children suspected of having the disorder whose diagnoses were confirmed by chromosomal analysis. These characteristics were brachycephaly, oblique eye fissure, nystagmus, flat nasal bridge, narrow palate, folded ear, short neck, incurving fifth finger, a gap between the first two toes, and hypotonia.

Health and Life Expectancy   Smith and Berg (1976) report a mortality rate during the first few years of life of 20 to 30% for Down Syndrome infants. This is attributable to a large extent to the congenital cardiac defects that occur in 40% of the children. Duodenal obstruction is another congenital abnormality occurring in greater frequency in Down Syndrome infants. With modern developments in cardiac surgery and the increasing tendency to perform necessary surgery on Down Syndrome children, greater numbers of Down Syndrome children with congenital heart defects are expected to survive.

A Down Syndrome child has an increased chance of developing fatal leukemia. Incidence of leukemia in young Down Syndrome cases is 10 to 20 times greater than that in the general population. With the use of antibiotics to combat infectious disease, and surgery to correct heart defects, leukemia may become a leading cause of death for Down Syndrome children.

After age five and up to age 40 mortality rates for Down Syndrome individuals are much like those of the general population. After age 40, Down Syndrome individuals seem to be somewhat more susceptible to the diseases associated with advanced age, indicating somewhat of a predisposition to premature aging (Smith and Wilson, 1973). For those Down Syndrome children without congenital heart defects and for those with corrected ones, physical care is essentially the same as for normal children. Down Syndrome children do show somewhat of a greater tendency toward upper respiratory infections and greater frequencies of conductive hearing losses attributed to a tendency toward otitis medea (Brooks, Wooley, and Kanjilal, 1972). For this reason Down Syndrome children should have periodic audiological examinations.

Thus, while a certain portion of Down Syndrome youngsters may require special medical and nursing care in their early years, the majority has no special needs and adequate care can be provided in a home setting.

Sensorimotor Development

Early Motor Development   Early motor development in the Down Syndrome infant is affected to some extent by his hypotonicity. Cowie (1970) assessed neurological and motor development in a group of Down Syndrome children residing at home during the first 10 months of life. She found a significant delay in the dissolution of primitive reflexes including the palmar and plantar, the moro, and the automatic stepping reflexes. Abnormal or deficient responses were seen in relation to the traction response, the position in ventral suspension, and in the patellar jerk. Cowie felt that these findings, together with the frequent strabismus that is seen in Down Syndrome children, might be related to the usual finding of hypotonia.

In a longitudinal study by Share (1975), motor milestones in a group of Down Syndrome children were close to normal during the first six months of life. From six months to a year the Down Syndrome children showed an increasing decline below the normal curve, such that at one year of age they showed delays of four or five months. During the next year this lag nearly doubled relative to chronological age. Share (1975) noted that, in time, motor skills improved such that, by age five years, motor development was one of the Down Syndrome child's areas of strength. By age five the children had adequate motor coordination for bead stringing and building block towers.

In Share's study, the Gesell Developmental Scales were used to assess several groups of Down Syndrome infants. One group consisted of Down Syndrome children from the Los Angeles area living at home. Share also gathered data on a group of New Zealand Down Syndrome children living at home and another group in a New Zealand institution. Both home-raised groups showed significantly earlier appearance of several motor skills, including holding the head up, sitting, crawling, and walking with support.

Carr (1970) using the Bayley Scales of Development found a similar pattern to that described by Share in Down Syndrome infant development. Carr noted close to normal functioning during the first six weeks. Thereafter, there was a rapid decline to 10 months and a less rapid decline to two years. Mean motor scores were below mean mental scores from six months to two years, but, at age three years, motor scores were higher than mental scores. The low scores on the Motor Scale for Down Syndrome children between ages one and two years may be attributed to a large extent to the delayed walking of most Down Syndrome infants.

Findings similar to those of Share and of Carr were obtained in other longitudinal studies by Dicks-Mireaux (1972) and Merlyn and White (1973). While all these studies note close to normal development up to six months, with developmental quotients 70 or above, and a decline after that, Smith and Berg (1976) point out that this decline does not represent a deterioration in functioning. The decline is rather an artifact derived from the computation of a test score that assumes a linear relationship between motor development and chronological age. Down Syndrome children continue to show progress, but at a much slower than normal rate, from age six months onward.

Contrary to the above studies, Connolly and Russell (1976) found significant motor delays to exist in their group of Down Syndrome children even before age six months, but this could be improved through an early stimulation program. Their early stimulation program, which is discussed later in this chapter, helped their Down Syndrome group achieve close to normal motor milestones through the first one-and-a-half years.

Acquisition of Motor Milestones in Down Syndrome   From these various studies, a general motor development pattern for the Down Syndrome child raised at home can be drawn (Table 1). For Down Syndrome children institutionalized at birth, the pattern of motor development is roughly the same for the first six months as for home-raised children. After six months, however, institutionalized children show much greater developmental delays than do Down Syndrome children at home (Carr, 1970).

General Cognitive Abilities

Most reports in the literature about early development and level of cognitive functioning in Down Syndrome have been based on assessments of institutionalized individuals who had been placed at an early age. It is only in recent years that reports have been made of intellectual skills of Down Syndrome children raised at home who have also had the opportunity of special educational intervention. Cognitive functioning appears better for those children raised at home than those who have received early institutionalization. It is therefore important for the health personnel discussing the child's prognosis with the new parent of a Down Syndrome child to be aware of recent studies of development in Down Syndrome children.

Cognitive Functioning in Infancy   Assessment of cognitive skills in infancy is usually done using an infant intelligence scale such as the Gesell Developmental Scales, Cattell Infant Intelligence Scale, or Bayley Scales of Infant Development. The tests yield a score known as a developmental quotient (DQ) rather than an IQ because it is not known whether infant tests are assessing the same skills that later contribute to

Table 1.   Approximate acquisition of motor milestones in months for Down Syndrome (DS) children (from combined studies)

Motor skill	Normal	DS child
Sits	8	11
Crawls	8	13
Pulls to stand	10	18
Stands unsupported	14	22
Walks unsupported	15	25

the intelligence quotient (IQ). Many of the items at the youngest levels of the infant tests are primarily sensorimotor items, and thus the pattern of DQ scores of Down Syndrome children is similar to their motor performance. As was noted in the discussion of motor development, intelligence scores for Down Syndrome children are found to be close to or within the average range up to six months of age but show a steady decline thereafter (Carr, 1970; Dicks-Mireaux, 1972; Merlyn and White, 1973; Smith and Berg, 1976).

The fact that development is close to normal during the first six months can in fact cause some parents to question the diagnosis. It is hard for them to believe that their child is retarded when they see his development moving along at a fairly normal rate. After age six months, however, DQ scores decline such that Carr (1970) found a mean DQ of 34.72 for her home-raised Down Syndrome group at age two years. Koch et al. (1963) found Gesell DQ measures at age two years to correlate positively with later Stanford-Binet IQ scores. Thus, the developmental level at age two years is more predictive of ultimate outcome than scores obtained in the first six months.

Institutionalized Down Syndrome Individuals   In the past, measures of intellectual functioning in Down Syndrome children were based on institutionalized populations. Studies over a 30-year period from 1938–1969 were fairly consistent in finding mean IQs that ranged from 22 to 28 in institutionalized Down Syndrome individuals (Smith and Berg, 1976). This placed the majority of Down Syndrome people raised in institutions in the range of severely to profoundly retarded.

Home-Reared Down Syndrome Children   More recent studies on home-reared Down Syndrome children have yielded different and more promising results. Goldman and Pashayan (1976) found IQs of noninstitutionalized Down Syndrome children to range from untestable to 78 with a mean of 46.9. Fishler, Koch, and Donnell's (1976) group of patients with trisomy 21 had IQs ranging from 18 to 75 with a mean of 53. Fraser and Sedovnick (1976) compared a group of home-raised Down Syndrome children with an institutional population. These investigators found those children at home to have IQs ranging from 30 to 80. This placed their ranges of intellectual functioning from severely retarded to borderline retarded. The institutionalized group, on the other hand, had IQs ranging from 17 to 40.

More current assessments of IQ in home-reared Down Syndrome children demonstrate that, although individuals with Down Syndrome can vary widely in intellectual functioning, the majority falls within the moderately retarded range and some even perform at the mildly retarded to borderline level.

Relation of Offspring with Down Syndrome to Parental Intelligence   It is not clearly understood just how the genetic disorder in Down Syndrome affects brain functioning other than that the result is mental retardation (Smith and Berg, 1976). A question of interest is whether or not a correlation still exists between parental IQ and IQ of a Down Syndrome offspring, as it does between parent and normal offspring. Will the more intelligent parents have higher functioning Down Syndrome children?

Two recent studies shed some light on this question. Goldman and Pashayan (1976) assessed IQ in a group of Down Syndrome children living at home. They also divided the parents into groups based on educational level obtained. These investigators noted a trend in which the mean IQs of children whose parents had a high school education or better fell at the lower end of the mildly retarded range. The IQ of children of parents from the lowest education group fell in the lower range of moderate retardation.

Fraser and Sedovnick (1976) found that parents with higher IQs had Down Syndrome offspring that also were higher functioning if the child was raised at home. It was also found that the IQs of the home-raised group were normally distributed as were their parents' IQs, with the children's IQs ranging from 30 to 80. Fraser and Sedovnick then looked at an institutionalized Down Syndrome group and found that their IQs were skewed toward the lower end of the distribution, which ranged from IQs of 17 to 40. In that this group had been placed shortly after birth, it is unlikely that the reason for their placement was because of low functioning, which might have explained the skew. These researchers hypothesize that an institutional setting does not provide the stimulation the child needs for his true functioning level to be expressed.

It is impossible to separate out in these studies the full effects of innate inheritance versus environmental factors on intelligence in the Down Syndrome child. There is support from both studies, however, for the expectation that Down Syndrome children raised at home, with parents of higher IQ or at least a high school education, will have IQs that fall close to or within the mildly retarded range. Institutionalized children on the other hand, irrespective of their parental background, will have IQs in the low moderate to severely retarded range.

Other Cognitive Deficits   Many Down Syndrome individuals may show deficits in visual-perceptual abilities. Poor pencil and paper skills are seen often (Fishler, Koch, and Donnell, 1976).

Cognitive Functioning in Mosaic Down Syndrome   Because the mosaic Down Syndrome individual has some normal cells, he may show fewer of the characteristics of Down Syndrome and may have higher intellectual ability (Rosecrans, 1968). Penrose (1967) evaluated a group of mosaic Down Syndrome individuals and found their IQs to range from 35 to above average. Mean IQ for this group was 70, in the borderline retarded range. Fishler, Koch, and Donnell (1976) found a group of mosaics to have an IQ range from 43 to 89, with a mean of 67, at the high mildly retarded level. Fishler et al. noted that the higher functioning individuals in the group had better speech quality, lacking the hoarse, unclear speech of the typical Down Syndrome person. The higher IQ mosaics also showed better vocabulary, comprehension, and number concepts. Some of the mosaics had adequate visual-perceptual ability. Those mosaics who showed poor visual-motor skills also had lower IQs.

Because mosaicism can arise at any point after cell division has begun, the number of normal cells will vary from one mosaic individual to another. Thus, it is difficult to predict the level of functioning of that particular individual once the diagnosis of mosaicism has been made. One can only say that there is a better probability that the mosaic individual will function higher intellectually than if he were classic Down Syndrome. However, as was found in the studies mentioned, many mosaic individuals still displayed moderate retardation as do the majority of individuals with Down Syndrome.

Language Development

Language is a specific area of cognitive functioning in Down Syndrome that develops at a much slower rate relative to other skills. While normal children begin saying words at about age one year, most Down Syndrome children do not begin saying words until two years (Merlyn and White, 1973; Smith and Berg, 1976). Language acquisition also shows much variability from one Down Syndrome child to another, and, although a few children may say words close to the normal time, others do not until close to six years. Language usually remains the most limited area of functioning, with motor and social skills being much more advanced.

In addition to very slow development of language, the majority of Down Syndrome children have very poor speech articulation, to the extent that their speech is difficult to understand. Whether this is attributable to the properties of the voice structure, to hypotonia of the oral musculature, or to poor auditory discrimination is not known. Speech therapy can be helpful in improving intelligibility. Share (1975) noted that, although the expressive language of most Down Syndrome children is usually limited, their receptive language seems to be at a considerably higher level. None of Share's group of children were able to use the prepositions *in, under,* or *on top of,* but they could carry out instructions that involved comprehension of these same prepositional relationships. Share suggests that, because the children understand these concepts, with special language training they most probably can learn to express them, as well. This is a variation from the normal child who is able to employ prepositions in speech by having heard them in his language environment. With the Down Syndrome child the capacity is there, but special intervention is needed to bring it out.

Share also found that the higher functioning Down Syndrome child with an expressive deficit often develops a very extensive gesture language to express his thoughts. The lower functioning child with the same degree of deficit does not develop a similar gesture system. It is this use of gesture that perhaps has contributed to the Down Syndrome individual's reputation for mimickry.

In an earlier study (Bilovsky and Share, 1965), the discrepancy between the Down Syndrome individual's receptive and expressive language had been documented by use of the Illinois Test of Psycholinguistic Abilities (ITPA). Cornwell (1974) also explored the discrepancy between verbal comprehension versus expressive skills in Down Syndrome children ranging in mental age from 0.1 to 5.10 years. She, too, noted that comprehension is much superior to expressive language. However, in terms of comprehension skills, the Down Syndrome children did show a severe deficit in conceptual ability. Use of numbers, in particular, was extremely impaired. Most children, with or without expressive language, were unable to deal with numerical symbols. Some of the children were able to learn counting skills, but they could not learn number manipulation. Cornwell also found that many of the children showed through mime that they understood what was asked of them although they often could not express it verbally. Cornwell suggests that the deficiency may be a combination of inherent problems with expressive language as well as articulation.

Social Adaptive Functioning and
Personality Development in Down Syndrome

Social adaptive functioning is the ability of the individual to cope with demands of daily living. These demands would include self-care skills, such as grooming and toileting, and independence skills, such as the ability to travel on one's own. Social adaptive functioning and measured cognitive functioning are not always at the same level in any particular individual. When social-adaptive skills are at a higher level than measured cognitive abilities, they may in fact be even more important than IQ in planning for the retarded individual's future. This is because IQ is a measure of academic potential, and academic abilities do not play as large a part in the employment and living opportunities for retarded individuals as do social-adaptive abilities.

The degree of self-help acquisition of Down Syndrome individuals is often above that that one would have expected on the basis of measured IQ. While this is often the case with retarded individuals, it is particularly true of the Down Syndrome person. An early study by Pototzky and Grigg (1942) had found social quotients (SQs) for an institutionalized Down Syndrome group to be nearly three-and-a-half years above their mental age. Another group of non–Down Syndrome retarded individuals were found to have SQs only two years above mental age. These early findings were supported in a more recent study by Grotz, Henderson, and Katz (1972), who found institutionalized Down Syndrome individuals much more capable of bathing, dressing, toileting, and feeding than other institutionalized retardates. Cornwell and Birch (1969) found that home-reared Down Syndrome children also showed SQs consistently higher than IQs obtained on the Stanford-Binet.

Although institutionalized Down Syndrome individuals can acquire a level of self-care significantly above that of most other retardates, their level of functioning still remains behind that of Down Syndrome children raised at home (Share, 1975).

Social development in the early years presents a picture similar to that of motor development for the Down Syndrome child. The milestones in the first six months occur at close to the expected age norm. The Down Syndrome infant smiles by age 12 weeks, only a few weeks behind a normal baby. The other social behaviors in the first few months, such as cooing and recognition of parents, also are delayed only slightly and follow the same sequence as in the normal infant (Cytryn, 1975).

After age six months the degree of delays in acquisition of social skills becomes increased. Share (1975) found that beginning feeding skills for his group of home-reared Down Syndrome children were not seen until 17 to 24 months, whereas for normal children they begin at nine months. The skills for putting on one's own clothes usually begin at 24 months for normal children, but for the Down Syndrome group they did not emerge until about 44 months. The Down Syndrome children were not toilet trained until age three, a skill achieved by normal children by age two. Although the delays are significant, Share's study does support the belief that Down Syndrome children can learn basic self-care functioning. The degree of skill acquisition can be enhanced by the use of behavior-shaping techniques.

Social Adjustment and Temperament   In his original description of the syndrome, Langdon Down noted that Down Syndrome individuals tended to be humorous, amiable, and given to mimickry. This has developed into the common stereotype attributed to the Down Syndrome individual. Several studies have explored personality in Down Syndrome more systematically. Domino, Goldschmid, and Kaplan (1964) and Silverstein (1964), in looking at institutionalized Down Syndrome individuals, in general found support for the belief that they tended to be sociable and easy going. Schlottman and Anderson (1975) assessed social behavior in institutionalized Down Syndrome children as compared to non–Down Syndrome children. These investigators found that the Down Syndrome children were more likely to participate in toy play activities with other children. The Down Syndrome boys displayed more social smiling, positive social vocalization, and less solitary toy play than did non–Down Syndrome boys. Down Syndrome girls' scores were not significantly different from controls. Schlottman and Anderson felt their findings tended to support a stereotype of cheerfulness, gregariousness, and friendliness for Down Syndrome children. Cytryn (1975) assessed social behavior in home-reared Down Syndrome children as compared to non–Down Syndrome retarded children living at home. The non–Down Syndrome retarded group was found to show greater withdrawal, lack of relatedness, impulsivity, and irritability than the Down Syndrome group. No differences were found with respect to hyperactivity, aggression, or lack of cooperation. Cytryn felt there was thus some support for believing that Down Syndrome children are better adjusted than other retarded children but that they do not differ completely.

Cytryn (1975) also classified his group of Down Syndrome children into general personality types and found that they formed three categories. The majority of children were found to be alert to their environment and displayed friendly social interaction. A minority formed a second category and tended to be dull and listless. A very few of the children formed a third group that could be characterized as negativistic, restless, and irritable. When Cytryn looked at maternal interaction of the Down Syndrome children, he found no differences among the mothers of the three groups of children. Thus, the personality differences did not appear to be related to child-rearing techniques but rather to innate differences in the children themselves.

These studies taken as a whole have found Down Syndrome children to show generally better social adjustment than other groups of retarded individuals. On the other hand, Baron (1972), in comparing the temperaments of young Down Syndrome children living at home to normal children, found the Down Syndrome group to be the same as normals in terms of adaptability, mood, distractability, and persistence. Baron concluded that there was no evidence for the stereotype of Down Syndrome children being better socially adjusted than normal. What may, in fact, be the explanation is that Down Syndrome children display fairly normal social adjustment and that this does not fit with the stereotype of the retarded individual.

Implications of Social Functioning in Down Syndrome   The greater social adjustment and adaptive functioning of Down Syndrome individuals in comparison to the majority of other retarded persons have important implications for potential for greater independent functioning as adults. Given that the Down Syndrome person can learn to a large degree to take responsibility for his personal care, the need for extensive supervision is not as great as for the majority of institutionalized retardates. This broadens the possibility for alternative living arrangements for most Down Syndrome individuals. In childhood it means that most Down Syndrome youngsters can be managed adequately in a home setting. For the Down Syndrome adult, it means that the custodial care provided by large residential institutions for the retarded is not necessary. Many Down Syndrome adults could function quite effectively in a small group home for retarded adults. Such homes are usually within the general community where several retarded adults live together, taking charge of their own personal needs and the day-to-day maintenance of the home, under the supervision of a director of the home.

Informing Parents of the Diagnosis

The birth of an infant is a time of high emotion for the new parents. Because of this, they are unusually vulnerable to stress. The stress of the birth of an abnormal child is a very harsh one, and the family's ability to make well thought out decisions around that child is much impaired. The family is in need of the support of a variety of health-related professionals, who can help them cope with the crisis.

In deciding when to tell the parents of the diagnosis, the experience of other clinicians may be of help. In an examination of parental preferences on the handling of the diagnosis of Down Syndrome, Gayton and Walker (1974) found that most parents would have preferred being told in the first week following delivery. Pueschel and Murphy (1975) suggest that parents should be informed as soon as a definite diagnosis has been made. If a definite diagnosis requires a chromosome analysis, then the parents should be told of the suspicion that the child has Down Syndrome. Usually the chromosome analysis can confirm or deny this in four to six days. The parents should have an opportunity to see the baby before being informed to avoid their being afraid to contact or look at the child.

By informing the parents shortly after birth, several unfortunate circumstances can be avoided. For one, as Gayton and Walker (1974) discovered, parents found it hard to tell other people that the baby had

Down Syndrome after they had told everyone that the baby was fine. By early informing, one also limits the chance that the parents will learn of the diagnosis in a distorted or incomplete fashion from an inappropriate source.

Who should be present at the session is another issue about which parents expressed feelings. Parents in the Gayton and Walker (1974) study expressed a wish that they had received the news while they were together to give each other emotional support. This procedure avoids the situation in which defensive hostility later is directed at the informing spouse or in which the informing spouse is bombarded with questions that he or she cannot answer.

The preferred informant might be either the family's obstetrician or pediatrician. It might also be helpful for both these physicians to meet together with the family. Pueschel and Murphy (1975) suggest that a social worker and physician together might serve as an informing team.

The Informing Session   The emotion with which the parents receive the news of the diagnosis will interfere to some extent with their ability to absorb all the information conveyed. The first information session should be fairly brief with provision made for a return session.

During the session, the physician might himself hold the infant during the interview in a caring way to model for the parents the normal affectional needs of the baby. It may be useful to demonstrate the physical findings directly on the baby. If other abnormalities exist, such as a heart defect, it is perhaps beneficial to have a medical specialist present to answer questions in relationship to the problem and what can be done about it (Golden and Davis, 1974). The genetic abnormality should be explained to the parent as well as the risks for future pregnancies. The parents should be made aware that genetic counseling is available to them.

Parents should understand that the child will develop although his development will be slow, relative to normal children. It might be explained that at birth it is impossible to predict what any child will be like and that this is also true for the Down Syndrome child. Retardation should be discussed, but parents should be told about variations in functioning and that both the child's innate endowment and the environment in which he is raised play a role in his ultimate level of functioning.

In discussing the baby, it is important to stress that the Down Syndrome baby has much the same needs as a normal infant, those of warm, loving parents. He will also be able to return that love and will be alert and responsive to those who care for him.

After encouraging questions, the informing team might end the first session with a second meeting planned for the next day. The baby should be allowed to remain with the parents as much as possible. Nursing staff might be alerted to provide support and information to the family if needed.

On the second visit more information can be provided in terms of the child's long-term prognosis. It can be stated that Down Syndrome children do not outgrow or catch up their delays in development. While as adults they will have limitations in development, it cannot be determined at birth what the family can expect from their child; but, regardless, the child will be in need of special education services throughout his school years and he will always require some degree of supervision. Parents should feel that they will not have to deal with this alone, however. Support services in the hospital should be made available to them, and the support team should be aware of community resources as well. Openness with siblings and other family members should be encouraged so that parents can get support from other individuals to whom they are close.

The Issue of Institutional Placement   Attitudes around early institutional placement of Down Syndrome children have changed considerably in the last decade. Gayton and Walker (1974) report that most parents of children born before 1963 were encouraged to institutionalize the child immediately, but since 1963 this is not as widely done.

The recommendation for institutionalization was usually based on the health-related professional's concept, frequently an erroneous one, of what the outcome for a Down Syndrome child is. Giannini and Goodman (1970) found that the parents of Down Syndrome children with whom they worked had been told by physicians such things as the child would die before he was two years old, the child would never achieve self-care ability, and the child's presence would have a harmful effect on the family. Another almost universal dictum was that the child's condition was hopeless and that he should be institutionalized before the parents got attached to him. Contradicting this, Golden and Davis (1974) point out that the attachment to an infant begins long before his birth, and, once a family has tried to raise the child, even if a later decision is made for placement, there will be fewer and less destructive guilt feelings than if the parents had never tried to cope with the child at home. An additional reality when considering the issue of institutionalization is that most institutions have long waiting lists and frequently will refuse admission to the young Down Syndrome child because he can be cared for in a home setting.

Unless there are complications that require continual nursing care, the family should be told that Down Syndrome infants do best when cared for at home and that in the past those children who were placed in institutions were denied a chance to reach their full potential. Because the needs of a young Down Syndrome child are the same as those of a normal child, there is no reason why his presence should place undue demands on other family members.

Parents can be assured that placement can be arranged at a later time if they find they cannot manage the child, but that for the early years it is critical for the child and important for them that infant and parents be together.

There are those families that, despite professional support, are under such stress that they cannot cope with the child at home. In those circumstances alternative, perhaps temporary, placement should be sought in a setting such as a foster home.

Planning for the Down Syndrome Child

To plan effectively for any Down Syndrome child, one must have a comprehensive picture of that child's strengths and weaknesses in a variety of areas of functioning. This can be performed most effectively through an interdisciplinary developmental evaluation.

The interdisciplinary team might consist of members from psychology, communications disorders, physical and occupational therapy, special education, pediatrics, nursing, and social work. After individual evaluations by the disciplines, the team would meet as a whole to plan for the total child and his family.

The use of a developmental team can be helpful in providing ongoing support to the family of the Down Syndrome child. The family will be in need of guidance in planning at different times throughout the child's lifetime. Families may be in need of supportive counseling services in times of stress. Having had an affiliation with a developmental team means that the parents will be able to find the type of professional support needed in a particular situation and that a trusting relationship hopefully will have been established already.

Psychological Assessment   To enable the planning of an educational program, the level of intellectual functioning of the individual child must be determined. As mentioned earlier in this chapter, in evaluating intelligence in mentally retarded individuals, one must consider both the child's measured IQ and his social adaptive skills.

Plans for the child will differ to an extent, depending on the child's degree of retardation. The retardation classification system (Table 2) most widely used is that of the American Association of Mental Deficiency (AAMD).

During at least the first two years, assessing intellectual development in the Down Syndrome child will require use of an infant develop-

Table 2.   American Association of Mental Deficiency classification of mental retardation

	Standard deviation	Wechsler IQ score	Binet IQ score
Mildly retarded	3 below the mean	55–69	52–67
Moderately retarded	4 below the mean	40–54	36–51
Severely retarded	5 below the mean	25–39	20–35
Profoundly retarded	6 below the mean	Below 25	Below 20

ment scale. Those used most widely are the Bayley Scales of Mental Development, the Cattell Infant Test, and the Gesell Developmental Scales. These tests yield a score called a DQ (developmental quotient) that is not considered to be equivalent to an IQ score. Infants' tests focus on sensory perceptual acuity, object permanence, memory, learning and problem solving, and early language skills. These skills are not felt to be the same as the more abstract reasoning tasks that are included on regular IQ tests. Measurement of abstraction is not yet possible in infancy. Therefore, it is important to remember that scores on infant tests, especially in the early months, are not necessarily predictive of later IQ.

As noted earlier in the chapter, Down Syndrome children tend to achieve higher DQs than later obtained IQs. However, DQs obtained on Down Syndrome children between 14 and 24 months of age do begin to correlate with Stanford-Binet IQs obtained at age five (Koch et al., 1963).

As the Down Syndrome child nears age three, it is possible to administer tests that do yield an actual IQ score. These tests include the Merrill-Palmer Scale of Mental Tests and the Stanford-Binet Intelligence Test. The Stanford-Binet has some drawbacks in use with the preschool-age Down Syndrome child. The Stanford-Binet has a heavy language focus among the tasks, and this puts the majority of Down Syndrome children at a disadvantage. This may explain why Down Syndrome children have been found to have a level of self-help skills above that of measured IQ. If the standardized IQ test used has been the Stanford-Binet, one has not fully assessed the child's potential in terms of nonverbal cognitive skills. The Merrill-Palmer may be the better instrument for use with the preschool Down Syndrome child because it has fewer items that require verbal expression than the Stanford-Binet and many more items that require nonverbal reasoning.

As the child with Down Syndrome reaches school age, the intellectual test of choice would be the level of the Wechsler Intelligence Test appropriate for his age. In the four- to six-and-a-half-year range this would be the Wechsler Preschool and Primary Scale of Intelligence (WPPSI) and

from six years to 16 years the Wechsler Intelligence Scale for Children—
Revised (WISC-R). The Wechsler tests consist of a verbal scale and a
performance scale, the latter being nonverbal reasoning items. Thus, one
can get a picture of the Down Syndrome child's level of language functioning but also can measure nonverbal intellectual ability.

As mentioned previously, in assessing cognitive ability in a retarded
individual, one must consider both measured IQ and social adaptive
functioning. To assess the latter the instruments that might be used
include the Vineland Scale of Social Maturity and the Adaptive Behavior
Rating Scale. These scales rate the person's level of performance of such
self-care independence skills as feeding, dressing, and mobility.

Family Intervention

Parents can be helped to deal with the crisis of the birth of the Down
Syndrome child through a variety of supports. Peer support in the form
of other parents of Down Syndrome children can be especially beneficial
(Gayton and Walker, 1974). Within the community there is usually an
organization for retarded citizens that can provide additional peer support as well as information about community services available to
families of retarded children. These might include educational opportunities, recreation programs, and respite care services.

Counseling   The counseling needs of the family of the Down Syndrome child are of several types. Among these are family counseling and
genetic counseling. Family counseling is needed to help the members of
the family with the feelings engendered by the birth of a handicapped
child. The birth of a defective child must necessarily be followed by a
grieving process by the parents for the loss of the expected normal child
(Solnit and Stark, 1962). These feelings must be acknowledged, but the
counseling psychologist or social worker must also help the family see
that there is still a child who needs them. The interest and concern of the
psychologist or social worker are evidence to the family that others are
available to help them in the task of meeting that child's needs and that
this is not a burden that they must carry alone. By providing specific
information about community resources, financial aid, and educational
programs, the family may be helped to mobilize for action. Action often
serves as an effective defense mechanism and it may lay the foundation
for the family's learning to cope with the disorder.

Counseling services may need to be extended to include the siblings
of the Down Syndrome child. Murphy et al. (1976) note that the siblings
are usually fully aware of their parents' emotional distress and concerned
about it, and yet the parents may be so preoccupied with their own feelings that they are not emotionally available to the other children. The
sibling at home, not having a good understanding of what has transpired,

may have frightening fantasies about his own responsibility for the parents' distress. The time required to take a handicapped child to any necessary medical specialists or to provide a home stimulation program may result in a sibling feeling excluded and angry.

Other reactions of siblings to the Down Syndrome child include concerns about peers taunting them because of their sibling who is different.

Murphy et al. (1976) describe an ongoing treatment program for Down Sydrome children at their center that attempts to include normal siblings in the treatment. Parents are encouraged to bring siblings along to observe the activities of the clinic. Group sessions are set up for the siblings to give them information about Down Syndrome. A physical therapist describes activities they could do with their Down Syndrome sibling to develop his muscle tone. A pediatrician discusses chromosomes in Down Syndrome, and a psychologist explains about mental retardation. The group meetings enable the siblings to meet with other siblings of Down Syndrome children, and they are able to share feelings and experiences in the same way their parents do in the parent group.

The psychological adjustment of the siblings is something most parents are concerned about in making the decision for a retarded child to remain at home. Gath (1973) evaluated the adjustment of school-age siblings of Down Syndrome children living at home. Gath found evidence of more antisocial behavior among the sisters of the Down Syndrome children but no differences in the behavior of the brothers compared to controls. Gath hypothesized that this discrepancy might be because of the girls' reaction to having to "help unduly" at home. If this is so, it is important for siblings not to feel that they are under pressure to care for their handicapped sibling, but rather that any contribution they make is valued and that their assistance is part of a total family involvement in helping the Down Syndrome child.

Contrary to the findings of Gath, Wolfensberger (1968) found no effect of having a handicapped sibling in producing psychological adjustment problems in the normal siblings.

Educational Programs

As yet, there is no medical cure for Down Syndrome. There is no way to correct the genetic defect and no medication that will enhance cognitive functioning.

Based on the theory that the hypotonia seen in most Down Syndrome infants is caused by an enzyme deficiency, an attempt was made to see if muscle tone could be improved with doses of 5-hydroxytryptophan. At first, reports indicated that there was improvement in muscle tone and also early developmental milestones. However, with later double-blind studies, no improvement was found in Down Syndrome children administered the drug. In fact, some of the treated infants began showing more convulsive and EEG abnormalities (Smith and Berg, 1976).

Although Down Syndrome cannot be cured, the Down Syndrome child can be helped to achieve his maximal potential through educational intervention. It is to this form of treatment that the health-related professional must turn.

Infant Stimulation Programs The hypotonia common to most Down Syndrome infants can to some extent contribute to the delays in early developmental milestones shown by children. Because Down Syndrome can be identified at birth, it is possible to begin a stimulation program almost immediately for the infant to enhance developmental progress.

One such program (Hayden and Dmitriev, 1975) focused on improving developmental progress in Down Syndrome infants from five weeks to 18 months of age. Parents brought their infant to class once a week and received 30 minutes of individualized training in early motor-sensory development. Initially the program focused on teaching basic skills such as head lifting, back arching, pulling to sitting, and turning head to visual and auditory stimuli. As the child matured, exercises were given to develop eye-hand coordination, depth and size perception, discrimination of color, shapes, and objects, and more advanced motor skills such as rolling over, crawling, standing, walking, and language.

In evaluating progress at the end of one school year, Hayden and Dmitriev (1975) found their group of children, ranging in age from three to 18 months, showed a mean difference of only one month of mental age from chronological age. This was in contrast to the report of Dicks-Mireaux (1972), who reported a lag of one year for his group of Down Syndrome children aged 19.5 months. Dicks-Mireaux's group resided at home but did not participate in a stimulation program.

Another infant stimulation program is described by Connolly and Russell (1976). Connolly and Russell began stimulation for one Down Syndrome group before age six months and for another after six months. The best gains were noted for the group begun earlier. Stimulation was provided in home sessions and group sessions at the clinic. Activities focused on gross motor development, including muscle strengthening and range of motion, and on sensory stimulation. The infant stimulation group was found to demonstrate milestone delays of zero to three months during the first two years, while the control group showed delays ranging from three months to one year. Connolly and Russell note that no evaluation could yet be made of alterations in intellectual capabilities as a result of early stimulation.

Bidder, Bryant, and Gray (1975) trained mothers of Down Syndrome children in behavior modification techniques to encourage acquisition of language, manipulative, and self-help skills in their children. Significant gains in language development and manipulation skills were demonstrated by the experimental group, while locomotion milestones were the same as for the control group.

It would appear from the results of the above studies that early stimulation programs can help the development of the Down Syndrome infant to approximate more closely that of the normal child than if the Down Syndrome child were not in such a program.

Preschool Educational Programs   In many states it is now mandatory that developmentally disabled children be provided with a publicly supported educational program in the preschool years. Many such nursery programs are thus becoming available within the public school setting or under contractual services to private school settings.

That preschool programs can be beneficial to Down Syndrome children has been demonstrated impressively by Hayden and Dmitriev (1975). After a year in the program all the children were demonstrating skills that would classify them as educable. The children were in fact beginning to read at age four and five and had reading vocabularies of over 30 words. Objectives of the preschool program ranged from a focus on gross motor skills, such as walking in the early years to tricycle riding in the later years. Activities to enhance fine motor development, concept formation, communication, and self-help skills were also provided.

With preschool programs being provided for Down Syndrome children on a wider basis, it may be that an even greater number of children will be found to be of educable potential than has been found in the past.

Elementary School Programs   Programming in the primary school years will depend to a large extent on the level of intellectual functioning of the Down Syndrome child. Public schools are now providing programs for retarded children of all levels of functioning (Barnard and Powell, 1972).

Public school programs for mildly retarded children are generally called "educable mentally retarded" (EMR) classrooms. These are classes that focus on the development of basic reading, arithmetic, and handwriting skills. The academic subjects are usually taught in self-contained classrooms, but the EMR children may be mainstreamed with normal peers for nonacademic subjects such as art, music, and social studies. Academic attainment for this group would be expected to be at a third to fourth grade equivalent.

Classrooms for moderately retarded children are usually called "trainable mentally retarded" (TMR) groups. The focus for these children is on independence skills. Trainable children are taught to recognize important signs and learn basic counting skills but do not usually have functional reading or arithmetic skills. These groups are usually held in self-contained classrooms in the public school.

The minority of Down Syndrome children found in the severe to profound category of retardation often have physical limitations as well as intellectual deficits. Many public schools provide classes for these children through programs for the multihandicapped in special education centers. The educational focus for the severely and profoundly retarded child is on maximal development of self-care skills such as feeding, dressing, and toileting. Development of communication skills to at least express needs is also attempted.

Vocational Opportunities for Down Syndrome Individuals   In the adolescent years, educational programs for the mildly and moderately retarded Down Syndrome individual would focus on vocational training.

Some mildly retarded adults are capable of holding a job in a regular employment situation. Other mildly retarded Down Syndrome individuals and many moderately retarded adults are capable of functioning in a sheltered workshop situation in which more supportive supervision is available than would be in regular employment (Zaetz, 1971).

The Down Syndrome Individual and the Future

With the current emphasis on home rearing and the increasing number of special education programs available beginning at birth for the Down Syndrome child, it can be expected that these children will show greater capabilities than they were considered in the past to possess. More opportunities for independent living are now available for the Down Syndrome adult in the form of sheltered workshops and community group residences. Contrary to the dictum that the Down Syndrome child's condition is hopeless, the Down Syndrome individual can now look forward to a meaningful life with many more opportunities for growth and independence.

PHENYLKETONURIA

Phenylketonuria (PKU) represents a remarkable success story in the fields of inherited disorders and mental retardation. Like Down Syndrome, the PKU condition is identifiable shortly after birth and has significant repercussions for both the child and his family. Unlike Down Syndrome, however, PKU is treatable, and retardation, which was once the usual outcome, is no longer inevitable. For normal development to be achieved, careful treatment management and family support must be provided by a variety of health-related professionals.

History of PKU

In 1934, A. Følling, an Oslo physician, described several sibships of patients who had been referred because of slow development. One mother had noticed a peculiar musty odor common to her affected offspring. Følling determined that a high level of phenylpyruvic acid was excreted in the urine of these patients. In the following years the work of G. Jervis, an American physician, added much to the understanding of the disease. Jervis discovered that patients with PKU had a metabolic error such that phenylalanine was not metabolized in these individuals and large amounts of phenylalanine thus accumulated throughout their body tissues. Jervis noted that the disease had a familial pattern. He determined that the condition was inherited through an autosomal recessive gene carried by each of the parents.

In an effort to sidestep the metabolic error, a special diet substitute was developed that was low in phenylalanine but supplied other proteins needed for growth. When a PKU infant was started on this diet soon after birth, he was able to achieve normal intelligence. Widespread screening programs soon developed for early identification of PKU infants (Knox, 1972).

Enzyme Error in PKU

In the normal metabolic chain, phenylalanine, an essential amino acid found in most proteins, is broken down into tyrosine. Phenylalanine metabolism is catalyzed by the liver enzyme phenylalanine hydroxylase.

In the PKU individual, there is no active phenylalanine hydroxylase and the unmetabolized phenylalanine continues to accumulate from protein ingestion. Phenylpyruvic acid is excreted in the urine and also in the sweat as a result of the overaccumulation. Excretion of the phenylalanine from sweat glands is the reason for the unusual odor that was noted by Følling in his discovery of the disease.

The high levels of phenylalanine have a toxic effect on the central nervous system, and the symptoms of PKU including mental retardation are produced.

Genetic Factors in PKU

Jervis (1954) determined that PKU is inherited through an autosomal recessive gene from each of the parents. This gene is defective in its ability to control phenylalanine hydroxylase. In the heterozygote state some reduction in phenylalanine hydroxylase can be detected, but the condition does not produce retardation or other characteristics of PKU. Because both parents carry one normal gene and one PKU gene, the chance of producing a PKU child is one in four. There is a 50% chance of producing a heterozygote offspring and a one in four chance of producing a child who does not carry the PKU gene. Both sexes are equally affected by PKU; thus, there appears to be no sex linkage.

Incidence of PKU appears to be about one in 18,000 births, making it a rare disease but one of the more commonly occurring inborn errors of metabolism.

The disease is found chiefly among populations of Northern European derivation, but it is also found among Oriental and Near East peoples. PKU is extremely uncommon among Jews and Blacks (Jervis, 1937).

Characteristics of the Untreated Disease

It is generally agreed that the PKU infant is clinically normal at birth. Because the mother carries on phenylalanine metabolism for the developing fetus, the enzyme defect in the fetus does not affect prenatal development. Following delivery, the neonate must begin phenylalanine metabolism for himself; for the PKU infant, this results in a rapidly escalating level of phenylalanine in his body.

If left untreated, the high levels of phenylalanine have profound effects on the development of the neurological system, the cognitive abilities, and the behavior of the affected individual.

Abnormal neurological functioning is seen in the majority of untreated PKU individuals. EEG abnormalities may be detected as early as one month (Dobson et al., 1968). While abnormal EEGs are the most frequent abnormality seen, many PKU individuals also show abnormal reflexes and muscle tone. Development of spasticity in lower extremities and of increased tendon reflexes has been noted to occur in the second and third decade of life (Pederson and Birket-Smith, 1974). Tremor and problems with fine motor abilities are found frequently among untreated or late-treated individuals (Sutherland, Berry, and Shirkey, 1960; O'Grady, Berry, and Sutherland, 1971).

Although the specific mechanism is not known, the continued high level of phenylalanine begins to produce progressive mental retardation. Developmental milestones are often delayed with 35% of untreated PKU children showing delayed walking and 63% delayed speech. In other instances children who were walking and talking began to show deterioration of these abilities. Epileptic seizures developing after age six months are also a common feature (Knox, 1972). Intelligence appears to decline precipitously during the first 10 months of life and more gradually up to age three (Koch et al., 1967). After age three, IQ tends to remain stable and this remains so throughout adulthood (Bruhl, Arnesan, and Bruhl, 1964).

Scriver and Rosenberg (1973) report that the majority of untreated PKU individuals have an IQ less than 20, and the remainder usually have IQs less than 50. The mean IQ for the population they evaluated over three years was 40.2. Four percent of the group did show IQ scores greater than 60. Smith and Wolff (1976) report that a group of children who were referred because of developmental delay and found to have PKU, had a mean IQ of 40 with a range of below 30 to 57. Siblings of these children, who were found to test positive for PKU as well, had a mean IQ of 45 with a range of less than 30 to 81.

Untreated PKU thus appears to result most often in severe retardation and less commonly in moderate retardation. A few individuals may even fall in the mildly retarded range.

Serious behavioral disturbances are common among untreated and late-treated PKU individuals. As infants they may be inactive and unresponsive, but as they become older irritability is usually seen. Some of the untreated individuals show autistic-like features (Hackney et al., 1968). Pederson and Birket-Smith (1974) found most of their group of untreated PKU individuals to be uncooperative and highly anxious. A few were aggressive. Psychotic personality characteristics have also been described (Rapoport and Richardet, 1975).

For a time, a question of whether or not undetected individuals existed in the population who had PKU but still exhibited normal intelligence remained unanswered. Levy et al. (1970) screened the normal population in Massachusetts for PKU on the basis of blood samples submitted for adult syphilis screening. Three samples out of 250,000 tested were positive for PKU. In evaluating these individuals who had positive PKU blood tests, all were found to have IQs in the mildly retarded range although they were leading independent lives. This study thus found no evidence for undetected PKU with normal intelligence. Smith and Wolff (1976) found some evidence for IQs in the normal range for PKU-affected individuals. They believe the incidence of this occurring to be about one in every six or seven cases of PKU. The IQs of these normal functioning individuals tend to be low average, however, and their unaffected relatives exhibit significantly higher levels of intellectual functioning. High levels of phenylalanine thus show a general effect of retarding intellectual functioning, although in a few individuals the deterioration may be mild.

Screening and Treatment for PKU

Once it had been determined that the cause of PKU lay in a metabolic error, attempts were made to bypass the error for more normal growth and development. The principle for this was to provide only enough phenylalanine necessary for growth but not enough to allow a build-up in the system. A diet formula of casein hydrolyzate with phenylalanine removed was developed to serve as the primary nutritional source for PKU children. Normal growth could be maintained and phenylalanine levels kept low by diet maintenance. Determining the effectiveness of the diet in producing normal intelligence in children begun on treatment at an early age has required large numbers of children over a period of time for validation (Knox, 1972). In the United States, The Collaborative Study, representing the joint effort of 15 metabolic clinics, was initiated to evaluate treatment effectiveness for PKU children across the county.

Screening for PKU   The early identification of the PKU child was a necessary factor if diet treatment were to be successful in producing normal intelligence. In that phenylalanine is excreted in the urine of the PKU infant, the earliest screening was to use a $FeCl_3$ test on the urine of newborn infants. Later it was found more effective in diagnosis to use a blood screening for elevated plasma phenylalanine in the newborn. In the 1960s most states in the U.S. instituted mandatory screening of newborns for PKU. Follow-up screening at the first well-baby visit was also recommended as a procedure for pediatricians to follow.

Screening allowed for children with abnormal levels of phenylalanine to be evaluated carefully for PKU within the crucial first weeks of life so that diet treatment could be instituted. Whereas most children had been referred previously for treatment because of delays that were already evident, the identification of newborn PKU children allowed the effectiveness of the diet to be tested on children who had not yet shown retardation.

The Low Phenylalanine Diet   A low phenylalanine formula, Lofenalac™ (Mead-Johnson), is the major source of protein for the PKU infant. Small amounts of phenylalanine necessary for growth are provided by the addition of evaporated cow's milk to the Lofenalac formula. Lofenalac is supplied as a powder to be mixed with water to the desired consistency. For the young infant the mixture is made similar to other infant bottle formulas. With the addition of smaller quantities of water, the Lofenalac forms a paste that can be used to introduce spoon feeding and the transition to solids.

Frequent adjustments are necessary in the first six months to supply sufficient protein, phenylalanine, and calories to meet the rapid growth demands of that period.

Parents are encouraged to introduce the cup, solids, finger feeding, and utensil use at the usual times. Lofenalac does not provide the normal chewing and tongue manipulation necessary for normal development of stages of the eating process or for the development of speech. It is thus important for the child to be provided with a variety of natural foods of different textures to provide these necessary developmental experiences. The clinic nutritionist carefully works out with parents the types and quantities of natural foods that can be provided on the basis of phenylalanine content.

The diet is usually not difficult to maintain during infancy, but, during the toddler stage and later, children tend to develop a dislike of the special foods, and many tensions around feeding develop in the family.

The psychologist and other members of the team can help the parents to understand that it is not necessary for the child to eat every spoonful at each meal. In young children there are normal periods of slowing down of appetite, and, if the parent is aware of this, a battle around eating can be avoided. Food jags and strikes are especially common in the two- to four-year-old period and this is true for the PKU child as well.

Parents need to be helped to use consistent discipline. Many parents feel compelled to be oversolicitous to the child, to bribe him or give extra treats to alleviate their guilt feelings over depriving the child of certain foods (Umbarger, 1964).

The young child continues to consume Lofenalac as a beverage but continues to get his source of phenylalanine from an increasing array of natural foods. It is important that foods such as meat and eggs be introduced in very small quantities so that the child learns to accept these foods with an eye toward diet termination (Hunt, Sutherland, and Berry, 1971).

It is suggested that the child's foods be drawn from those served to the rest of the family. This is to help the PKU child feel a part of the family unit and not excluded from it by his separate diet.

Effectiveness of Diet Treatment

Cognitive Functioning in Treated PKU Children   In the later 1960s, reports began to appear about cognitive functioning in PKU children who had been screened at birth and put on the low phenylalanine diet within the first few months of life. Hackney et al. (1968) reported on a group of PKU children treated before two months of age with resultant IQs all above 70. However, half these children exhibited neuropsychological problems such as short attention, distractibility, and poor motor coordination. These difficulties presented handicaps in terms of school learning. Hackney et al. (1968) hypothesized that some of these children may have been "overtreated" in the first year of life by rigorous maintenance of very low levels of phenylalanine at a time when the physiological need for phenylalanine for growth is high.

Additional studies have found that early-treated children had IQs in the low average range, but they tended to be 10 to 15 points lower than

IQs of unaffected parents and siblings (Dobson et al., 1968; Berman and Ford, 1970; Hudson, Morduant, and Leahy, 1970). The Collaborative Study in a 1973 report (Williamson, Koch, and Dobson, 1973) compared early-treated PKU children to untreated. The treated children had a mean IQ of 98.7 and the untreated children had a mean IQ of 65.5. This is a highly significant comparison and gives considerable strength to the effectiveness of early diet treatment. In a recent report (Dobson et al., 1976), a group of early-treated PKU children were found to have a mean IQ of 94, while their unaffected siblings had a mean IQ of 99.

The efficacy of diet treatment is demonstrated impressively in terms of PKU individuals admitted to residential institutions for the retarded. No PKU admissions have occurred of children born where screening of newborns was being performed at the time of birth (MacCready, 1974).

The importance of beginning the diet in early infancy has been demonstrated through several investigations. Dobson et al. (1968) found that children placed on diet treatment within the first month after birth had IQs in the low average range, but for the children started after that time IQs were progressively lower with later treatment dates. Hansen (1975) reports that treatment begun within the first 30 days resulted in a significantly higher IQ (mean IQ = 89).

While IQ level in early-treated PKU children appears to fall within the average range, there is a question of whether or not the children suffer more subtle deficits in specific areas of cognitive functioning not reflected in the global IQ measure.

The early-treated children studied by Hackney et al. (1968) were found to have deficits in attention, space perception, language development, and speech articulation.

Scores of early-treated PKU children on the Illinois Test of Psycholinguistic Abilities (ITPA) were found to be lower than those of unaffected siblings by Dobson et al. (1968). However, O'Grady, Berry, and Sutherland (1971) found no difference in overall score on the ITPA for early-treated PKU children and unaffected siblings. O'Grady et al. (1971) did find their PKU group to be deficient on one subtest of the ITPA, that of verbal expression (vocal encoding). These investigators speculated that the deficit in verbal expression might be related to an inhibition on the part of these children generalizing from the restrictive dietary regime to the area of verbal interaction.

Effects of the Diet Regime on Psychosocial Development   The study of O'Grady et al. (1971) had raised the notion that the restrictive diet experience might itself have an effect on the psychological development of the child.

Wood, Friedman, and Steisel (1967) had found that mothers of early-treated PKU children inhibited the child's exploratory behavior in a food-play situation. These mothers also tended to distort the food aspects of the situation and hindered the child from making realistic discriminations. Restrictiveness was also found to be characteristic of maternal interaction with the PKU child in a non-food teaching situation. The mothers of PKU children, who were on the diet at the time of the study, tended to use more verbal controlling statements and more physical intrusion than control mothers (Katz, 1972).

A restrictive child-rearing experience is felt to affect the development of certain cognitive perceptual skills (Witkin et al., 1962; Dyk, 1969). In a study by Katz (1975), early-treated PKU boys were found to be poorer in a perceptual disembedding task than matched controls. No differences were found for PKU girls. Perceptual disembedding is a cognitive task considered to relate to restrictiveness of child rearing, with more restricted children showing poorer disembedding ability (Dyk and Witkin, 1965). That an effect was shown for PKU boys but not for PKU girls was hypothesized to reflect a differential effect on the sexes of the restrictive diet regime. The study by Katz (1975) also raised the notion that studies of cognitive abilities of PKU children should be done with boys and girls considered separately.

The PKU Child and His Family

The Initial Diagnosis Most PKU children are identified at the present time through screening in the newborn nursery. The positive laboratory report is often received by the hospital after the infant's discharge and the family is referred to the regional PKU clinic for further investigation of the infant's metabolism.

The regional PKU clinics usually receive state and federal support, and minimal charges are made to the families. Most clinics use a team approach in the identification and treatment of the disease. The team might consist of pediatrician, nurse, psychologist, social worker, nutritionist, and biochemist.

At the time of identification, the infant might be hospitalized for diagnostic procedures, or, if the family is able to make frequent visits to the clinic, testing might be on an outpatient basis. The infant initially is put on adequate protein intake for sufficient phenylalanine to be ingested to determine irregularities in metabolism. Laboratory tests including blood counts, serum phenylalanine and tyrosine levels, and urinary amino acids are run. The infant receives a physical examination, and a family history is taken. Particular attention is given to the family history because of the hereditary nature of the disease. For the child to have PKU, each parent must be a recessive genetic carrier. Careful note is made of the incidence of mental retardation or slow development on both sides of the family.

If the biochemical tests are negative as is often the case, the child is discharged with perhaps a brief follow-up plan. Some children with mildly elevated levels of phenylalanine have been found to have a variant of PKU called hyperphenylalaninemia. These children are at less risk for retardation, but some diet modifications are often made (Berman and Ford, 1970).

Children with normal phenylalanine levels at follow-up would be expected to have completely normal development. The event of a false positive test, however, may have repercussions in terms of parental reactions. Rothenberg and Sills (1968) found that parents of children who had had false positive PKU screening tests experienced acute and chronic anxiety ranging from mild periodic concern to acute anxiety hysteria. Some parents continued to believe that their child would become mentally retarded despite test results that were completely normal. There thus appears to be a need for the team to provide reassurance and counseling even in the event of a false positive.

When the biochemical tests are confirmatory for PKU, an attempt is made to lower the level of serum phenylalanine to below 10 mg/dl within one week if possible. Care must be taken not to make the level too low or phenylalanine deficiency results with a breakdown and release of phenylalanine from the body's own cells (Acosta and Wenz, 1977). Phenylalanine level is reduced by means of a special low phenylalanine formula, Lofenalac, which serves as the main nutritional source for the infant and young PKU child.

A "challenge" is usually offered by an increase in phenylalanine to confirm the diagnosis at this point. Further "challenges" may be made again at three to six months and again at 12 months to assess if the deficit in phenylalanine metabolism has been of a transitory nature or represents true PKU (Koch et al., 1970).

The team approach is helpful at the inception of diet therapy. The nutritionist explains to the family the principle of the low phenylalanine diet. The social worker may evaluate family structure to assess the family's ability to carry out diet maintenance. The psychologist may do developmental testing of the child to monitor cognitive growth. After the first week, the nurse often makes a home visit to advise the parents on home care. The nurse often reiterates the pediatrician's instructions and demonstrates the technique for collecting blood samples at home to mail to the clinic. The family is asked to send blood samples and three-day food records to the clinic periodically for monitoring. Weekly visits to the clinic continue through the first year and less frequently thereafter.

Helping the Family after Diagnosis   The period following the confirmation of the diagnosis of PKU is marked by emotional ambivalence of the parents. Frequent distortions and misunderstandings are found in their knowledge of the disease despite careful information given by the clinic team. Some parents go through a period of disbelieving the validity of the diagnosis. Others experience marked anxiety and confusion (Keleske, Solomons, and Opitz, 1967; Wood, Friedman, and Steisel, 1967). The period following diagnosis is one in which the parents will need much support from the clinic team. This will usually require an ongoing counseling relationship. Further support may be provided by meeting with other parents of PKU children and by seeing the successful results of diet treatment in the older PKU child.

Because PKU is a hereditary disorder, parents should be provided genetic counseling. With an understanding of the principle of transmission of the disease, the parents may be helped to avoid the common tendency to look for whose side was to blame. Genetic counseling should also be provided around family planning. Parents must understand that there is a one in four chance of a future pregnancy producing a PKU child and a one in two chance of a child being a carrier of the disease. Unfortunately diagnosis of PKU by amniocentesis is not yet possible; thus, the option of preventing the birth of an affected child is not open to parents. Keleske et al. (1967) report that 84% of the parents of PKU children in their group did not plan to have more children. This was not, however, because of their concern about another child being born with PKU. Rather, parents cited limited financial resources and ability to care for their existing children as reasons to limit family size.

Diet Management   A major focus in counseling new parents of PKU children is helping them gain an understanding and feeling of competence in diet management. Without support from the clinic team, the necessity of maintaining the rigorous diet regime can have devastating effects on the family. Nurturing is so basic to the developing parent-child relationship that it cannot help but be a heavily emotion-laden issue. That parents must deny most common foods to their child can create much tension and anxiety in the family.

There is a tendency for many parents to overprotect the child and stifle his attempts at independence. This attitude in itself can lead to serious behavior problems and strains in the parent-child relationship. There is a concern among professionals working with PKU children that the restrictiveness of the dietary regime itself may produce handicaps in the child's adaptive abilities although his intelligence may be normal (Sutherland, Umbarger, and Berry, 1966; Bentovim et al., 1970; Lonsdale and Faust, 1970; Katz, 1975). The psychologist can help parents become aware of normal developmental stages and support them in allowing the child to develop self-help and independence at the appropriate stages.

As the PKU child grows it is important for him to learn to make acceptable food discriminations on his own. In order for him to do this he must have some understanding of the nature of his problem.

It is not considered wise to inform the child that if he eats certain foods they will make him sick. There is, in fact, no physical sensation apparent to the child when high phenylalanine foods are consumed. Many children when told that they will get sick will try a food just to find out, and, upon experiencing no aversive reactions, they may feel their parents have not been truthful.

It is probably better to tell the child that he is on a special diet that will help him and provide a simple explanation about the problem of too much phenylalanine. Members of the Collaborative Study have developed a film for children, "Phe and me," which provides children with an understandable description of the problem (MLK Film Productions, 1973). The better understanding the child has, the less chance there will be for the snitching of forbidden foods and similar problems that frequently occur with the older child.

It is not as yet known what the long-term effects of termination of the diet are or at what age this can safely be done. This question is under current investigation by the Collaborative Study (Acosta and Wenz, 1977).

Recent controlled studies of termination of diet in early-treated children have had conflicting results. Holtzman, Welch, and Mellits (1975) terminated the diet at age four years in one group of PKU children and found no differences in IQ at age six years from a matched group of PKU children who remained on diet. Brown and Warner (1976) report that a group of PKU children taken off diet at age six years showed significant decreases in Wechsler and Stanford-Binet intelligence test scores as compared with a group remaining on diet and a group of normal controls. Several recent studies have reported on neurological deterioration in the second and third decade of life in PKU individuals off diet. This is hypothesized to result from demyelinization caused by a pathological process separate from the retardation seen in the early years. These investigators have raised the possibility that diet maintenance may be necessary to prevent this process in adolescence and early adulthood (Pederson and Birket-Smith, 1974; Wood, 1976).

A further question about diet termination concerns the necessity for diet treatment during pregnancy for PKU girls reaching adulthood. The chances of causing fetal damage are very high for the pregnant PKU woman off diet. The high levels of phenylalanine in the mother appear to have a toxic effect on the developing fetus, which itself most often does not have PKU (Hansen, 1975).

Arthur and Holme (1970) attempted to avert fetal damage by putting a pregnant PKU woman on a low phenylalanine diet at 22 weeks gestation. The infant delivered with low birth weight but showed improved growth, and at two years of age showed normal developmental progress. With greater numbers of early-treated PKU girls reaching adulthood with normal potentials for fulfilling adult roles, the question of the advisability of pregnancy for these women will require greater knowledge than we currently have. But the fact that this represents a real problem in the near future is in itself a mark of the success of PKU treatment.

SUMMARY

Our knowledge about chromosomal and other genetic disorders has increased greatly in the past decade. Among those syndromes for which there are now well recognized chromosomal abnormalities and distinguishing physical characteristics are the sex chromosome disorders of Klinefelter Syndrome and Turner Syndrome. Down Syndrome represents a chromosomal abnormality involving an imbalance in chromosome number. The disorder has many characteristic physical features including mental retardation. Phenylketonuria is also an inherited disorder although no particular chromosomal pattern has been identified with the disease. PKU is a metabolic disorder which, left untreated, results in severe mental retardation. PKU, like Down Syndrome, can be identified within the first days of life. Unlike Down Syndrome, however, mental retardation can be prevented for the PKU child by a special diet treatment if begun soon after birth. Both Down Syndrome and PKU, then, have important implications for the affected child and his family from the outset of life. For both disorders there is an overriding need for support services from a variety of health professionals. Support services might include genetic counseling, family counseling, and educational planning. Through proper psychological management the family of the child with an inherited disorder can be helped to gain a healthy acceptance of the child and his disorder, and the child may be helped to achieve his full potential.

REFERENCES

Acosta, P., Fiedler, J., and Koch, R. 1968. Mothers' dietary management of PKU. J. Am. Diet Assoc. 53:460–464.
Acosta, P., and Wenz, E. 1977. Diet management of PKU for infants and preschool children. U.S. Department of Health, Education and Welfare Publication No. (HSA) 77–5209.

Antley, R., and Hartlage, L. 1976. Psychological responses to genetic counseling for Down's Syndrome. Clin. Genet. 9:257–265.

Arthur, L., and Holme, J. 1970. Intelligent, small for dates baby born to oligophrenic phenylketonuric mother after low phenylalanine diet during pregnancy. Pediatrics 46:235–239.

Barnard, K., and Powell, M. 1972. Teaching the Mentally Retarded Child: A family care approach. The C. V. Mosby Company, St. Louis, Mo.

Baron, J. 1972. Temperament profile of children with Down's Syndrome. Dev. Med. Child Neurol. 14:640–643.

Bentovim, A., Clayton, B., Francis, D., Shepherd, J., and Wolff, O. 1970. Use of amino acid mixture in treatment of phenylketonuria. Arch. Dis. Child 45:640–650.

Berman, J., and Ford, R. 1970. Intelligence quotients and intellectual loss in patients with phenylketonuria and some variant states. J. Pediatr. 77:764–70.

Bidder, R., Bryant, G., and Gray, O. 1975. Benefits to Down's Syndrome children through training their mothers. Arch. Dis. Child. 50:383–386.

Bilovsky, D., and Share, J. 1965. The ITPA and Down's Syndrome: An exploratory study. Am. J. Ment. Defic. 70:78–82.

Brooks, D., Wooley, H., and Kanjilal, G. 1972. Hearing loss and middle ear disorders in patients with Down's Syndrome. J. Ment. Defic. Res. 16:21–29.

Brown, E., and Warner, R. 1976. Mental Development of PKU children on or off diet after age six. Psychol. Med. 6:287–296.

Bruhl, H., Arnesan, J., and Bruhl, M. 1964. Effect of a low phenylalanine diet in older phenylketonuric patients. Am. J. Ment. Defic. 69:225–230.

Carr, J. 1970. Mental and motor development in young Mongol children. J. Ment. Defic. Res. 14:205–220.

Clow, C., Reade, T., and Scriver, C. 1971. Management of hereditary metabolic disease. The role of Allied Health Personnel. N. Engl. J. Med. 284:1292–1298.

Connolly, B., and Russell, F. 1976. Interdisciplinary early intervention programs. Phys. Ther. 56:155–158.

Cornwell, A. 1974. Development of language, abstraction and numerical concept formation in Down's Syndrome children. Am. J. Ment. Defic. 79:179–190.

Cornwell, A., and Birch, H. 1969. Psychological and social development in home-reared children with Down's Syndrome. Am. J. Ment. Defic. 74:341–350.

Cowie, V. 1970. Study of Early Development of Mongols. Pergamon Press, Oxford, England.

Cytryn, L. 1975. Studies of behavior in children with Down's Syndrome. In E. Anthony (ed.), Exploration in Child Psychiatry, pp. 271–285. Plenum Press, New York.

Dicks-Mireaux, M. 1972. Mental development of infants with Down's Syndrome. Am. J. Ment. Defic. 77:26–31.

Dobson, J., Koch, R., Williamson, M., Spector, R., Frankenberg, W., O'Flynn, M., Warner, R., and Hudson, F. 1968. Cognitive development and diet therapy in PKU children. N. Engl. J. Med. 278:1142–1144.

Dobson, J., Kushida, E., Williamson, M., and Friedman, E. 1976. Intellectual performance of 36 phenylketonuric patients and their unaffected siblings. Pediatrics 58:53–58.

Domino, G., Goldschmid, M., and Kaplan, M. 1964. Personality traits of institutionalized mongoloid girls. Am. J. Ment. Defic. 68:498–502.

Down, J. L. 1866. Observations on an ethnic classification of idiots. Clin. Lect. Rep. London Hosp. 3:259–262.

Dyk, R., 1969. Exploratory study of mother-child interaction related to development of differentiation. Am. Acad. Child Psychiatry 8:657–691.

Dyk, R., and Witkin, H. 1965. Family experiences related to the development of differentiation in children. Child Dev. 36:21–55.

Fishler, K., Koch, R., and Donnell, G. 1976. Comparison of mental development in individuals with mosaic and trisomy 21 Down's Syndrome. Pediatrics 58:744–748.

Fraser, F., and Sedovnick, A. 1976. Correlation of IQ in subjects with Down Syndrome and their parents and sibs. J. Ment. Defic. Res. 20:179–182.

Gath, A. 1973. School age sibs of mongol children. Br. J. Psychiatry 123:161–167.

Gayton, W., and Walker, L. 1974. Down's Syndrome: Informing parents. Am. J. Dis. Child. 127:510–512.

Giannini, M., and Goodman, L. 1970. Counseling families during the crisis reaction to Mongolian. In R. Noland (ed.), Counseling Parents of the Mentally Retarded, pp. 110–121. Charles C Thomas, Springfield, Ill.

Golden, D., and Davis, J. 1974. Counseling parents after birth of an infant with Down's Syndrome. Children Today 3:7–11.

Goldman, W., and Pashayan, H. 1976. The effect of parental education an eventual mental development of non-institutionalized children with Down's Syndrome. J. Pediat. 89:603–605.

Grotz, R., Henderson, N., and Katz, S. 1972. A comparison of the functional and intellectual performance of phenylketonuric, anoxic and Down's Syndrome individuals. Am. J. Ment. Defic. 76:710–717.

Hackney, I., Hanley, W., Davidson, W., and Linsao, L. 1968. PKU, mental development, behavior, and termination of low phenylalanine diet. J. Pediatr. 72:646–655.

Hanley, W., Linsao, L., and Netley, C. 1971. The efficacy of diet therapy for phenylketonuria. Can. Med. Assoc. J. 104:1089–1092.

Hansen, H. 1975. Prevention of mental retardation due to PKU: Selected aspects of program validity. Prev. Med. 4:310–321.

Hayden, A., and Dmitriev, V. 1975. The multidisciplinary preschool program for Down Syndrome child at the University of Washington model preschool center. In B. Friedlander, G. Sterritt, and G. Kirk (eds.), Exceptional Infant, Vol. 3. Assessment and Intervention, pp. 193–221. Brunner/Mazel, New York.

Holtzman, N., Welch, D., and Mellits, E.D. 1975. Termination of restricted diet in children with PKU: A randomized controlled study. N. Engl. J. Med. 293:1121–1124.

Hudson, F., Morduant, V., and Leahy, I. 1970. Evaluation of treatment begun in first three months of life in 184 cases of PKU. Arch. Dis. Child. 45:5–12.

Hunt, M., Sutherland, B., and Berry, H. 1971. Nutritional management—PKU. Am. J. Dis. Child. 122:1–6.

Jackson, J., North, E., and Thomas, J. 1976. Clinical diagnosis of Down's Syndrome. Clin. Genet. 9:483–487.

Jervis, G. 1954. Phenylpyruvic oligophrenia (phenylketonuria). Res. Publ. Assoc. mental deficiency. The genetics of phenylpyruvic oligophrenic. Proc. Am. Assoc. Ment. Defic. J. Psycho-asthenics 64:13–24.

Jervis, G. 1954. Phenylpyruvic oligophrenia (phenylketonuria). Res. Publ. Assoc. Res. Nerv. Ment. Dis. 33:259–282.

Katz, K. 1972. Effects of maintaining a controlled diet on the teaching strategies and speech patterns of mothers of children with PKU. Unpublished master's thesis, Rutgers University, New Brunswick, N.J.

Katz, K. 1975. Effects of early diet treatment on cognitive abilities of children with PKU. Diss. Ab. Int. 35(10-B):5116.

Keleske, L., Solomons, G., and Opitz, E. 1967. Parental reactions to PKU. J. Pediatr. 70:793–798.

Knox, W. 1972. Phenylketonuria. In J. Stanbury, J. Wyngaarden, and D. Fredrickson (eds.), The Metabolic Basis of Inherited Disease, pp. 266–295. McGraw-Hill Book Co., New York.

Koch, R., Acosta, P., Fishler, K., Schaeffler, G., and Wohlers, A. 1967. Clinical observations on phenylketonuria. Am. J. Dis. Child. 113:6–15.

Koch, R., Share, J., Webb, A., and Graliker, B. 1963. The predictability of Gesell Developmental Scales in Mongolism. J. Pediatr. 62:93–97.

Koch, R., Shaw, K., Acosta, P., Fishler, K., Schaeffler, G., Wenz, E., and Wohlers, A. 1970. An approach to management of PKU. J. Pediatr. 16:815–828.

Levy, H., Karolkewicz, V., Houghton, S., and MacCready, R. 1970. Screening the normal population in Massachusetts for PKU. N. Engl. J. Med. 282:1455–1458.

Lillienfeld, A., and Benesch, C. 1969. Epidemiology of Mongolism. The Johns Hopkins Press, Baltimore.

Lonsdale, D., and Faust, M. 1970. Normal mental development in PKU. Am. J. Dis. Child. 119:440–446.

MacCready, R. 1974. Admission of PKU patients to residential institutions before and after screening programs of the newborn infant. J. Pediatr. 85:383–385.

Merlyn, M., and White, D. 1973. Mental and developmental milestones of non-institutionalized Down's Syndrome children. Pediatrics 52:542–545.

MLK Film Productions. 1973. "Phe and Me." 837 Jennifer Street, Madison, Wisconsin 53703.

Murphy, A., Pueschel, S., Duffy, T., and Brady, E. 1976. Meeting with brothers and sisters of children with Down's Syndrome. Child Today 5:20–23.

O'Grady, D., Berry, H., and Sutherland, B. 1971. Cognitive development in early treated PKU. Am. J. Dis. Child. 121:20–23.

Pederson, J., and Birket-Smith, E. 1974. Neurological abnormalities in PKU. Acta Neurol. Scand. 50:589–598.

Penrose, L. 1967. Studies of mosaics in Down's anomaly. In G. Jervis (ed.), Mental Retardation, pp. 3–18. Charles C Thomas, Springfield, Ill.

Penrose, L., and Smith, G. 1966. Down's Anomaly. Little, Brown & Co., Boston.

Pototzky, C., and Grigg, A. 1942. A reversion of the prognosis in mongolism. Am. J. Orthopsychiatry 12:503–510.

Pueschel, S., and Murphy, A. 1975. Counseling parents of infants with Down's Syndrome. Postgrad. Med. 58:90–95.

Rapoport, D., and Richardet, J. 1975. Concerning PKU: The contribution of clinical psychology to the complete understanding of the disease. Rev. Neuropsychiatr. Infant. 23:111–127.

Rosecrans, C. 1968. The relationship of normal/21 Trisomy mosaics and intellectual development. Am. J. Ment. Defic. 72:562–565.

Rothenberg, M., and Sills, E. 1968. Iatrogenesis: The PKU anxiety syndrome. J. Am. Acad. Child Psychiatry 7:689–692.

Schlottman, R., and Anderson, V. 1975. Social and play behavior of institutionalized mongol and non-mongol retarded children. J. Psychol. 91:201–206.

Scriver, L., and Rosenberg, L. 1973. Amino Acid Metabolism and Its Disorders. W. B. Saunders Co., Philadelphia.

Share, J. 1975. Developmental progress in Down's Syndrome. In R. Koch and F. de la Cruz (eds.), Down's Syndrome (Mongolism) Research, Prevention and Management, pp. 78–86. Brunner/Mazel, New York.

Silverstein, A. 1964. An empirical test of the mongoloid personality. Am. J. Ment. Defic. 68:493–497.

Smith, D., and Wilson, A. 1973. The Child with Down's Syndrome. W. B. Saunders Co., Philadelphia.

Smith, G., and Berg, J. 1976. Down's Anomaly. 2nd Ed. Churchill, Livingston, N.J.

Smith, I., and Wolff, O. 1976. History of PKU and influence of early treatment. Lancet 2:540–544.

Solnit, A., and Stark, M. 1962. Mourning and the birth of a defective child. Psychoanal. Study Child 16:523–537.

Sutherland, B., Berry, H., and Shirkey, H. 1960. A syndrome of PKU with normal intelligence and behavior disturbances. J. Pediatr. 57:521–525.

Sutherland, B., Umbarger, B., and Berry, H. 1966. Treatment of PKU. Am. J. Dis. Child. 111:505–523.

Umbarger, B. 1960. PKU—Treating the disease and feeding the child. Am. J. Dis. Child. 100:908–913.

Umbarger, B. 1964. PKU diet treatment. Am. J. Nurs. 64:96–99.

Williamson, M., Koch, R., and Dobson, J. 1973. PKU Collaborative Study—Current Status Presented at Third IASSMD Congress, September, The Hague, The Netherlands.

Witkin, H., Dyk, R., Faterson, H., Goodenough, D., and Karp, S. 1962. Psychological Differentiation. John Wiley and Sons, New York.

Wolfensberger, W. 1967. Counseling parents of the retarded. In A. Baumeister (ed.), Mental Retardation; Appraisal Education, and Rehabilitation, pp. 329–400. Aldine Publishing Co., Chicago.

Wood, A., Friedman, C., and Steisel, I. 1967. Psychosocial factors in PKU. Am. J. Orthopsychiatry 37:671–679.

Wood, B. 1976. Neurological disturbance in a PKU child after discontinuation of dietary treatment. Dev. Med. Child Neurol. 18:657–665.

Zaetz, J. 1971. Organization of Sheltered Workshop Programs for the Mentally Retarded Adult. Charles C Thomas, Springfield, Ill.

6

Toilet Training, Enuresis, Encopresis

C. Eugene Walker

TOILET TRAINING

Few subjects in the area of child development evoke more concern and produce more firmly held opinions than the area of proper toilet training. Ilg and Ames (1962) have noted that only school problems evoke more questions from parents who seek advice from the Gesell Institute of Child Development. Similarly, Mesibov, Schroeder, and Wesson (1977) reported that questions about toileting were second only to concerns about negative behaviors in a parents' call-in, drop-in clinic conducted by mental health workers in connection with a private pediatric clinic. Parents want to know when to train, how to train, and how to deal with problems along the way. They worry about the effects of too early or too strict or too late or too lax training. However, a review of the popular literature written by "experts" to guide parents in this area (Shaw, 1976), as well as a review of medical and pediatric textbooks (Matthews, 1976), indicates a scarcity of even basic information of a factual nature. In addition, the "experts" differ greatly in recommendations made. The area obviously is one that involves considerable confusion among parents and professionals.

Over the years, attitudes toward toilet training have changed dramatically. In previous generations it generally was considered important to train the child at a very young age. Early and strict training was recommended. The child that developed early control of toileting functions was thought to be showing developmental progress and precociousness. It was often assumed by parents that progress in this area was highly correlated with intellectual ability and was a precursor of numerous achievements by the child in other areas. Parents further tended to regard early training as evidence of superior parenting. It was a source of pride to the mother to have trained her child at a younger age than the children of friends and neighbors. When this approach to child rearing and toilet training was prevalent, boasts were made to the effect that, "My child was always trained . . . right from birth," or, "I was able to train my child by three months. I never had any trouble with him." However, research has indicated that the child is not able to control the bowels until around the second year of life and the bladder until around the third year of life sufficiently well to actually be trained. Those who claim training from the very start or at very young ages really represent cases of training of the parents rather than the child. Many parents learn the child's schedule and learn to recognize signs that the child is about to have a movement. They then rush the child to the toilet at the right time. Eventually some degree of conditioning takes place and still later the child gains conscious control over toileting. Thus, it seems as though the child were trained at a very young age. However, in reality he was not trained in the usual sense until much later than the parents report.

In more recent times, particularly through the influence of Dr. Spock's famous child care book (1957), parents have been encouraged to take a much more lenient and relaxed attitude toward toilet training. In fact, going to the opposite extreme, many parents and experts believe that no effort need be made to toilet train a child. The rationale given for this is that control of bowel and bladder is a developmental skill that will occur when the child is ready and is sufficiently uncomfortable by urinating and defecating in his clothing. Any attempt to speed this process up or retard it will have very little influence on the child. Advocates of this position state that they know of no adults that are not trained. However, data are presented later in this chapter that indicate that some adults do have difficulty with enuresis and encopresis.

Stehbens and Silber (1971) studied the attitudes of parents at the birth of their first child with respect to the age at which they expected their child to be toilet trained and to whom they would turn for advice should there be problems. Fifty percent of the parents stated that they expected to begin training before 16 months and to have the child completely trained by the age of two. The parents stated that they would seek the advice of physicians should difficulties develop. In a later study (Stehbens and Silber, 1974) the parents were asked about their actual experience with training their first child. As might be expected, there were significant differences between their attitudes before training a child and those following their first experience. Actually only 20% of the parents began bowel or bladder training by 16 months. However, 58% had initiated training by two years of age. Seventy percent of the children were not trained successfully until after the age of two. Those who sought advice sought the advice mainly from friends and relatives rather than physicians. About 20 to 30% thought they might do things differently with subsequent children. Some stated they would take a more relaxed approach, and a few said they would start later with subsequent children.

Numerous disorders are attributed by various experts to ill-advised toilet-training methods. The disorders identified include such things as discipline and delinquency problems, neurosis, sexual disturbances, enuresis, and encopresis. Unfortunately, none of these has been substantiated by careful research and they are as often attributed to too strict or too early training as to too late or too lax training. Thus, the parent and professional are confronted with a situation in which there are few data to guide them, opinions often of a contradictory and confusing nature abound, and dire consequences are assumed to result if the "right thing" is not done. It would appear that a great deal of overreaction and exaggeration surrounds this area of child rearing. The following comments are offered as a middle-of-the-road approach to the problem, with full appreciation for the fact that a greal deal of this is based on the author's own clinical and personal child-rearing experience rather than substantiated fact. The two major questions addressed are when to train and how to train.

When to Toilet Train

Before a child can be trained, it is necessary for certain developmental-maturational processes to occur. In the newborn infant, bowel and bladder emptying are reflexive actions. As the child develops and matures, more conscious control becomes possible for these functions. However, there is a strong maturational element in this, and the ability to suppress these reflexes, as well as the ability to initiate the involved processes on demand, requires considerable neurological development (Harper, 1962). As Knobloch and Pasamanick (1974) comment,

> In order to be completely "toilet trained," the child must: consciously associate the excretory act with certain internal sensations, with a particular and appropriate place, and with certain words; voluntarily inhibit relaxation of the sphincters, and terminate that inhibition (release) voluntarily; verbalize or otherwise indicate the need; differentiate between stimuli from bladder and bowel and inhibit or release the appropriate sphincter; and foresee sufficiently the urge to urinate or defecate—a formidable series of tasks, the complexities of which are not always appreciated (p. 204).

Too early training is physiologically out of the question. Later, appropriately timed training should result in rapid success.

Girls tend to establish control earlier than boys. However, it is extremely important to keep in mind that, as with all maturational characteristics, there are wide individual differences. Thus, while some children may be trained successfully before two years of age and most may be trained between two and three years of age, there will be a significant number of children who are not ready to be trained and cannot be trained until later than three years of age. A longitudinal study of 900 children (Harper, 1962) indicated that two-thirds achieved full bowel control by two years, 90% by three years, and 95% by four years. Over half of this group had daytime control of urine by two years of age, 85% by three years and 90% at four years of age. Nighttime urine control was established by approximately two-thirds of the children at three years of age, 75% at four years, 80% at five years, and only 90% by eight-and-a-half years. Thus, attempts to train children at two years of age (which is generally recommended) are likely to fail in a significant percentage of cases. Even at four years of age, 5 to 10% will still be having problems.

In addition to having the physical ability to control the bowels and bladder, the child should be of sufficient maturity to be able to follow instructions and cooperate with parents in the training. Numerous signs are cited in the literature as indicators that the child may be ready to be trained. Some authors cite the ability to walk alone as indicating that sufficient muscle tone has been achieved to make it possible to toilet train a child (Brazelton, 1969; Homan, 1970). Others (Salk, 1972) suggest that the ability to communicate verbally with the parent and to understand and follow instructions is crucial. Many authors also suggest watching the child until some degree of regularity in the function of his bowels becomes apparent. This regularity indicates that training may be possible and allows the parent to capitalize on this regularity in training efforts. Gruenburg (1968) and others suggest looking for signs of discomfort or displeasure on the part of the child following soiling, indicating that he may be amenable to training. These signs are usually assumed to occur between 18 and 24 months of age.

As indicated, bladder control comes somewhat later, between two-and-a-half to three years of age. Signs that the child may be ready to proceed with bladder control are such things as having achieved bowel control, being dry for periods of at least two hours during the day, waking up dry from naps, and beginning to show discomfort and displeasure with being wet. Azrin and Foxx have done considerable research on the toilet training of normal and retarded youngsters. In their book *Toilet Training in Less Than a Day* (1976), they suggest considering beginning of bladder training at 18 to 20 months of age. The present author would consider this somewhat young to begin. However, they suggest tests in three areas to determine readiness. First, they propose a brief survey of the child's current bladder control. They suggest that the parent ask himself the following questions:

> 1) Does my child urinate a good deal at one time rather than dribbling throughout the day? 2) Does he often stay dry for several hours? 3) Does he appear to know he is about to urinate as indicated by his facial expressions or by special postures he adopts? If he does all three, he is aware of his bladder sensations and has enough bladder control to begin training. If he does

only the first two, he may still be ready for training, since not all children give this visible indication of their desire to urinate.

They then go on to consider physical readiness as follows:

Does he have enough finger and hand coordination to pick up objects easily? Does he walk from room to room easily and without the need for assistance? If he does, he is sufficiently developed physically.

They then propose 10 tests with respect to instructional readiness:

To determine if your child has sufficient social response and understanding, ask him to carry out the following ten actions. Ask him to show you (point to): 1) his nose, 2) his eyes, 3) his mouth, 4) his hair. Ask him 5) to sit down on a chair, 6) to stand up, 7) to walk with you to a particular place, such as another room, 8) to imitate you in a simple task, such as playing patty-cake, 9) to bring you a familiar object, such as one of his toys, 10) to place one familiar object with another—for example, "put the dolly in the wagon." If he carries out eight of these ten instructions, he should be considered intellectually ready for training (pp. 36–37). (Copyright © 1974 by Nathan H. Azrin and Richard M. Foxx; reprinted by permission of Simon & Schuster, a Division of Gulf & Western Corporation.)

How to Train the Child

Using the above tests, parents may be guided as to when to make an effort to toilet train. However, the maturational and individual difference aspects of developing this control should be kept clearly in mind in the early attempts to train. Thus, the best approach to first attempts to train is to allow the child to observe other family members toileting and to encourage him to try to do the same. Any signs of success or cooperation should be greeted with modest signs of pleasure and reinforced with mild praise or recognition that the child is becoming a grown-up person and is just like his brothers, sisters, and parents. If the child is ready to be trained, such efforts will often have quite rapid success. However, if the child does not show signs of succeeding, it is best to cease such efforts and to show no signs of dismay or displeasure. After waiting a period of two or three months, another similar effort may be made. It is not wise to become overly enthusiastic about such efforts, to use excessive pressure or aversive methods, nor to show signs of distress if success is not forthcoming. Likewise, it is well to avoid excessive praise and recognition when there is success. The training should be handled in a relatively low-key, matter-of-fact manner with an underlying expression of confidence that the child will learn and will start toileting the way others in the family do when the time is right.

Efforts along these lines may be made until around age five or six, when the child is ready to begin school. By this time, most children will have learned the proper toileting habits, and no further difficulties should be encountered. However, if the time at which the child will be enrolled in full days of classes at school is approaching and toilet training has not been successful, a more rigorous approach may need to be taken.

Azrin and Foxx have described an ingenious, creative, and highly successful method for training in bladder control. The same basic principles can be applied to bowel training. Their method has been researched carefully and is based on principles of operant conditioning. The details are spelled out in several articles (e.g., Foxx and Azrin, 1973) as well as in their book *Toilet Training in Less Than a Day* (Azrin and Foxx, 1976). Basically, they recommend that the mother arrange to spend several hours uninterrupted and undistracted with the child. This means that the rest of the family either is out of the house for the day or stays in another area of the home so that the mother and child will not be disturbed. The child is dressed in loose fitting pants to facilitate removing them, and a supply of snacks, drinks, and treats are on hand. The procedure begins by using a doll of the type that wets. All of the basic procedures in toileting are carried out as a game by the child and the mother, using the doll as an example. The doll is given fluid, then wets, and is scolded if the wetting takes place in the pants or praised if it takes place in the toilet. The child helps the doll check her pants and go to the toilet properly when she has to. During this period of time, and following, the child is given large quantities of his favorite beverages to ensure that the child will need to urinate. After the doll is trained and the child understands what is expected, he begins to practice on himself. Dry pants inspections are made every five minutes and a reward (praise and/or treat) given if they are dry. There are then prompted potty trials approximately every 15 minutes in which the child goes through the motions of potting whether or not he actually has to urinate. During these times, he removes clothing, sits on the potty, and stays there for five to 10 minutes. Following this, he is able to dress and leave. A child-size potty chair is used to make mounting and sitting easy. Azrin and Foxx also favor the type of chair that plays a little tune when urine strikes it. This signals that urination has begun and is an additional reward for the child. Eventually, the child will urinate on one of the potty practice trials. Approval is shown and a reward is given for this. Next, the child is encouraged to go to the potty on his own when he feels the need to urinate. Early in the training, the child is instructed to go to the toilet for practice, later he is asked if he wants to go to the toilet and is asked to indicate where he would go if he had to go potty, and, finally, he is simply reminded that his pants should be dry and asked if they are. This process shifts the responsibility for toileting from the parent to the child.

When the child begins to go to the bathroom on his own, the parent stops prompted potty practice trials and checks for dry pants every 15 minutes instead of every five minutes. If the child has an accident during the training, the parent shows verbal displeasure, makes him feel the wet pants, and then has him carry out a series of "positive practice trials" in which he starts from where he was when the accident occurred and walks rapidly to the toilet, lowers his pants, and sits on the toilet. He then does the same thing starting from other points, until a total of 10 trials are completed. The clothing is then changed and the child cleans himself. The child is reminded that pants should be dry and wetting should be done in the toilet. One additional feature of this program is the "friends who care" technique. A list of friends and relatives whom the child admires is made up. During the day their names are worked into the instructions (e.g., "Your brother, Bob, will be so happy when you tell him what you have learned today," or, "You did it just like Daddy. Good for you."), and later in the day some of these people talk with the child to indicate their pleasure at his accomplishment. A written certificate can also be given to mark completion of training if the parent and child wish. Additional accidents are handled by means of positive practice trials.

Azrin and Foxx report that the average child can be trained with this method in less than four hours. However, it should be pointed out that independent studies of this method (Butler, 1976; Matson and Ollendick, 1977) have reported only minimal success unless the mothers have access to professional supervision in addition to the book. They also report that for younger children more time is required and emotional reactions (tantrums and avoidance behavior) are common, especially with unsupervised mothers.

Azrin and Foxx (1971) have reported good success with a modified version of the above procedure in training institutionalized children. The major adaptations of the program involve: 1) use of wet-alarm pants, which signal with a beeping sound when a wetting or soiling accident occurs, 2) carrying out the program over a longer period of time, and 3) an elaborate clean-up program involving a shower, cleaning the floor, the clothes, etc., which constitutes a mildly aversive overcorrection consequence for toileting accidents.

Problems Encountered in Toilet Training

Homan (1970) has presented the following list of practices to avoid when toilet training.

> It is not advisable to 1) leave him on the toilet so long that he begins to hate the lesson, 2) play with him while on the toilet, 3) praise him excessively if he manages to have a bowel movement on the john, 4) frighten him by flushing the toilet while he is on or near it, 5) exhibit disgust or distress at the sight or odor of the bowel movement, 6) continue to put him on the toilet if he cries at

the experience or is physically pained by the passage of a hard stool, or 7) if he usually has loose movements, which would be virtually impossible for him to control, or 8) if he is sick or out of sorts for some reason, or 9) if he is involved already with learning several other lessons in behavior, or 10) if he has recently had a frightening change in his environment, such as a change in homes, a new bed, the advent of a sibling, or the sickness or absence of a parent; finally, 11) he should not be left alone on the toilet at first, lest he associate the bathroom with lonely imprisonment (p. 110). (Reprinted by permission.)

Numerous problems and difficulties are commonly encountered in toilet training. Often the parents report that the child will sit on the toilet for long periods of time without evacuating, only to have an accident in his clothes immediately after leaving the toilet area. This is sometimes interpreted as hostility or passive-aggressiveness. However, more commonly, the problem is that the child feels under pressure while on the toilet and the anxiety inhibits sufficient relaxation to permit urination or defecation. However, as soon as he is removed from the toilet he relaxes and the process that had been inhibited by the tension now takes place. When this happens, it is necessary to reduce the pressure to perform and to be patient until the child learns to relax on the toilet. Also, teaching the child to place both feet firmly on the floor or on a stool enabling him to have the proper posture and to be able to exert pressure in the desired direction sometimes results in success.

Many children have accidents with some frequency long after they have seemingly learned to control their toileting functions. These accidents appear to happen particularly when the child is engrossed in play and does not wish to be interrupted. If the accidents are relatively infrequent, simple encouragement and patience will result in the child eventually eliminating the accidents on his own. However, if the accidents occur with sufficient frequency that the parent wishes to do something about it, the best advice is to have the child come into the house and toilet at regular intervals that precede the times when the accidents usually occur. For example, a child can be brought in to the toilet after lunch and make an attempt to have a bowel movement and urinate. He can be called in at mid-afternoon for another trip to the toilet, which can be followed by a cookie and a glass of milk or something to make the visit pleasant rather than aversive. Or, any other time during the day when the child is likely to have a bowel movement, the parent can have him come into the house and toilet before the most likely time of the accident.

During the toilet-training years some children begin to engage in what parents become concerned about as bizarre toileting behaviors. Such things as showing an inordinate interest in the bowel movement, refusing to allow the parent to flush the stools down the toilet, playing with the material and smearing it on the body or walls in the house, urinating and defecating in unusual places such as in the middle of the floor or on the wall, excessive curiosity about the bathrooms at other families' homes and at public places such as restaurants, attempts to observe other children and adults toileting, excessive talking or teasing among peers with respect to toilet habits, and, with girls, attempts to urinate standing up are all common. If the child is otherwise undisturbed, these behaviors may be disregarded and are not a matter for concern. Most children show one or more of these behaviors during their developmental years. They should only be considered serious if they persist for an unreasonable length of time, particularly after the child is of school age, or if they occur in connection with other symptoms of emotional disturbance. Generally, if the parents take a matter-of-fact attitude in teaching proper toileting habits and ignore the seemingly bizarre behaviors, the child will adapt to appropriate behavior in this area. It is best to avoid amusement or unusual interest with regard to the inappropriate behaviors or to make any strenuous effort to eliminate them. Ignoring the unusual behavior along with mild corrective reminders regarding the appropriate behavior is almost always sufficient. In general, toilet training should be a relaxed and normal process with as little stress for the parents and the child as possible. Calmness, patience, and understanding along with normal maturation and development will in most cases get the job done.

ENURESIS

Enuresis is a word of Latin and Greek origin that means literally "to make water." In clinical usage it refers to urination in the clothing or bed beyond the time at which the child should have been toilet trained and in the absence of organic pathology. There are several different patterns of enuresis. Diurnal enuresis refers to daytime wetting in the clothing. A child is usually considered enuretic in this sense if he is still wetting beyond the age of three or four. However, some would set the age at as late as five or six. Nocturnal enuresis refers to wetting the bed at night. Because nighttime control of urination generally is achieved a year or two later, on the average, than daytime control, most clinicians would not make the diagnosis of nocturnal enuresis in a child until the child is approximately four or five. However, some would make it as young as three while others would be hesitant to make such a diagnosis until the child was six or seven or older (deJonge, 1973; Henderson, 1976). Enuresis is also described as being primary or secondary. In the case of primary enuresis, bladder control has never been accomplished. In the case of secondary enuresis, control was accomplished and then lost. Enuresis may also be described as regular (several times per week) or irregular (sporadic accidents). Crosby (1950) has proposed a distinction between "essential" enuresis (attributable to *lack* of training in infancy) and "complicated" enuresis (attributable to *faulty* training practices). The frequency with which a child must have wetting accidents before he is called enuretic has not been established. Different authors use different criteria ranging from once or twice per month to once or twice per week. Some children wet as often as several times per day or night. None of the above distinctions has been consistently found to be related to any characteristic of the child or to response to treatment, with the possible exception that the older child (particularly females) with diurnal and nocturnal enuresis is more likely to show signs of emotional disturbance and be difficult to treat (Lovibond and Coote, 1970; Shaffer, 1973).

Estimates of the frequency of the problem vary from research report to research report and figures appear to vary from country to country (deJonge, 1973). A good deal of the variance is artificial because different researchers use different standards of frequency and duration to determine whether or not a child will be labeled enuretic. For example, if a child wets one time after being trained, should he be labeled enuretic? If not, how many times and how close in succession must these occasions occur before the child is labeled enuretic? Differences in child-rearing techniques and tolerance of wetting accidents and parental willingness to report accidents from one culture or subculture to another also undoubtedly contribute to the differences. However, all studies are relatively consistent in indicating a significant proportion of children experiencing diurnal and/or nocturnal enuresis through the first five years of life. Lovibond and Coote (1970) estimate that, at age four to five years, approximately 20% of children are enuretic. Boys are about twice as likely to have the problem as girls (Doleys, 1977). The proportion decreases constantly until in teenage and adult years the percentage is extremely low (1–2%) (Doleys, 1977). Figure 1 presents incidence data prepared from several sources by Yates (1970).

That there are a significant number of adults with this problem is clear. For example, as many as 1 or 2% of recruits for military service during World War II were rejected at various recruiting centers because of enuresis. An additional 1% were terminated from the service for this problem. Approximately 20 males were discharged for this reason for every female. Enuretic recruits are generally described as younger, immature for their age, slightly lower in intelligence and educational accomplishments, and having more emotional problems than nonenuretic recruits (Plag, 1964). However, they generally adjust adequately to military life if given the chance (Harris and Firestone, 1957), and

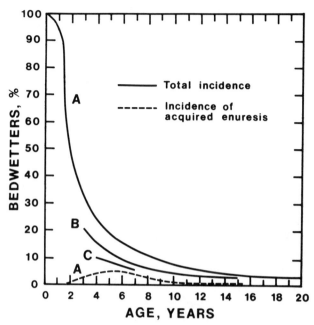

Figure 1.   Incidence of bed-wetting (from Yates (1970), modified from Jones (1960)). A = results from Crosby (1950); B = results from Bransby, Blomfield, and Douglas (1955); C = results from Hallgren (1956). (Reprinted by permission of John Wiley & Sons, Inc.)

psychotherapy has been reported as helpful (Kriegman and Wright, 1947), while drugs such as imipramine have not been found to be helpful (e.g., Hicks and Barnes, 1964). Cooper (1973) has also described the problem of giggle micturition in adults in which the person uncontrollably urinates during times of laughing and giggling, although he is fully continent at other times.

Etiology

Suspected causes of enuresis fall into three categories: organic disorder, emotional disturbance, and learning problems. Organic disorder may be in the form of bladder or urinary tract infection. Symptoms such as fever, pain, a burning sensation when urinating, diurnal dribbling, excessive frequency or urgency, a small or irregular stream, or passage of blood may signal presence of disease or infection.

Organic disorder may also be in the form of central nervous system impairment (particularly spinal cord lesions), which can be evaluated by proper medical and psychological examination. For example, a wide variety of acquired and congenital lesions of the spinal cord as well as anomalies of nerve innervation of the bladder produce what has been variously called neurogenic bladder, subclinical neurogenic bladder, occult neurological bladder, isolated neurogenic dysfunction, reflex neuropathic bladder, and uninhibited neuropathic bladder. The common feature in these conditions is a spastic bladder, which results in involuntary voiding of urine (Kelalis, King, and Belman, 1976). Ditropan (PDR, 1977) is often prescribed in these cases to inhibit spastic contractions of the detrusor muscle.

Structural problems in the urogenital system cause some cases of enuresis. Urinary incontinence also occurs in various chronic diseases, particularly diabetes mellitus and diabetes insipidus. Epilepsy and even food allergies are mentioned by some authors as causes (Henderson, 1976). While estimates vary, it is generally agreed that 90% or more of the cases of urinary incontinence are caused by other than organic factors (Pierce, 1972). Thus, the term enuresis is customarily restricted to disorders of nonorganic origin. Organic pathology should be ruled out by competent medical examination.

A second major suspected causal factor in enuresis is emotional disorder of a psychodynamic nature. Many clinicians believe that enuresis is in itself a symptom of emotional disturbance, and it is generally assumed to occur in the neurotic child. Analytical therapists frequently relate enuresis to sexual conflict and disturbance, with the process of urination being symbolic of suppressed masturbation, ejaculation, or sexual identity confusion (e.g., Fenichel, 1946). Imhof (1956) regarded it as an expression of a need for more love and conceptualized it as "weeping through the bladder." Robertiello (1956) stated that bedwetting was an agent of the super-ego and represented a cooling off of the genitals, thus reducing sexual fire. Other authors stress the passive-aggressive and hostile aspects of the act in disrupting the family and causing the mother extra work (Solomon and Patch, 1969). In spite of the fact that this approach to the causation of enuresis is a commonly recited theory among child psychologists and psychiatrists, there are virtually no data to substantiate it. It would appear that when this type of causation is involved it is a rare exception rather than the rule.

The third view regarding the cause of enuresis and the one that has the broadest support from investigations of 1) the normal development of control of urination in children, 2) characteristics of enuretic children, and 3) response to treatment is the behavioral or learning approach. Normal urination in the infant at birth is basically reflexive. The main components of the urinary system are the kidneys in which the urine is generated, the ureters which are the tubes that transport the urine from the kidney to the bladder, and the urethra which is the tube that extends from the bladder through the genitals to the outside of the body where urine is discharged. The bladder is a round sac-like structure that has much the shape and characteristics of a small balloon. The walls of the bladder are broadly innervated by the detrusor muscle, while the opening between the neck of the bladder and the beginning of the urethra is surrounded by two sets of muscles, the internal sphincters, and the external sphincters. As urine passes from the kidney to the bladder, the walls of the bladder expand gradually. The detrusor muscle does not respond to increased volume in the bladder until the volume exceeds approximately 200 ml. At this point, the detrusor begins to contract rhythmically. This motion leads eventually to the urination reflex, which consists of strong contractions of the detrusor muscle along with relaxation of the internal and external sphincters, resulting in expulsion of urine with considerable force. In the infant and young child this process occurs without interference and results in regular discharge of urine. For the child to adopt appropriate adult behavior in this area, it becomes necessary for him to establish cognitive control over this basically reflex action. It is during the period of time when the child is attempting to learn to control this reflex cognitively that the problems surrounding toilet training and enuresis occur. However, the basic problem appears to be one of *learning* in the vast majority of the cases rather than psychodynamic conflict or organic disease.

It is well known that even in the well-trained adult this reflex can be inhibited only within certain tolerance limits. Yeates (1973) has pointed out that mature bladder function is "made up of a series of phases: *filling, desire to void, postponement, initiation of 'sphincter' relaxation and bladder contraction, maintenance of both these until the bladder is empty, filling, etc.*" In bringing this reflex under control it is necessary to learn both to postpone the urination process and to be able to initiate it and complete the emptying of the bladder at the appropriate time and in the appropriate place. This proves to be a relatively difficult and complex task for many youngsters.

Characteristics of Enuretic Children

Numerous characteristics have been attributed to enuretic children over the years. It is important to keep in mind that establishing a correlation between a characteristic and enuresis does not imply causation. However, because some of the characteristics (if established by data) might have an influence on the method of treatment employed, a brief review of these characteristics and their current status are included in this section.

As indicated earlier, there is a widely prevalent belief that enuresis is a symptom of emotional disturbance. Some reports have indicated a higher degree of emotional disturbance in children who are enuretic. However, careful examination of these studies indicates that many of them are reports from medical clinics and/or centers offering psychiatric and psychological care for children. Often the main presenting symptom was not enuresis. The presence of enuresis was discovered by interview. This, therefore, represents a biased and unreliable sample in terms of determining the incidence of emotional disturbance in enuretic children (Shaffer, 1973). In addition, many of the studies were poorly controlled, and the bias of the experimenter may well have influenced data collection techniques, since "everyone knows that enuresis is a symptom of emotional disturbance."

Extensive studies of large numbers of children have failed to confirm wide prevalence of emotional disturbance among enuretic children. For example, Cullen (1966) studied 1,000 families in an effort to evaluate the prevalence of various behavior disorders in relation to the child's medical history and environment. In all, 3,440 children were included in the sample from these 1,000 mothers. Nocturnal enuresis occurred frequently among these children but was found to be unrelated to behavior disorders or emotional disturbance. A similar study by Tapia, Jekel, and Domke (1960) included 830 children who were evaluated and rated with respect to overall adjustment. These ratings were then compared with the frequency of nocturnal enuresis. Of the 830 children, 167 were determined to be well adjusted, 429 were determined to have no significant problems, 166 were marginally disturbed, and 68 clinically were disturbed. Six cases were eliminated because of insufficient information. No relationship between adjustment and the symptom of nocturnal enuresis was found in this study.

Shaffer (1973) carefully reviewed the literature having to do with the association between enuresis and emotional disorder and concluded that there was evidence of a relationship between the two. As previously discussed in this section, many researchers and clinicians would question this, and Shaffer goes on to qualify this conclusion in such a way that it is almost retracted:

> Although emotional disorders are more common in bedwetters than in children who are dry, most children who wet the bed are, nevertheless, psychiatrically normal. When enuretics do display a psychiatric abnormality, there is no consistent pattern of disturbance, and the evidence for a syndrome of habit disorders, such as thumb-sucking, nail-biting or tics, in association with enuresis is unconvincing. There is some suggestion that enuretic children are slower to lose and acquire other age-related behaviours, and are more acquiescent and less outgoing and confident, than non-enuretics.
>
> The nature of the association between emotional disorder and enuresis remains uncertain (pp. 133–134).

Careful examination of the literature in this area indicates that in general the type of disturbance found in enuretic children revolves around anxiety, situational stress, family disruption (divorce, death of a parent, etc.), and early stressful life events such as accidents, hospitalization, birth of a younger sib, etc. (Douglas, 1973).

Thus, the following general conclusions may be drawn in this area. First, while it is true that emotional disturbance is slightly more prevalent among enuretics, it is clear that most enuretics are not suffering from emotional disturbance. In addition, there is no association between any specific type of emotional disturbance such as neurosis or psychosis and enuresis other than a tendency for increased situational stress and family disruption to be common. Thus, it is clear that enuresis should not be regarded as a symptom of emotional disturbance. Considering the nature of the process of learning urination control, it is probable that the majority of children who are enuretic simply have not learned to control the reflex adequately. The minority of enuretics who are emotionally disturbed may have been exposed to less adequate rearing in general (including urine control) or may be more preoccupied and distracted, resulting in their paying less attention to toileting habits than the average child. In addition, it is well known that the normal physiological reaction to increasing anxiety and tension is increased frequency of urination. This may strain the limits of the control learned by children of younger ages.

Developmental Delay   Developmental delay is frequently suggested in connection with enuresis. Because there is a strong maturational component to gaining control of the bowels and bladder, it is only natural that many would assume that children who have difficulty gaining control might suffer from a failure or delay in the development of the neuromuscular system. Thus, Oppel, Harper, and Rider (1968) have reported that lower birth weight is associated with achieving bladder control later in life. Finley (1971) has reported that the sleep patterns of enuretic children suggest immaturity, specifically in terms of the greater amount of time spent in Stage 4 sleep. In addition, some studies have reported greater behavioral immaturity in enuretics (e.g., Macfarlane, Allen, and Honzik, 1954). However, whether this latter precedes the enuretic problem or is a result of it is difficult to determine.

MacKeith (1972) has argued that developmental delay may be employed in two senses. One is in the sense of description. That is, the child is enuretic beyond the age at which statistically most children have achieved control. A second sense uses the term in such a manner that it implies a causative mechanism such as failure of the neuromuscular system to develop normally. MacKeith and others argue that it is accurate descriptively to note that certain children develop control later than others and are, therefore, delayed in this function. However, they point out that there is very scant evidence to suggest any kind of mechanism involving the nervous system and feel that the overwhelming amount of evidence is that very few cases of enuresis can be accounted for on this basis. Therefore, while some children may be slow in acquiring control, by the time they are five years old most of the children (98.5% according to MacKeith) can be assumed to have sufficient neuromuscular development to control the bladder. If the child is still wetting, the problem probably is elsewhere. In the view of the present author, however, the possibility of developmental delay would suggest that in stubborn cases which appear to resist treatment effects it might be well to wait a year and try again after allowing time for additional maturation.

Organic Pathology of the Brain   Somewhat related to the concept of developmental delay is the idea that enuresis may be related to organic pathology of the brain. As indicated earlier in this chapter, certain lesions, particularly in the spinal cord, as might be involved in such disorders as spina bifida occulta, are related to incontinence. However, many other investigators have speculated that higher centers may be involved. For example, numerous investigators have reported abnormal EEG patterns among enuretics, some suggesting that enuresis may be an epileptic equivalent producing minor seizures at night that result in release of urine. However, the data in this area are conflicting and many of the studies are poorly controlled. In two careful studies by Poussaint (Poussaint and Greenfield, 1966; Poussaint, Koegler, and Riehl, 1967), it was found that enuretics do not have a higher than usual incidence of EEG abnormality and that children with EEG abnormalities do not have a higher than usual incidence of enuresis. In a recent review of this literature, Salmon, Taylor, and Lee (1973) point out that the research is very conflicting and no conclusion can be drawn at present. They further indicate that, if such an association were found to exist, it would be able to account for only a small number of the cases.

Intelligence and Enuresis   While an occasional article has indicated a lower mean IQ for enuretics than nonenuretics, the general consensus of the literature in this area is that there is no difference between intellectual ability for enuretics and nonenuretics. The only exception to this appears to be for older enuretics. Bjornsson (1973) found that 10- to 15-year-old enuretics in his study of 1,098 children, ages five to 15, had a mean IQ of 87.83 while the nonenuretics had a mean IQ of 100.3. As noted earlier in this chapter, adult enuretics in the military service were reported to score lower on the military General Classification Tests (Plag, 1964).

Enuresis is known to be common in severely retarded children. However, moderately retarded children appear to learn as readily as normal children when given the same training. In addition, severely retarded children learn quite rapidly in many cases when subjected to careful training (Azrin, Sneed, and Foxx, 1973). Thus, it is not likely that cerebral impairment accounts for the majority of toilet-training problems of retarded children (except in cases of severe retardation). It appears more likely that less effort is made to train them and more tolerance is shown for their failure to learn.

Genetics Since enuresis is frequently clinically observed to run in families, some have suggested that there may be a genetic basis for enuresis. Numerous studies have reported that a high percentage of the parents, siblings, and relatives of bed wetters were also bed wetters themselves when they were children (e.g., Crosby, 1950; Poulton and Hinden, 1953; Young, 1963). Percentages of family history of enuresis in children under treatment for the problem vary from study to study but generally range from 40 to 55% (Baller, 1975). However, other studies such as Crosby (1950) report much lower incidences—in the neighborhood of 17 or 18%. Of course, the definitions employed and the extensiveness of the interviews involved could well account for the discrepancies. Bakwin, a leading proponent of the genetic theory of enuresis, has assembled the data available so far (1973). He finds a 68% concordance of enuresis for monozygotic twins and a 36% concordance for dyzygotic twins in the data available. He also notes that 77% of children with two parents having a history of enuresis are enuretic themselves; approximately 43 to 44% of the children with one parent enuretic are also enuretic; and 15% of the children with neither parent enuretic are enuretic. Thus, there does seem to be evidence suggestive of a hereditary factor in enuresis. However, to date, no specific mechanism for the transmission of this characteristic has been demonstrated, and most studies have not ruled out environmental influences (such as family attitudes and training procedures) on the problem.

Sleep Patterns The depth of sleep of enuretics and the sleep cycle in which bed-wetting takes place have been of interest to a number of investigators. One of the most persistent complaints of parents attempting to work with their bed-wetting child is that the child appears to sleep extremely deeply and is very difficult to arouse at night. If the enuretic child is one who sleeps more soundly than other children, this would be a partial explanation for the problem he has. However, the data are conflicting. Bostock (1958) reported an experiment in which seven enuretic and 12 nonenuretic children were awakened at intervals during the night, using a buzzer. The enuretic children took an average of 418 seconds to awaken, whereas nonenuretic children took only 319 seconds on the average. On the other hand, Boyd (1960) examined 200 children between the ages of five and 15. Half were enuretic, the other half were not. They were matched for age and sex. The children were awakened by calling their names and by shaking them gently. The enuretic children took an average of 16 seconds to awaken, whereas nonenuretics took 20.5 seconds.

Studies of the stage of sleep indicate similar confusion. Some studies report that nocturnal enuresis occurs in deep sleep, while others suggest that it occurs in light sleep or wakefulness. Finley (1971) studied children from age five to 15 and reported a possible resolution of this problem. He found that as age increases the depth of sleep in which enuresis occurs becomes progressively lighter. Five-year-old enuretics most frequently wet their beds during deep sleep, while the 15-year-olds wet exclusively during brief periods of semiwakefulness during the night. Ten-year-olds were as likely to wet during deep sleep as wakefulness. In this study Finley also tested arousal thresholds for the children in the morning. Enuretics were found to be much more difficult to arouse in the morning after the experiment. This was particularly true for the younger enuretics. Studies of sleep stage indicated that enuretics tended to spend significantly more time in Stage 4 deep sleep than did nonenuretics. A further interesting finding of this study was that the time of onset of the first postenuretic rapid eye movement (REM) was related to the depth of sleep at the time of the enuretic episode. When enuresis occurred in a light sleep or wakefulness, the postenuretic REM occurred within three to 15 minutes. However, when enuresis occurred during deep sleep the next postenuretic REM occurred approximately two hours and 15 minutes later. Finley, in commenting on the data in this study, suggests that it is tempting to assume that enuretics are children who have a high nighttime threshold for external stimuli as well as the internal stimuli of bladder distention, resulting in bed-wetting. As the enuretic child gets older, enuresis begins to occur in lighter stages of sleep or during wakefulness.

> [This] suggests that the CNS shows a progressive tendency to "respond" to a sensory input from the distended bladder. Thus, as age increases there develops an increasing tendency towards arousal prior to and during the moment of enuresis. Ultimately, this eventuates in complete physiological and behavioral arousal preceding micturition so that enuresis is voluntarily checked. When this occurs the patient is considered to have "outgrown the problem of bed-wetting" (Finley, 1971, p. 38).

Thus, Finley speculates that enuretics may suffer from a maturational defect in the sleep-arousal system. However, he recognizes that this would not be a sufficient explanation for all problems of enuresis.

Socioeconomic and Ethnic Factors Some studies have shown socioeconomic and ethnic factors to be related to enuresis. Enuresis has been found to be more prevalent in lower socioeconomic groups, in larger families, and in families in which the mother has less education

(Bakwin and Bakwin, 1972; MacKeith, Meadow, and Turner, 1973). The incidence of enuresis varies from country to country and among racial and ethnic groups (deJonge, 1973). However, attitudes toward child rearing, including toilet training, tolerance of, and willingness to report enuresis, vary with the cultural and socioeconomic background of the individuals included in investigations. Because virtually all of the studies are based on self-report, it is difficult to interpret these data and they may be largely artificial.

Time of Training   Enuresis is sometimes thought to be related to too early or too late as well as to too strict or too lax training methods (Bakwin and Bakwin, 1972). However, Lovibond (1964) and Dimson (1959) could find no support for these notions. The data in this area would have to be regarded as inconclusive at present.

Bladder Size   Finally, several researchers have reported that enuretics have smaller functional bladder capacities than normal children (e.g., Hallman, 1950; Muellner, 1960; Starfield, 1967). It should be noted that this refers to *functional* capacity rather than actual size. Esperanca and Gerrard (1969) found that children with smaller bladder capacities urinate more frequently both during the day and at night. They, then, pass the same amount of urine as other children but do so in smaller quantities and at more frequent intervals. They are enuretic during the day as well as the night, unless they go to the toilet frequently, which many of them do. However, Doleys (in press) has pointed out that not all enuretic children appear to have smaller capacities (smaller functional capacity seems to be more frequent in primary enuresis), and it has not been demonstrated convincingly that increased bladder capacity is necessary or sufficient to produce a reduction in enuresis. Nevertheless, the fact that some enuretics have a smaller functional bladder capacity may have implications for treatment.

Treatment of Enuresis

Over the centuries numerous treatments have been attempted (Glicklich, 1951). From existent medical writings we know that enuresis has been considered a problem since at least 1550 B.C. A medical text of that date recommends juniper berries, cyprus, and beer as medication for enuresis.

During the middle ages numerous concoctions were prepared for this problem, as they were for most medical disorders of the day. One physician of the time wrote as follows,

> I myself know from experience that the flesh of a ground hedge-hog checks the flow of urine, so that if it be frequently administered, it prevents the passage of urine, although in this matter there seems to be controversy, because Avicenna asserts that the flesh of a hedge-hog softens the bowels and provokes urine; so to Rasis. Yet if one considers their dicta, he will

understand that what is said is true; the experiment is true and has been proved by me (as cited by Glicklich, 1951, p. 861).

In 1554 Thomas Phaer published the first pediatric textbook of medicine entitled *Boke of Children.* There is in this text a paragraph entitled "Of pyssying in the bedde." Among the remedies prescribed for this problem are the following:

> Many times for debility of vertus retentive of the reines or blader, as wel olde men as children are oftentimes annoyed, whan their urine issueth out either in theyre slepe or waking against thery wylles, having no power to reteine it whan it cometh, therfore yf they will be holpen, fyrst they must avoid al fat meates and drynkes.
>
> Take the wesande (trachea) of a cocke, and plucke it, than brenne it in pouder, and use of it twise or thryes a daye, The stones of an hedge-hogge poudred is of the same vertue.
>
> Item the clawes of a goate, made in pouder droken, or eaten in pottage.
>
> If the patient be of age, it is good to make fyne plates of lead, with holes in them, and lette them lye often ot the naked backe (as cited by Glicklich, 1951, p. 862).

In the nineteenth century considerable attention was given to the problem of enuresis because it posed numerous economic and social hazards. Children of higher social station were ineligible for boarding schools of the day if they were enuretic. In addition, children, particularly girls, who were enuretic were unsuitable for work as maids because of their bed-wetting. Injections were often made and external medications applied to the sacral area of the back to stimulate the nerves in this area. One of the more barbaric treatments involved burning blisters in the area. Originally it was thought that the blistering would stimulate the sacral nerves, thus preventing bed-wetting. However, the same treatment was used to prevent children from lying on their backs because it was thought that warmth from the bed on the sacral nerves might cause bed-wetting. Because it was thought by many that allowing the child to lie on his back resulted in bed-wetting, various instruments including spikes, knotted ropes, etc. were used to prevent children from lying on their backs during sleep. Various other kinds of rotation of the body at different angles (such as elevating the feet, pelvis, or genitals) were felt to be beneficial in retaining urine.

Cauterization of the opening of the urethra with silver nitrate was thought to make this portion more tender to the passage of urine, forcing the child to retain the urine. One physician, Dominick Corrigan, employed a treatment in which he poured collodian into the prepuce of males, hermetically sealing it.

Trousseau developed a very popular treatment in the nineteenth century. His description is as follows:

An apparatus which consists of a sort of small cone made of ivory or vul-
canized caoutchouc fixed by a "T" bandage, which bandage is applied
around the loins and kept in its place by a cincture to which are attached in
front, bands passing under the thighs. The stem-pessary of my apparatus is
longer and more bulky than that of the bandage used for compressing
hemorrhoids as it is requisite to be introduced higher up in the rectum so as
to reach the situation of the vesiculae seminalis. I now use a simpler
apparatus in that it does not require a bandage, an apparatus consisting of a
sort of metallic bung of the form of a very elongated olive varying in size
between a pigeon's egg and small hen's egg. This bung diminishes
downwards, taking the form of a neck, the diameter of which does not
exceed 5 mm. so that once introduced into the rectum, it is retained there by
the natural constriction of the sphincter of the anus. The bung-like
compressor is soldered upon a flat stem of the same metal about 3–4 cm. in
length and ½ cm. in breadth; the anterior one-half of the stem is intended to
be applied to the perineum and the other one-half to the coccygeal region.
Size varies with the individual's age and manner of tolerance. The junction
of the compressor and stem forms an acute angle of 75° on one side and an
obtuse angle of 125° on the other. The obtuse angle looking toward the coccyx
and the acute angle toward the pubis with the superior part of the bulge rest-
ing on the prostate (cited by Glicklich, 1951, p. 868).

Various primitive tribes have employed measures such as beating
and ridiculing. For example, one West African tribe pours a mixture of
water and ashes on the head of the child. The child is then driven out into
the street where the other children of the village clap their hands and run
after him singing "adida ga ga ga ga," which translates to "urine
everywhere." The Navajo Indians were known to use a treatment during
which the child stood naked with his legs spread over a burning nest of the
phoebe. This was thought to help because birds don't wet their nest.

In their classic article on the use of the pad and bell for the treatment of enuresis, Mowrer and Mowrer (1938) review the variety of treatments that have been employed over the years. They note that these
include:

Innumerable drugs and hormones; special diets (including fresh fruit, caviar,
and colon bacilli); restriction of fluids; voluntary exercises in urinary control; injections of physiological saline; sterile water, paraffin and other inert
substances; real and sham operations (passage of a bougie, public application of cantharides plasters, cauterization of the neck of the bladder, spinal
punctures, tonsillectomy, circumcision, clitoridotomy, etc. high-frequency
mechanical vibration and electrical stimulation of various parts of the body;
massage,   bladder and rectal irrigations; Roentgen and other forms of
irradiation; chemical neutralization of the urine; sealing or constriction of
the urinary orifice; hydrotherapy; local "freezing" of the external genitalia
with ice or "chloratyl"; elevation of the foot of the patient's bed; sleeping on
the back; not sleeping on the back; and the use of a hard mattress (p. 436).

While a couple of these methods are still in use today and appear to have some merit, most of them are without merit—many obviously dangerous and harmful.

In view of this long history of unwise and harmful treatment of enuresis, many physicians and psychologists currently recommend an attitude of patience and restraint, allowing the child to develop control of his own functions without coercion or exposure to possible danger. In general, this would appear to be a wise approach. However, as the child becomes older, and particularly when he enters school, there may be good reasons for introducing appropriate treatment. The child who is wetting after the age of seven or eight is likely to be restricted in various kinds of school and peer activities such as overnight parties, trips, etc. In addition, he generally begins to feel different and peculiar with respect to his peers who do not have this problem. Other children, when they discover it, often tease and ostracize the bed wetter. The anxiety and concern of the parents about the "problem" often color their view of the child and produce considerable conflict in the family. As a result of these factors, treatment may be more required at this age than at earlier ages. In the sections below the basic forms of treatment that have been found to be safe and effective are reviewed.

Support and Encouragement   Most textbooks of pediatric medicine suggest some degree of support and encouragement as a first step in treatment. The general recommendation is to talk with the child and attempt to increase his motivation by having him realize that his doctor wants him to work on the problem and see if it can be eliminated. Advice is then given to the parents regarding being patient with the child and praising him when he does well. This, along with the fact that most children will spontaneously cease wetting over a period of years, is a very conservative but sensible treatment in many cases. Few careful studies have been done on the effectiveness of this approach. However, Dische (1971) reported cessation of wetting in 32% of 126 patients treated by this method.

Restricting Fluids   Restricting fluids after supper and having the child urinate just before going to bed are often suggested. However, unless the child is drinking excessive amounts of fluid or diuretics, such as iced tea, certain soft drinks, etc., just before bedtime, this method appears to have little effect. Studies indicate that enuretic children do not produce more urine than normal children (Troup and Hodgson, 1971). They either urinate in response to minimal pressure in the bladder or fail to respond to the need to urinate by waking. Restricting fluids and encouraging urination before bedtime may be of minimal benefit in very mild cases, but have virtually no effect on the more problematic cases.

Drug Treatments   Numerous drug treatments have been attempted for enuresis. For example, parasympatholytic agents such as atropine or belladonna have been administered in attempts to decrease the tone and reactivity of the detrusor muscle. Sympathomimetic agents such as dextroamphetamine sulfate have been administered to produce a lighter sleep pattern so that the child will awaken when there is an urge to void. Diphenylhydantoin has been found to have an effect in controlling some enuretic children who have abnormal electroencephalograms (Halverstadt, 1976). Anticholinergics have been used in attempts to increase bladder retention. Sedatives have been given to reduce tension and to calm the child. Benadryl has been administered on the theory that an allergy may underlie the inability to control urine. Antidiuretics have been administered to decrease urine output, and caffeine has been administered during the day to increase daytime urination (Henderson, 1976). However, these treatments have been found to have minimal to no effectiveness with most cases.

By far, the most popular drug treatment in current use is the administration of antidepressants such as imipramine (Tofranil). The drug is usually given after supper starting with 10 mg each night for one week. If there is an improvement, this dosage is continued for up to several months. If there is no improvement, or only minimal improvement, the dosage is increased by weekly increments of 10 mg to a maximal dose of 40 mg for younger children, gradually increasing to 75 mg for teenagers (McKendry and Stuart, 1974).

The mechanism by which imipramine has its effect is unknown. Its effectiveness has been attributed to a variety of actions including anticholinergic effects on the bladder, which inhibit urination. However, more recent research has concentrated on the effects of this drug on sleep patterns that may be related to wetting incidents at night. According to a recent review by Stewart (1975), the results of several major investigations in this area show a remarkably similar pattern. Only a very small number of children cease wetting the bed completely as a result of the medication. However, somewhere between 25 to 40% of the patients show significant improvement in terms of wetting only two or three nights per week rather than almost every night. This effect usually comes approximately two weeks after the treatment has begun. Unfortunately, most patients become discouraged and cease using this treatment, because there is only a reduction rather than a cessation of wetting. Studies of relapse rates following this treatment suggest that the majority of children treated in this manner return to wetting as soon as the medication is discontinued. The percentage who do not is no higher than would be expected to have grown out of the problem with increasing age.

Forsythe and Merrett (1969) found that there was little difference between continuation of treatment with the drug or with placebo. In addition, Shaffer, Costello, and Hill (1968) found it made no difference whether the drugs were withdrawn suddenly or gradually.

Serious side effects from the use of the imipramine are said to be unusual. However, since the drug only reduces wetting, continuation of this treatment over a long period of time should be approached cautiously. There is a need for much more information regarding the long-term effects on children at different developmental ages. Stewart (1975) has expressed concern about the psychological effects on the child including changes in sleep, morale, nervousness, irritability, and concentration. Excessive doses of imipramine administered to children either through errors of prescription or by overzealous parents are known to depress respiration, as well as induce cardiac irregularities and hypotension. In Great Britain, 22 deaths from overdoses of imipramine were reported over a four-year period (McKendry and Stewart, 1974). Currently there is a trend to use Elavil rather than Tofranil because it is thought that there are fewer side effects with the former (Halverstadt, 1977, personal communication).

The use of drugs in the treatment of enuresis would appear to have only very modest success and to be accompanied by numerous undesirable side effects. Studies of the use of drugs in adolescents and adults with enuretic problems have failed to support their effectiveness with these age groups to any degree (Hicks and Barnes, 1964; Blackwell and Currah, 1973).

Psychotherapy Psychotherapy or family therapy is often suggested as a treatment for enuresis. However, no carefully gathered data have indicated any significant effectiveness of psychotherapy over the general rate of spontaneous remission (Lovibond, 1964). Studies that have compared psychotherapy with other forms of treatment have generally found psychotherapy to be the least effective treatment (e.g., DeLeon and Mandell, 1966). Although psychotherapy may be of great benefit to the child and family in changing patterns of interaction within the family, there is no convincing evidence that it will significantly affect the specific symptom of enuresis.

Hypnotherapy Hypnotherapy has also been used in the treatment of enuresis. The procedure generally employed is to give the child positive suggestions, under hypnosis, that he will retain urine and not wet the bed at night or that, if necessary, he will get up in the middle of the night and go to the bathroom rather than wet the bed. This is generally coupled with some degree of insight and supportive therapy also done under hypnosis. Collinson (1970) reported on 11 cases treated in this manner. The ages of his cases ranged from five-and-a-half to 38 years of age, and follow-up ranged from one to five years. In nine out of the 11 cases, the child was dry at the time of follow-up. Interestingly, Collinson noted that four of the children were phobic to water. He used insight-oriented therapy as well as systematic desensitization to reduce their fear of water. Correction of the bed-wetting problem did not occur until their fear of water was eliminated.

Olness (1975) has reported on the use of self-hypnosis in the treatment of nocturnal enuresis. The child is first trained in a hand levitation method of hypnotizing himself, which involves painting a clown on the thumbnail and holding a quarter between the thumb and finger. The child stares at the clown and imagines the quarter becoming heavier and heavier. As the quarter falls, the child becomes hypnotized. After the training in self-hypnosis, the child is instructed to hypnotize himself at night and to say something along the following lines before going to sleep, "When I need to urinate I will wake up all by myself, go to the bathroom all by myself, urinate in the toilet, and return to my nice dry bed. I will go back to sleep. If I need to urinate another time, I will wake up all by myself, go to the bathroom, all by myself, urinate in the toilet, and return to my nice dry bed. When I wake up, my bed will be dry and I will be very happy." Using this approach, 40 children (20 boys and 20 girls) ranging in age from four-and-a-half to 16 years were studied. At the time of the published report, the 40 children had been followed for between six and 28 months and were still being followed by the project. Of the 40, 31 had stopped bed-wetting and six had reduced the frequency of wetting. Three were unimproved. Of the 31 who had completely stopped bed-wetting, 28 had done so within the first month of treatment.

Behavioral Techniques   In a recent review of the literature, Doleys (1977) has pointed out that some improvement in enuresis has been noted by merely having the child self-record wetting incidents over a period of time. While this method alone is seldom sufficient, it may be used with benefit in connection with other treatments.

Reinforcement for a dry bed each morning is often used, but generally in connection with other forms of treatment, rather than alone. However, Atthowe (1972) has reported a study in which incontinent, lobotomized, and severely disturbed adults were placed on a token economy program in which continence was rewarded and incontinence was punished mildly. After seven months of treatment, all patients became continent and remained so through a 42-month follow-up. Johnson and Thompson (1974) have reported a case study on the combined use of modeling via a younger sibling and reinforcement in eliminating wetting accidents in a five-year-old boy.

Punishment is frequently reported by parents as a method they have tried without success, but is seldom reported as a part of professional treatment. However, Tough et al. (1971) reported a case study of two brothers who were punished by means of a cold bath if the buzzer was triggered to sound by the pad in their bed. Examination of their results does not indicate any effectiveness beyond what the pad and bell would be expected to produce.

Periodic Waking   Periodic waking of the child throughout the night to go to the bathroom and attempt to urinate has been found effective in eliminating enuresis in some cases. While this method has not been subjected to extensive research it appears to show promise. Young (1964), in a study of 58 children, found that over a period of four weeks the staggered waking procedure resulted in 10 children becoming completely continent. A total of 67% showed some improvement. Creer and Davis (1975) used this method with nine subjects in an institutional setting. All subjects showed a decrease in the frequency of bed-wetting, and four subjects became completely free of wetting. The staggered waking procedure is one that should be carried out over a period of weeks when used.

The implementation of the program can be made by the parents and the child. Parents can be instructed to awaken the child at intervals throughout the night and have him go to the bathroom to urinate. These intervals can be randomized to some extent, but also should include awaking at times at which the child generally will need to urinate. The method may also be employed by having the child take responsibility for awaking himself. This can be done by providing him with an alarm clock, which he sets to awaken at intervals. It would be possible, of course, to reward the child for a dry bed each morning along with the staggered awakening, thus making it a more pleasant experience. Some researchers (Lovibond, 1964; Morgan and Young, 1972) have cautioned that use of this method may result in increasing the frequency of urinating at night rather than learning to sleep through the night with a full bladder. However, it would appear that the danger of this is relatively minimal and could be corrected should the therapist note its occurrence.

The mechanism by which this procedure works has not been defined. However, the method does result in increased attention to the cues that urination is about to take place. There may also be some desire to avoid the aversive characteristics of being awakened during the night.

Bladder Retention Exercises   Over the years, various clinicians and researchers have used an exercise that has a dual effect of increasing the child's control over the urination reflex as well as increasing functional bladder capacity, which, as noted earlier in this chapter, is deficient in some enuretic children. This method seems to have first been described by Muellner (1960). The basic procedure in employing this technique is to have the child go to the bathroom area when he has the urge to urinate (fluid intake may be increased during training to facilitate the process).

The child is then requested to retain the urine as long as possible before urinating. When the child no longer feels able to retain the urine, he is instructed to urinate in the toilet. At the beginning, some children can retain the urine only for a few seconds. However, with training they generally get to the point where they can retain it several minutes or even hours. Starfield and Mellits (1968) used this method with 83 enuretic children. The results were that 66% showed improvement and an additional 19% were reported to be cured.

Vincent (1964) has described a device that exerts pressure on the perineum between the anus and the genitals. Pressure in this area results in cessation of urination. While this device has not been researched sufficiently to judge its worth, it may prove useful in connection with bladder-retention training. Some clinicians advise patients to exert pressure in that area with their finger when they are practicing retention.

Kimmel and Kimmel (1970) have reported use of the bladder retention method along with reinforcement for retaining urine. The child is asked to retain the urine longer and longer until he is able to hold the urine 45 minutes or longer. This generally takes 15 to 20 days. During the training period, the child is rewarded with trinkets and small gifts for increasing the length of the time that he can retain urine. He is expected to increase by approximately two to three minutes per day. If the child urinates in the toilet, he is also reinforced for that. In addition, the child is reinforced for dry-bed nights. In a study by Paschalis, Kimmel, and Kimmel (1972) of 31 children, 15 were found to be completely free of bed-wetting and another eight showed significant improvement on the basis of 20 days' treatment, with the follow-up data gathered three months later. Stedman (1972) successfully applied this method with an adolescent patient.

Sphincter-control exercises are also often found helpful in connection with bladder-retention training. To do these exercises, the child is simply instructed to practice starting and stopping the stream of urine while toileting. Rewards may be offered as reinforcement to enhance the process.

Care should be taken when using the bladder-retention methods not to force excessive amounts of fluid or to attempt to retain the urine for unusually long periods of time. Although uncommon, complications such as loss of muscle tone of the bladder and, in rare cases, rupture of the bladder are possible. Generally a cup or two of fluid per hour with retention encouraged up to one or two hours will be well within safe limits. However, if the child shows signs of distress, the requirements should be lowered.

Pad and Bell Without a doubt, the most effective treatment for cases of nocturnal enuresis is the use of the pad and bell. This method was discovered serendipitously by a German physician named Pfaundler and reported in a paper in 1904 (Costello, 1970). Pfaundler was attempting to alert nurses in an institution for children to the fact that a wetting had occurred so that the bed and clothing could be changed, preventing skin irritation and rashes. He developed a device that would ring a bell when moistened by urine. This was the signal to the nurse to change the child's diaper or clothing. The staff at the institution began to notice that when this device was used the children began to stop wetting. Thus, the therapeutic effects of the procedure were noted. The next major development occurred in 1938 when Mowrer and Mowrer reported employing this technique with considerable success. In 1939, Morgan and Witmer independently reported similar results. Although found to be extremely effective in early studies, the method had only sporadic use until recent years. Even today relatively few people responsible for the care of children are familiar with the technique.

The basic procedure is to place a pad in the bed that is sensitive to urine. This pad is attached to a bell or buzzer and in some cases to a light. When the child urinates, the buzzer and/or light are activated, awakening the child, who then goes to the bathroom to complete the process of urination. The child then cleans the bed, resets the equipment, and returns to sleep. Over a period of time this training, properly carried out, results in cessation of bed-wetting for as many as 80 or 90% of the cases (Costello, 1970; Yates, 1970). A primitive and questionably effective version of this treatment described by Torrey (1972) is a procedure used by witch doctors in which a toad is tied to the penis. If the child wets, the water causes the toad to croak, thus awakening the child.

Numerous articles in the literature provide detailed instructions for constructing the pad and bell apparatus (e.g., Fried, 1974; Kashinsky, 1974). Keeping the pad, which is subjected to much abuse from the child's sleeping and urinating, in working order is a difficult task. However, a highly resilient and effective design has been developed by Finley and Smith (1975). If the therapist does not wish to construct equipment, inexpensive equipment may be purchased for around $25 to $30 through medical aid sections of department store catalogues such as Sears' or Montgomery Ward's. It is also possible for parents to lease equipment from several commercial companies who make the equipment available. The use of equipment from commercial companies, however, is not advised because the cost of leasing the equipment is generally excessive, there is some question about the safety of the equipment that is produced by some of the companies, and the staff who supervise the use of the equipment are generally not trained properly. Lovibond and Coote (1970) have presented a description of a particularly poor procedure used by one commercial firm.

At first interview the child-patient is greeted with the remark that he is both stupid and dirty. If response to treatment is slow the parent is exhorted to "belt him all the way to the toilet and all the way back again each time the alarm rings." Next day he is to be dressed in a diaper, stood in a corner and the family is to gather round and jeer at him. Failure or relapse is ascribed to laziness or defiance, and a thrashing is prescribed (p. 387).

One of the most sophisticated pieces of equipment that is available can be obtained from Dr. William Finley at Children's Medical Center in Tulsa (Research, Children's Medical Center, Post Office Box 35648, 5300 Skelly Drive, Tulsa, Oklahoma 74135). The medical center leases the equipment for patient use. This equipment has been determined to be completely safe and is supervised by competent psychological and medical staff at the center. The equipment can be mailed to the patient for use in other parts of the country.

In the case of the simple equipment available from the mail order catalogues or that is often described in the literature, the general procedure is to use two pieces of tinfoil-coated paper, the top one of which has holes in it. These are separated by absorbent paper and connected by electrical cord to the buzzer and light. The pad is placed in the bed, and, when urine wets the paper, this completes the circuit, ringing the buzzer and turning on the light. A problem inherent in this equipment is that, if the equipment is battery operated, the buzzer and light are relatively low intensity and often do not awaken the child. However, if the equipment is plugged into the wall to provide a louder sound and to turn on a brighter light, this involves the danger of having the child lying in a pool of urine while attached to an apparatus that is plugged into the wall. The danger of shock and, in a rare instance, possibly death is not to be denied. The equipment available from Children's Medical Center has solved this problem by using a very safe pad that is hooked up only to a small battery. When urine touches the pad the result is that a small battery-operated light, similar to a flashlight, is turned on. This beam of light crosses the baseboard of the equipment and activates a second part of the equipment that is plugged into the wall. This makes a loud sound and turns on a spotlight that is trained on the child's face, thus awakening the child. Thus, the child is never connected to anything but a small battery. This arrangement is completely safe and highly effective.

The pad and bell apparatus is generally agreed to work on a conditioning model. However, the exact nature of the conditioning taking place has been in question since the development of the apparatus and is not yet resolved. One explanation assumes a simple classical conditioning paradigm in which distention of the bladder becomes associated with the sound of the bell that awakens the child, the result being that bladder distention eventually becomes the cue to awaken the child before he wets the bed. However, this model suspiciously resembles backward conditioning and fails to account for the fact that most of the children eventually learn to sleep through the night without wetting or awakening to go to the bathroom. The problem with regard to this model is how does the transition from being awakened by a full bladder to simply staying asleep and retaining the urine take place.

A model that does take this into account was developed by Lovibond (1964). Lovibond assumes that the sound and light are aversive stimuli. The learning taking place, then, is based on aversive conditioning. The basic model is that the sleeping child, not wishing to be awakened by the sound and the light, will either awaken on his own and go to the bathroom or, as is most often the case, retain the urine and sleep through the night undisturbed. Based on this model, Lovibond has developed an apparatus that gives a minimal hooting sound before triggering the loud sound and light. The purpose of this is to enhance the aversive conditioning process. This equipment has proved as effective as the more traditional equipment but does not appear to have the expected significantly higher success rate (Turner, Young, and Rachman, 1970). However, when dealing with a success rate of 80 to 90%, it may be difficult to improve upon this to any great degree.

Crosby (1950) has developed apparatus somewhat similar to the pad and bell in that a sound signal is delivered, but, in addition, his equipment has certain other characteristics. Electrodes are attached to the genitals, which, when activated by urine, result in a mild electric shock to the groin region. The shock is not delivered directly to the genitals but to the groin region. Other reports have appeared in the literature describing similar apparatus (e.g., McKendry et al., 1972). This treatment seems to have first been suggested in 1830 by a pediatrician named Nye.

> Attach one pole of an electric battery to a moist sponge or a metallic plate fastened between the shoulders of the patient and the other to a dry sponge attached to the meatus urinarius. When this has been done and arranged so as not to annoy the patient, let him be put to bed and the circuit of the bed completed. The sound of the battery will soon lull the patient to sleep. While the sponge is dry, no electricity passes through the body of the patient, and his slumber is undisturbed, but the moment the patient begins to urinate, the sponge is moistened and becomes a conductor of electricity. The circuit is completed through the body of the patient and he or she is at once aroused, awakened and caught in the very act and thus caveat is entered by the will as well as by the electricity against further proceeding at least for this time. A repetition of a like experience a sufficient number of times, ought, I am inclined to think, to cure the patient, but since this suggestion has occurred to me I have not had the opportunity of putting it to the test of practical experiment and submit it to the consideration of the profession for what it is worth (refer to Glicklich, 1951, p. 870).

However, the available data do not indicate any significant improvement in success rate for this method (Yates, 1970) and the possibility of harm to the child either directly as a result of the shock or indirectly in terms of sexual disturbance or dysfunction later in life would appear to make it unwise to use this method.

One of the persistent problems in the use of the pad and bell technique has been the relatively high relapse rate. This generally ranges between 20 and 40% (Doleys, 1977). When relapse occurs, the general procedure is to apply the method again and to do so repeatedly if further relapses occur. However, the Finley apparatus mentioned above provides for use of intermittent reinforcement. On some of the trials the child is awakened, while on others an alarm is sounded in the parent's room 20 minutes after the wetting has occurred. This is to allow the parents to go to the child's room in order to have him change his clothes, clean up the bed, and reset the equipment. However, these trials represent nonreinforced trials. The intermittent reinforcement schedule has shown much more resistance to extinction, which reduces the relapse rate. In one study the relapse rate for this procedure was found to be only 12% (Finley et al., 1973). Overlearning has also been reported as an effective means of reducing relapse rates (Young and Morgan, 1972).

As indicated earlier, extensive reviews of the literature reveal a high degree of effectiveness for the pad and bell. Studies comparing the pad and bell with psychotherapy (e.g., Werry and Chorssen, 1965; DeLeon and Mandell, 1966) and with drugs (Turner, 1973; Wright and Craig, 1974) have indicated superior performance for the pad and bell. The apparatus has been found to be effective with children, adults (e.g., Seiger, 1952), institutionalized retarded patients (Turner, 1973), and geriatric patients in a nursing home (Collins and Plaska, 1975).

Some clinicians have been concerned about symptom substitution when enuresis is treated with conditioning procedures. However, as with other areas of behavioral treatment, extensive reviews have failed to confirm any significant amount of symptom substitution (Doleys, 1977). It appears to be a relatively rare case when anything occurs that might be called symptom substitution. When a second symptom does appear, many times the new symptom is less offensive and more easily dealt with than the original problem. There is, in addition, good evidence that the problem of enuresis can induce stress in the child and in the family, producing emotional disturbance by its very presence (Baller, 1975). Thus, the generation of symptoms by the problem of enuresis may be a far more important concern than the problem of symptom substitution following conditioning treatment. Sacks, DeLeon, and Blackman (1974) found that children who learn to be continent through conditioning procedures also show general improvement in functioning and personality following.

Two dangers that have been discussed in the use of conditioning equipment are: 1) the possibility of shock, which, as noted earlier, can be eliminated with carefully constructed equipment, and 2) superficial burns as a result of equipment malfunctioning. Burns are uncommon but have been reported in the literature when the child fails to be awakened by the stimuli and is in contact with the equipment while the current is still on (Greaves, 1969). The current passes through the skin and produces small superficial burns in a pattern corresponding to the openings in the foil pad. This may result if the batteries for the equipment are weak or if the child is an unusually sound sleeper. The burns can be treated with topical dermatological medications but may leave scars. However, if the equipment is functioning properly and the patients are instructed carefully, this danger can be avoided. The pad design described by Finley and Smith (1975) appears to greatly reduce the likelihood of burns (Neal and Coote, 1969), as does placing the pad under the bedsheet or inside a pillowcase. Additional safety precautions involving the design of the equipment are discussed by Meadow (1973). However, burns are quite rare and with reasonable caution most therapists will never encounter them in practice.

Combination of Procedures It should be pointed out that the methods reviewed so far have been used in combination and clinically often produce the best results when used in combination. For example, Azrin, Sneed, and Foxx (1974) have presented a training method, which they refer to as "dry-bed training." The method is quite complicated and involves sending a trainer-technician to the home for a night. The interested reader should refer to the original article for full details. Basically, the method begins with positive practice trials, forced fluids, and mild expressions of displeasure about wetting before the child goes to sleep. A pad and bell apparatus is used to signal wettings. In addition, the child is awakened every hour, goes to the bathroom, engages in a bladder-retention exercise, and is reinforced for retention, proper toileting, and a dry bed. Accidents during and following the first night of training result in reprimands, additional positive practice trials, and cleanliness training (child cleans self and bed). The program is phased out as the child develops control. Azrin et al. (1973) compared this method with a control group using the standard pad and bell procedure and found their method produced superior results. It is possible to use drugs in connection with any of the other treatments including the pad and bell. The drug effect of changing the sleep pattern sometimes enhances the conditioning process (Doleys, 1977). As might be expected from other studies of learning under drug-induced conditions, relapse rates have been found to be higher when drugs are combined with conditioning (Young and Turner, 1965). However, gradual withdrawal of the drug while continuing the conditioning process might reduce this problem. Helpful information on this phase of treatment is provided by Ciminero and Doleys (1976). Samaan (1972) reported successful use of waking the child at two- to three-hour intervals along with reinforcement with candy and praise for going in the toilet when awakened and having a dry bed in the morning. It is also possible to train bladder retention in connection with the pad and bell or to provide a reward for dry nights in connection with the pad and bell and so forth. Collins (1976) has proposed using reinforcement in a unique manner. Since one of the major problems with children who wet the bed is that they often do not awaken when the buzzer sounds, Collins recommends rewarding the child if he awakens and shuts off the alarm before the parents are aroused and arrive at the room. This added incentive often makes the procedure work better.

Clinical Application of the Pad and Bell Procedure

In recognition of the fact that the pad and bell procedure is the most effective treatment for nocturnal enuresis, the following instructions are given to facilitate use of this method by those who are not familiar with it.

The first step is to obtain a history from the parents and examine the child to determine whether or not use of the pad and bell is indicated. This method is generally not used for children under four, and the present author prefers to wait three or four years beyond this. If the child is severely emotionally disturbed, the more severe problem should be dealt with. The pad and bell may be used later. However, if only mild problems are present or the child is symptom-free, use of the pad may well contribute to better adjustment of the child. Care should be taken to rule out any organic pathology that may account for the problem. This can be done by proper medical examination and consultation. Baseline data on the frequency of wetting and size of the spots may be collected for a week or two before treatment, but frequently this is not feasible in routine clinical practice. If the history reveals that one or both parents were enuretic as children, the clinician will want to keep this in mind. Many times such parents are overly enthusiastic or excessively passive in pursuing the treatment program, depending on how their experience affected them.

The fact that the problem is basically one of learning to suppress the urination reflex and that this is sometimes difficult for children to learn should be explained to the parents and the child. Simple examples of reflexes, such as eye blink, can be used to get the point across. The parents should be reassured that the child is not being hostile or uncooperative when he wets. The child should be reassured that many people have this difficulty when they are young and that even adults can only control the urination reflex within certain limits. It should be explained to the child that the pad and bell will help him overcome the problem by helping him learn to control the reflex.

The equipment should be explained and demonstrated for the child. Most children find this very interesting and intriguing. They are generally cooperative, even eager to participate. However, should a child indicate that he does not want to participate, it is best not to attempt the treatment.

Assuming the child is willing, the equipment should be placed in the bed according to the instructions pertinent to the particular type of apparatus being used. Generally speaking it is wise to put the pad under a sheet or enclose it in a pillow case. This prevents direct contact between the child's body and the pad. The child should sleep in very light underclothing or no underclothing below the waist. If there is another child sleeping in the room, arrangements may be made for one or the other to temporarily sleep in a different room or on a rollaway bed in the living room. However, in many cases, the uninvolved child will sleep through the alarm undisturbed and no special arrangements will be needed.

There should be *no* restriction of fluids. Restricting fluids simply delays the process of conditioning. The parents and the child should be told that this is a *training* procedure and that it is expected that the alarm will go off several times in the first days or weeks of the treatment. Otherwise, many parents bring it back within a week and say that it rang almost every night and the child is still wetting the bed. Therefore, it must not be working.

Following a wetting, the pad should be cleaned with soapy water. It can be then placed in working order and put back in the bed. This should be the child's responsibility, but the parents may offer minimal, sympathetic help. The pad should also be cleaned from time to time with acetone or alcohol to remove any build-up of material on the pad that will interfere with proper functioning.

Because the child sleeps on the pad and frequently wets it, it will be necessary to check the connections from time to time to make sure they are intact and working. The batteries in battery-operated equipment need to be checked periodically to make sure they are charged. For pads that require absorbent paper, a large roll of paper picnic-table covering can be used.

A typical program might be to put the pad and bell in the bed, offer to reward the child if he wakes up in time to shut the alarm off before the parents arrive in the room, and to reward him for each day that his bed is still dry by morning.

The parents should be instructed to carry out the program in a very matter of fact manner without overpraising the child for success or showing disdain or displeasure for failures. A record may be kept each night of whether or not the child wet, how often, and the size of the spots. They should report to the therapist either in person or by letter or phone each week. At this time, further instructions and reassurance can be given. In this manner, the therapist will be able to follow the progress of the child.

The parents can be told that the first sign that the treatment is working will be that the spot will become smaller. Following this, there will be dry nights, and eventually dry nights will predominate.

Frequently children have trouble arousing themselves at night. When the alarm rings, they are to awaken and go to the bathroom to complete the urination process. Following this, they return to clean the equipment and reset it before they return to sleep. When the child has trouble awakening, the parents should be instructed to go into the room and either bounce him up and down gently or to wash his face with very cold water. If the signal is not loud enough, the alarm can be placed in or on a large metal pan, which will produce a louder sound. Brighter lights, including spotlights, can be employed. Medication producing a lighter sleep pattern may also be prescribed, if needed. Some conditioning can take place without the child awakening, but progress is usually more rapid if the child awakens.

Some children sabotage the program by shutting the equipment off or disconnecting it during the night. Generally discussing this with the child, moving the equipment out of reach, or taping the connection and switches in such a way that it is not easy to disengage them is sufficient. If not, the wisdom of continuing with the program should be considered.

Doleys (1977) as well as Werry and Chorssen (1965) has noted that careful and constant supervision of the parents and child in carrying out the program is a necessity for satisfactory results. Lax supervision is associated with poor results.

It should be explained to the parents and child that within two to three weeks some progress will generally be obvious and that, on the average, within six to eight weeks the child will probably be dry most every night. It is generally wise to continue with the treatment for a period of time after the child is dry. For example, following two weeks of consecutive dry nights, overlearning may be instituted by having the child drink an extra glass or two of fluids before bed. The child will often wet again at this point. Treatment continues until two weeks of consecutive dry nights are again achieved. If the child wets excessively and persistently with the additional fluids, they may be terminated and treatment continued again until two weeks of dryness are achieved. Some therapists recommend leaving the equipment in the bed, but disconnected, for an additional couple of weeks after that. The equipment is then withdrawn and the program complete.

The parents and child should be warned that relapses occur from time to time. If there should be a relapse, the program can be reinstituted. Additional relapses do occur sometimes but are not common.

Many parents and patients are skeptical about the effectiveness of the pad and bell device. Generally explaining some of the rationale to them and assuring them that it is effective in 80% to 90% of the cases are sufficient to obtain cooperation. While most children will be dry within two or three months with the above treatment, with more difficult cases it may be necessary to continue for several months or longer. It is also advisable to use combinations of treatment with the more difficult cases.

The most difficult part of the treatment generally is to keep the equipment in working order because it takes quite a bit of abuse from being slept on and urinated on repeatedly. Therefore, one should either be somewhat inclined toward working with electrical equipment or have someone available to them who is. The equipment, after some use, will require maintenance and repair to remain functional. Sometimes the equipment will fail to sound the alarm when a wetting has occurred. When this occurs: 1) be sure the parents and child understand how the equipment works and have it set up properly, 2) check to be sure that all connections, batteries, etc. are functional, 3) check to see if the child is turning it off, and 4) check to see if bedclothes or underclothing are too thick.

If the system sounds false alarms: 1) check for short circuits in the equipment, 2) be sure the paper separating the sheets of foil is thick enough and large enough to prevent contact, and 3) if perspiration is setting off the alarm, use thicker paper or lower the temperature in the room.

Additional practical instructions on the use of the pad and bell have been prepared by Dische (1973), Morgan (1974), and Taylor and Turner (1975).

ENCOPRESIS

Compared to the problem of enuresis, there are considerably fewer data and less is known regarding the problem of encopresis. As many authors have pointed out, researchers and clinicians seem to prefer to keep a respectful distance from the encopretic child. The term encopresis was first used in 1925 by Pototsky, and in 1926 Weissenberg suggested that it be used as a companion term to enuresis (Bellman, 1966). Encopresis is defined as involuntary fecal soiling by the child in his clothing beyond the age at which toilet training should have occurred, and in the absence of organic pathology. There are numerous organic conditions that result in fecal incontinence. Among these are such things as dietary factors, allergic reactions to food and other substances, infectious diseases of the large intestine, and anomalies of the intestinal tract and/or the nerve supply to the tract (Vaughan, McKay, and Nelson, 1975). Medical treatment for these conditions is required. Such organic factors should be explored thoroughly and ruled out before a diagnosis of encopresis is made. By definition, encopresis implies that the cause is psychogenic.

The digestive system is an enclosed tube running through the body with openings at the mouth and anus. As food is ingested through the opening of the mouth, the digestive process begins. This process continues in the stomach and small intestine. As the food is digested, needed nutrient is absorbed by the body. In the large intestine, additional absorption takes place and the waste material is formed into cakes or stools, which are excreted through the anus. The large intestine is situated in the shape of an incomplete square or rectangle in the midsection of the body (see Figure 2). The first structure of the large intestine is the cecum, which is attached to the small intestine and forms

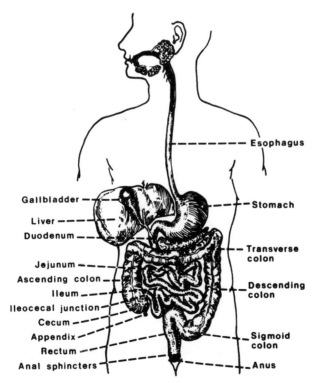

Figure 2.   Diagram of digestive system (liver and gallbladder have been turned upward and to the right for easier viewing of intestine).

a blind pouch slightly below the area where the two join. The ascending colon passes upward in the abdominal cavity to about the level of the liver, where it makes a right turn and crosses the cavity. The crossing portion is called the transverse colon. The transverse colon then makes a right turn and becomes the descending colon, which connects to the sigmoid colon, which is a short curved portion of the large intestine that attaches to the rectum. The rectum ends in the anus, which is composed of internal and external sphincter muscles.

Normally the fecal material is moved through the tract by a combination of peristalsis and mass movements. The rectum generally does not contain feces. However, as fecal material moves through the tract or is voluntarily forced through the tract by contraction of the thoraxic and abdominal muscles, a small amount of fecal material enters the rectum. The stimulation of the walls of the rectum, as well as the pressure from the material forced into this area, results in increased activity in the intestinal tract and relaxation of the internal and external sphincters. This expels the feces from the body. The process is enhanced by contraction of the thoraxic and abdominal muscles, the descent of the diaphragm, and efforts to further relax the sphincters. Defecation may be initiated by relaxing the sphincters and contracting these muscle groups, or it can be avoided by voluntary contraction of the external sphincter, which is under voluntary control.

Types of Encopresis

Various distinctions have been made in regard to different types of encopresis. For example, encopresis has been described as primary or secondary. In the case of primary encopresis the child has never achieved bowel control, whereas in secondary encopresis the child was trained at one time but has now begun to soil. The terms continuous and discontinuous are sometimes used as equivalent to primary and secondary. In addition, some children chronically and regularly soil while others soil only occasionally. Thus, distinctions are frequently made in terms of chronicity or frequency. Most soiling accidents take place during the day; however, nocturnal soiling has been reported. There are cases in which a child soils both day and night or one or the other—nocturnal soiling alone is rare but has been reported (Vaughan and Cashmore, 1954). Some children soil at relatively predictable times during the day. Others soil seemingly at random intervals. Still others appear to soil or not depending on social circumstances. For example, some children soil only at school while others never soil at school. Encopresis is sometimes described as retentive or nonretentive. In retentive encopresis there is evidence of constipation and/or obstipation. In nonretentive there are no signs of constipation present. Other authors have suggested combinations of these categories. For example, Easson (1960) has proposed four categories:

1. Primary infantile encopresis (never toilet trained and not constipated)
2. Primary reactive encopresis (never toilet trained, constipated)
3. Secondary infantile encopresis (toilet trained but now soiling with absence of constipation)
4. Secondary reactive encopresis (toilet trained, now soiling with presence of constipation)

None of the above categories has reached the status of commonly accepted and adopted nomenclature within the field. Different authors use different distinctions and different definitions for the distinctions that they employ. Most of the larger scale studies lump all cases together without distinction. This, of course, adds to confusion in the area and makes data difficult to compare from one study to another.

Examination of the literature suggests three broad categories, which are reflected in the writings and which may serve some purpose in facilitating discussion.

One category might be termed *manipulative soiling*. Numerous authors (e.g., Hilburn, 1968; Hoag et al., 1971; Lifshitz and Chovers, 1972) suggest that some children either consciously or unconsciously soil in a pattern that results in successful manipulation of their environment, such as avoiding school attendance, expressing hostility toward the mother, etc. However, careful study of encopretic children suggests that, as was the case with enuresis, relatively few cases actually follow this pattern even though it is a commonly held theory (Yates, 1970; Wright, 1973).

A second category may be made up of children who expel feces in a diarrheaic fashion. This has sometimes been referred to as *chronic diarrhea* or *irritable bowel syndrome* (Davidson, 1973). Basically, the child seems to react to stress and emotional upset with periods of incontinence. These periods tend to follow stressful life events, and the symptoms subside between events. If they do not subside, the situation can become life threatening as a result of dehydration and upset of the electrolyte balance.

The third category has to do with the child who develops *chronic constipation*, resulting in impaction and psychogenic megacolon (Ravitch, 1958). By far, the majority of cases fits into this category. It has been estimated that from 80 to 95% of the cases of encopresis are a result of constipation (Fitzgerald, 1975; Levine, 1975). While it may seem paradoxical that children who present with the problem of fecal soiling are really constipated, consideration of the basic process involved makes the reason for this clear. The problem generally begins with the child becoming constipated. The initial constipation may be a result of a number of factors. There is some thought that certain children may have an inherited tendency to become constipated more easily than others. The child may have been exposed to an unfortunate dietary choice that resulted in constipation. Painful bowel movements sometimes cause children to begin to retain feces. Also, there may be emotional factors, such as depression, that result in the initial constipation. But, for whatever reason, once the constipation starts, it is possible for this to become chronic and result in impaction. When material becomes firmly impacted in the intestine, the normal peristaltic and mass movements are not adequate to fully evacuate the bowel. As a result, material continues to build up and impact to the point where the intestine becomes stretched, loses its muscle tone, and the walls become relatively thin. This further inhibits the normal activity and motion of the bowel, resulting eventually in severe impaction and megacolon (a greatly enlarged colon). If this condition prevails, fluid material from the stomach and small intestine reaches the large intestine, but there is no area for the fluid to be absorbed, producing cakes and no room for the fecal material to be retained. As a result, it seeps out around the impacted material and stains the clothing. This soiling is usually a pasty and watery fecal material. The child frequently states that he was not aware of the need to defecate at the time the soiling occurred. This is usually regarded with great skepticism by the parents, but is entirely accurate. Because the material was simply seeping around the impacted mass, there was little sensation. In addition, the impaction and obstipation result in a lack of awareness of the need to defecate, which is present with the normal functioning colon. On occasion, when large amounts of the impacted material loosen, the child may have large bowel movements in his clothing or in the toilet. The parents are frequently amazed at the size of these movements, both in terms of the amount of the material and the diameter of the stools. There are reports of stools sufficiently large that they had to be broken into smaller pieces in order for the plumbing to accommodate them. There have also been reports of sufficiently severe impaction that manual removal of the material under general anesthesia was required (Nixon, 1961).

Chronic megacolon obviously poses numerous health hazards in terms of the general body functioning as well as specific damage to the intestinal tract. Thus, this is a condition that requires aggressive treatment. The age at which treatment should begin is not nearly as much of an issue with encopresis as it is with enuresis. This is because the majority of the cases are caused by constipation or diarrhea, which invites treatment. Of course, in some cases involving younger children, examination will reveal an absence of these factors. Advice on toilet training may be all that is needed in such instances.

Correlates of Encopresis

Before discussing treatment of these disorders, it might be well to look at the various correlates of encopresis. As indicated earlier, most studies do not classify the cases in any systematic way. Therefore, the various types are generally mixed together in the same study. Because most cases of encopresis appear to be accounted for on the basis of chronic constipation and megacolon, the data may be regarded as primarily relating to this disorder. However, because of the lack of specificity in definition, all of the data must be regarded with a degree of skepticism.

Most estimates of the incidence of encopresis suggest that about 3% of children will have this difficulty (e.g., Levine, 1975). However, because of the classification and definitional problems, no accurate incidence figures are really available. Reported rates have ranged from 1.5% (Bellman, 1966) to 5.7% (Olatawura, 1973). In addition, many researchers and clinicians feel that this is a very underreported disorder. The psychologist who inquires routinely regarding encopresis of his patients is generally amazed at the number of unreported cases that are uncovered in this manner. Males generally predominate by about five or six to one over females in the reports in the literature (Levine, 1975).

There is some speculation that certain children may have a genetic or constitutional predisposition to become constipated more readily than others and thus to be more susceptible to encopresis (Bell and Levine, 1954). While this is quite plausible, there are no real data to support this nor has any specific mechanism by which this might occur been established. Wolters and Wauters (1975) have studied, by means of a checklist, somatopsychic characteristics of 25 encopretic children and a control group of 25 nonencopretic children. Included in the checklist were numerous factors relating to the circumstances of the pregnancy, delivery, early development, general health, appetite, frequency of abdominal pain, gas, etc. They found no evidence of any constitutional predisposition to encopresis.

Some studies have suggested that there is considerably more turmoil and disturbance in the families of encopretics (Anthony, 1957; Bemporad, 1971; Hoag et al., 1971). The children and parents are described as having a variety of emotional problems ranging from minor to severe (Lehman, 1944; Shane, 1967; Collier, 1974). Mothers of encopretic children have been described as rigid, masochistic, lacking in warmth and love, overly concerned with cleanliness, and dominating and nagging. Fathers have been described as being weak, ineffectual, and uninvolved. The child is described as being shy, withdrawn, overly conforming, anxious, stubborn, compulsive, overly neat, and depressed (e.g., Shirley, 1938; Richmond, Eddy, and Garrard, 1954; Pinkerton, 1958; Hoag et al., 1971). Psychoanalytic formulations have focused on either the anal-erotic-pleasurable aspects of retaining the feces or the hostile, aggressive feelings supposedly being expressed toward the mother (Lehman, 1944; Shane, 1967; Lifshitz and Chovers, 1972). Fenichel (1945) sees fecal incontinence as a substitute for masturbation. However, there are not sufficient data to establish the actual incidence of emotional or family disturbance as related to encopresis. Nor have the personality charac-teristics mentioned above been convincingly shown to be significantly more prominent in encopretic than nonencopretic children. While encopresis and emotional disturbance do occur together on occasion and *appear* to be causally related, most encopretic children are not emo-tionally disturbed and the families appear to be stable. In addition, it is not clear how many unreported cases may exist in the general popula-tion, resulting in a biased sample when data are collected in clinics. There is the further problem that the presence of the symptom itself may cause upset and disruption in the child and family rather than resulting from it. Thus, no general conclusion may be drawn in this area.

In a similar vein, some authors (e.g., Olatawura, 1973) have sug-gested that encopresis occurs more commonly among lower socioeco-nomic level children. There may be a tendency in this direction; however, this also could easily be attributed to other factors, particularly biases in samples available for research or in willingness of parents to admit the symptom.

Some authors (e.g., Hushka, 1942) also suggest that early and/or coercive toilet training may result in encopresis at a later date. Anthony (1957), in commenting on the interactive relationship and power struggle between mother and child during toilet training, coined the term "the potting couple." However, the data in this area are confusing, and no connection between the two has been firmly established.

Immaturity, developmental delay, and similar type explanations for soiling have been mentioned (e.g., Bellman, 1966; Olatawura, 1973) but are not regarded by most authors as playing a significant role in the majority of cases because basic bowel control is generally achieved at a young age with relative ease by most children.

With the exception of severely retarded children or moderately retarded children who have not been subjected to adequate toilet train-ing, there does not seem to be a relationship between intellectual ability and encopresis. While an occasional study has reported low IQs for encopretics, more carefully controlled studies show no differences (Bellman, 1966; Wolters, 1974).

In a careful study of 102 cases of encopresis, Levine (1975) reported that various symptoms appeared to accompany encopresis. Among the more commonly reported symptoms for the children in this study were chronic abdominal pain, poor appetite, and lethargy. Thirty-two out of the 102 encopretic children were also enuretic. Other studies have reported similar ratios. In this study, 27 mothers of secondary encopretics noted that a stressful event seemed to occur just before the soiling. Among these events were loss of a parent, traumatic entry into school, and birth of a younger sibling. Other clinicians and researchers have also commented on the precipitating role of stressful or upsetting events. Levine did not find evidence of encopretic children being compulsively neat, having a tendency to amass large collections or to hoard objects, or having any other distinctive personality characteristics.

Finally, Garrard and Richmond (1952) have reported that encopretic children often refuse to defecate in the toilet (however, they do use it for urination) and frequently defecate in a standing or supine position rather than a sitting position.

Treatment

As was the case with enuresis, numerous relatively barbaric treatments have been applied to the encopretic child over the years. For example, Eduard Henoch, a physician in Berlin in 1881, is one of the earliest writers to describe the diagnosis and treatment of this condition. Henoch began with injections of ergotamine in the anal region. Finding this successful, he speculated that the cause was psychogenic and in future treatment used injections of distilled water. This appeared to work also. He then prescribed such things as a couple of strong blows with the hand in the "perineal tract." He also reported that he found it useful to threaten to mistreat the patient with a branding iron and electricity (Bellman, 1966).

Since the three broad categories of encopresis noted earlier in this section suggest different etiologies, different treatments seem advisable.

In the occasional case where a child is using soiling in a manipulative way, the most successful treatment would appear to be family counseling in which the child is taught to express himself in more effective ways and the family is given assistance in learning how to respond more appropriately to the child. This may be coupled with efforts to eliminate sources of reinforcement for the soiling and to reinforce not soiling. The basic principles involved in this type of treatment are no different from normal family counseling and behavioral treatment. Therefore, they are not discussed at length here.

Should the soiling be a result of diarrhea caused by tension and anxiety, the most effective treatment is to reduce sources of stress and anxiety by means of environmental manipulation, supportive psychotherapy, and in some cases appropriate medication. Antidiarrheal medications and diets may be prescribed by a physician. Long-term success seems to depend on helping the person learn more effective ways of coping with problems. Cohen and Reed (1968) as well as Hedberg (1973) have reported the successful treatment of chronic diarrhea patients by means of systematic desensitization. Byrne (1973) presented two case histories in which hypnosis and direct suggestion were used with irritable bowel syndrome. The patients, a 23-old female and a 43-old female, had been having numerous episodes of diarrhea brought on by stress. Under hypnosis, they were given the suggestion that they could control the nervous system, calm down the bowel, retard peristaltic motion, and that their bowel habits would return to normal. They were also taught self-hypnosis and were told to give themselves similar suggestions under auto-hypnosis. In both cases, the diarrhea was brought under control. Relaxation training (Bernstein and Borkovec, 1973; Walker et al., in press) and assertive training (Alberti and Emmons, 1974; Walker et al., in press) may also be effective with this type of disturbance. The basic treatment strategy is to reduce stress and increase ability to cope effectively with life problems.

The third category described above is that in which constipation is present. Frequently it is accompanied by megacolon. As with all of the disorders discussed here, it is essential to rule out organic causes for the condition before psychologically based treatment is begun. Organic causes for constipation may include diet, obstructions of the intestinal tract, and neurological disorders, notably Hirschprung's disease (Silber, 1969; Nixon, 1975). Hirschprung's disease is a condition in which a section of the colon is innervated insufficiently with nerve fibers to produce normal peristaltic motion. As a result, fecal material proceeds to this spot and then stalls, forming an impacted mass. As the impaction increases, megacolon results. Treatment for this disorder is surgical removal of the deficient tissue and reconnection of the two ends to form a properly functioning tract. Table 1 presents the distinguishing features for differentiating between aganglionic megacolon (Hirschprung's disease) and functional or psychogenic megacolon caused by chronic constipation (Vaughan, McKay, and Nelson, 1975). However, it should be pointed out that most cases that come to the attention of a psychologist are of the functional type. Hirschprung's disease is generally diagnosed much earlier, usually relatively soon after birth. This and other possible organic causes, however, must be ruled out.

In the absence of organic pathology, the standard medical treatment for encopresis caused by constipation consists of oral administration of one or two teaspoons of mineral oil twice a day for a period of three to nine months. This is often preceded by a series of enemas or laxatives to initially reduce the impaction. The mineral oil must be administered at a suitable interval (one to two hours) after meals or in connection with

Table 1.   Differentiating features of aganglionic megacolon and the common pattern of functional constipation

	Aganglionic megacolon	Functional constipation
Onset	Birth or neonatal period Symptoms of intestinal obstruction	About 60% in first year of life; most of remainder from 1 to 4 years
Course	Failure to pass formed bowel movements except by enema	Huge bowel movements at long intervals
Withholding efforts	Not present	Present
Soiling	None	At least two-thirds of cases
Growth	Impaired	Usually normal
Abdominal findings	Distended; large fecal mass remains in same site	Variable distention and masses
Rectal examination	Rectum not dilated and usually empty of stool	Cavernous rectum, often filled with soft feces
Roentgenographic findings	Colon dilated proximal to an area of normal caliber; postevacuation film shows poor evacuation of barium	Colon dilated to anus; postevacuation film shows effective evacuation
Rectal biopsy	Absence of ganglion cells, large nerve bundles	Normal

From Vaughan, McKay, and Nelson, 1975, p. 781; reprinted by permission.

multiple vitamin tablets because the mineral oil has a tendency to retard absorption of some vitamins. The mineral oil serves as a gentle laxative and produces a degree of regularity of evacuation while in use. Once regularity has been established, the mineral oil may be decreased gradually and withdrawn. In many cases the established habit of regularity will continue following withdrawal of the treatment (Vaughan, McKay, and Nelson, 1975; Nisley, 1976).

Numerous reports in the literature indicate successful treatment of encopresis by means of operant techniques involving reinforcement and punishment. However, the majority of these are reports of single cases and were relatively specific to the particulars of the case involved (e.g. Young and Goldsmith, 1972; Houle, 1974; Ayllon, Simon, and Wildman, 1975; Bach and Moylan, 1975). Some of the programs were based exclusively on positive reinforcement (e.g., Neale, 1963), while others used positive and negative consequences (Edelman, 1971). Conger (1970) reported successful treatment of a nine-year-old boy by manipulation of social consequences (attention and physical contact from mother). Doleys and Arnold (1975) used an overcorrection technique, "Full Cleanliness Training." Full cleanliness training originated with Foxx and

Azrin (1973) and involves three steps: 1) parents express displeasure about soiling, 2) child is required to scrub soiled clothes for 15 minutes, and 3) child must clean and bathe himself. Doleys and Arnold also had to deal with toilet phobia in this case. Toilet phobia is not present in most cases but is observed in some, and minor fears and resistances to the toilet are common. The toilet phobia was eliminated in one day of intensive training involving a type of in vivo desensitization, modeling, and reinforcement for successive approximations. Doleys et al. (1977), in a case study, reported an elaboration of this method that involves full cleanliness training, regular pant checks, and toileting, along with reinforcement for appropriate toileting behavior. This method was successful with the three children reported on in the case study. Nilsson (1976) has treated several cases successfully with a type of token economy, and Giles and Wolf (1966), as well as others, have treated institutionalized retardates with similar methods.

Some success has been reported in using biofeedback in the treatment of encopresis. For example, Engel, Nikoomanesh, and Schuster (1974; see also Schuster, 1974) reported on the use of operant conditioning and biofeedback in the treatment of six patients (five adults and one child) who had severe fecal incontinence as a result of external sphincter impairment caused by organic disorders. Using biofeedback, the subjects were taught to bring the internal and external sphincters under control, making it possible for them to retain feces and become continent.

Young (1973) has reported successful treatment of children with retentive type encopresis by means of a method that he refers to as gastroileal reflex training. Basically, the method involves evacuating the impacted material by means of enemas, giving the child a prescribed dose of Senokot before going to bed (this is to relieve colonic inertia and assist in the ready initiation of the gastroileal reflex), and placing the child on the toilet 20 to 30 minutes after meals, which is the time at which the gastroilealic and the gastrocolic reflexes generally occur. These reflexes occur shortly after the ingestion of food or fluid and serve to increase motility in the intestine, eventually resulting in defecation. The child was reinforced with signs of approval if he defecated. Of 24 children treated by this method, 19 were treated successfully in less than one year, with a mean of approximately five months. Three were treated successfully in more than one year, with a mean of 17 months, and two children did not respond. During a follow-up period ranging from six months to six years, the symptom recurred in four of the children.

Although systematic studies of large numbers of children are not available, some case reports (Baer, 1961; Goldsmith, 1962; Olness, 1976) have appeared involving the use of hypnosis in the treatment of retentive encopresis in children. The general procedure is to hypnotize the child and give him suggestions that he can control his bowel movements by having them regularly on the toilet and that he will be able to retain fecal material in between times. Allusions are sometimes made to intestinal reflexes to enhance the suggestive process. The supposed reasons for the soiling are sometimes explored under hypnosis as an additional part of the treatment. The child may also be encouraged along the lines of feeling that he is the boss and responsible for his own behavior. In some cases the child is taught self-hypnosis and is instructed to hypnotize himself while on the toilet (e.g., Olness, 1976). This approach has been found successful with children as young as three-and-a-half years of age.

Wright (1973, 1975) has reported a relatively substantial study of encopresis employing a treatment program that combines cathartics and contingency management techniques. This method has been used for several years in the Pediatric Psychology Service at the University of Oklahoma Medical School. To date, over 200 children have been treated with virtually 100% success (Wright, 1977, personal communication). There are approximately 10–15% of the families that do not cooperate in carrying out the program as prescribed, and there have been one or two cases in which it appeared that the program was carried out appropriately but failed. Approximately 15–25% relapses have been noted. However, they respond favorably to reinauguration of the program. Because this program appears to be one of the most successful reported, relevant clinical procedures are presented in the next section.

Clinical Application of the Wright Method

The basic method employed by Wright is described by Wright and Walker (1977) and involves the following steps:

1. A careful physical and any necessary tests are accomplished to rule out the possibility of an organic etiology to the problem.
2. Interview with parents and the child and in some cases psychological testing are completed to rule out the possibility of serious psychopathology or emotional disturbance. If the child is seriously disturbed, the more serious psychological disturbance is treated and the treatment of encopresis is delayed until some improvement in the more serious problem is realized. However, if the child appears to be symptom free or has only moderate personal problems, the encopresis is treated. Generally, improvement is seen in the general functioning and emotional stability of the child as a side benefit to treatment of encopresis.
3. The parents are instructed in the details of the program. They are the ones who explain it to the child. The child is given a brief explanation and is reassured that the program will help him overcome his problem. In the interview with the parents, the role that constipation

plays in the disorder as well as the fact that the child is unable to control his bowel and is not aware of the soiling is explained to alleviate concerns of the parents that the child is either severely disturbed or attempting to be hostile by soiling. It is further explained to the parents that in order to eliminate the soiling problem it is necessary to regularly evacuate the bowel over a sufficient length of time that the tissue has a chance to regain its normal shape and tone and begin to function normally. It is explained that it is also important to teach the child good toilet habits and to motivate him to begin to take full responsibility for appropriate toilet behavior. It is stressed that a) if the colon can be evacuated regularly over a sufficient period of time for it to begin to function normally, and b) if the child can be trained to take responsibility for his own toileting, these two in conjunction will result in resolution of the problem. If the colon is simply evacuated and good toileting habits are not taught, impaction will gradually develop again and the soiling will return. If good toilet habits are simply emphasized without proper evacuation, the child will be under pressure to perform physically in a way that is not possible because of the impaction and megacolon.

4. The treatment program consists of the following components:

   a. To begin the program, the child's colon is thoroughly evacuated. This is done with an enema or two the night before the program starts.

   b. The parents are instructed to follow a program of having the child go to the bathroom immediately upon awakening in the morning. Other times of the day can be substituted if the morning is impractical. However, this is a good time physiologically and in terms of the life-style of most people. Therefore, the morning is usually used. The parents supervise this attempt. If the child produces a reasonable amount of feces at this point (about ¼ to ½ cup), he is praised, given a small reward, and the day proceeds with breakfast and preparing for school, etc. The reward is used to reinforce the child for trying as hard as he can and is agreed upon in advance. Choice of rewards is discussed in Section 4e below.

   c. If the child does not produce a reasonable amount of feces on his own, the parent inserts a glycerin suppository and permits the child to dress, have breakfast, and prepare to leave for school. By the time the child is finished with breakfast, the suppository will usually have its effect and the child can be taken back to the bathroom where he makes another attempt to defecate. If he is successful this time, he receives a reward. This reward should be smaller than the one for defecating entirely on his own.

d. If shortly before time to leave for school arrives and no defecation has taken place, the parent gives the child an enema to produce defecation. It is important that the enema chosen be one that is safe for repeated administration and that side effects be watched and controlled should they occur. Children's Fleet enemas are very acceptable, but others can be employed. Enemas can be used safely every day for one to two weeks. After this, it is best to decrease them to every other day or even every third day if prolonged use is required. Seldom are enemas given with sufficient frequency to constitute a hazard. However, caution is required in cases in which they are necessary with any degree of frequency. No reward is given if an enema is needed to produce defecation. Essentially, defecation must occur every morning, or at the appointed time each day, during the program. While it is true that it is not necessary for a person to defecate every day, as a training technique during the program it must be ensured that the child defecates regularly and daily. This also ensures that the child's colon will regain its normal shape and tone. Following the morning training period and defecation, the child leaves for school. Sometimes a child has trouble getting started on regular evacuation on his own, requiring frequent enemas, or gets to the stage where suppositories are all that is needed, but they seem to be needed with considerable frequency. In such cases, dietary manipulation involving the addition of roughage (especially bran cereals, bran muffins, etc.), vegetables, fruit juices, etc., and decreasing dairy products (cheese, milk, ice cream) has proved helpful. Nisley (1976) has outlined additional dietary considerations for children with fecal impaction. Stool softeners, available without prescription, may also be needed on occasion.

e. At the end of the day, the child's clothing is examined. This is done at a specified time, e.g., after school or after supper, shortly before bedtime, or some other suitable time. If there is no soiling, he receives a reward. If there is soiling, he receives mild punishment. Proper use of rewards and punishments is *crucial* to the success of the program. The program requires three possible rewards (two for defecating and one for not soiling) and one punishment (for soiling). It often takes careful and astute questioning of the parents and child to determine suitable rewards and punishments. The old adage that one man's meat is another man's poison must be kept in mind during this process. Things that are very rewarding to one child are considered of no consequence by another or may actually even be punishment for another. Likewise, things that are punishing to one child may actually be rewarding to another child. Therefore, careful interviewing is required. It is also of great importance that the reinforcement be one that is very compelling, and that the punishment be one the child definitely wants to avoid. A gold star on a chart or something of that sort will generally not be sufficient. It must be something that the child wants and is willing to work fairly hard to get. Likewise, the punishment should be something that the child really wants to avoid, although it should not be excessively severe. Among the rewards that are most successful in this program are such things as money, candy, small toys, praise, extra privileges, tickets to recreation events, etc. One of the most effective rewards and one that is quite general in that it works with most children is allotting them a certain period of time, say 20 or 30 minutes at the end of the day, in which their parents will do anything they ask. They may want to play checkers or piggy-back ride, talk with the parents, have the parents read a book to them, or something of the sort. This type of reward is usually a very effective reward and one that obviously has beneficial side effects in promoting interaction and pleasant association between the parent and child.

As indicated, choice of the punisher should also be made carefully. Some of the punishments that have been found effective are restriction of television viewing, loss of privileges, being grounded, monetary fines, and having to do extra chores (especially chores of siblings). Thus, if the child does not soil during the day he may be allotted 20 or 30 minutes of parental time. On the other hand, if he does soil, he may have some privilege restricted for a day. The rewards and punishments, once selected, are delivered daily as indicated in the preceding steps of the program. Rewards are given in the morning for defecation (unless an enema is used), and a reward or punishment is given in the evening, depending on whether or not soiling has occurred. For example, a typical program might involve a small gift-wrapped toy (selected from a grab bag of other gift packages) if the child defecates on his own in the morning, a piece of gum or candy if a suppository is required, and thirty minutes of parental time (the child's name is often used to label this, e.g., "Billy Time") if no soiling occurs during that day. If soiling occurs, the child cannot watch TV for one hour after dinner.

f.   The above regime is continued on a daily basis without interruption. Because many parents are fairly discouraged about the chances of ever finding anything that will help with the problem, it is a good idea to let them know that you understand how they feel. Then, present the program to them in a very positive manner and explain that it virtually never fails, if carried out properly. It is also important to stress to the parents that they must be 100% consistent in this program and that it must be done whether or not they feel well, whether or not they are visiting friends, or regardless of any other activity that may be going on in the household. This is important because people frequently think of numerous reasons to depart from the program, and obviously the program will not work if it is not being employed. The parents are instructed to keep daily notes of exactly what was done and the result. These notes are mailed to the office at the end of each week.

   In addition, a phone call contact is made with the family each week. The phone call is generally timed to come a day or so after the written report has been received. On the phone it is possible to give additional support, encouragement, or advice and to deal with problems that may come up during the program.

   Basically, the main problem that occurs is that the parents for one reason or another begin to become lax in following the program. It is important to keep track of what they are doing on a day-by-day basis from their written report and the phone calls in order to encourage them to be consistent in following the program. If they have concerns or difficulties, these can be discussed and they can be reassured about them.

   Often parents fail to send in the written reports or fail to make the phone calls. If the therapist wants the program to be successful, he will have to depart from the standard procedure and place a phone call to the patient. Careful follow-up has been found to be essential. When the follow-up is exact and compulsively carried out, the program works. When the follow-up is lax, parents generally interpret this as permission to be lax in carrying out their part of the program with the child. In the end, the program is not carried out properly and does not work.

g.   After two consecutive weeks in which no soiling has taken place, the process of phasing out the program is begun. To do this, one day during the week is selected on which the cathartics will not be employed. The remainder of the program continues as usual. If no soiling occurs for one week following discontinuation of the cathartics for the day selected, an additional day off the cathartics is added for the following week. The days should generally be selected to be some distance apart, such as beginning with a Thursday and then adding a Monday, etc. Days can then be added to the program each week in which no soiling occurs by inserting days equidistant from the days already off the program. This is continued until the child is completely free of soiling and completely off cathartics. At this point the reward and punishment program is terminated. While this may seem abrupt, the habit is generally well established by this time and being free of soiling is sufficiently rewarding to maintain it.

If soiling occurs at any time during the phase-out period, the procedure used is to retreat one step and start over again. That is, if the child has worked his way up to three days off the program and soils, he then moves back to two days off the program and five days on. If another soiling occurs, he backs up to one day off the program and six days on, etc. Often, soiling persists during this period, with the child working up to four or five days off the program, then falling back to two or three, back up to four or five, etc. When this occurs, it frequently helps to give an enema the morning after each soiling. This program generally alleviates the encopretic problem in approximately 15 to 20 weeks. One benefit that seems to occur with most of the children in such a program is that they spontaneously begin to show improvement in other areas of their lives. That is, they begin to be happier, feel more self-confident, respond to discipline better, work better in school, and in various other ways show progress toward maturity.

Wright (1975) has reported a study of 14 patients using the above program. Twelve were male and two female, ranging in age from three to nine. Three of the 14 subjects had never achieved bowel control. Three began soiling after bowel training had been accomplished but also following a critical family incident such as divorce, a death, or the birth of a new sibling. The eight remaining subjects began soiling after bowel training had been achieved, but no critical incident could be identified. Results indicated that the average length of time to completion of the program for all 14 subjects was 16.93 weeks, with a range of from 10 to 38 weeks. Although one subject required 38 weeks to completely stop soiling, only four of the subjects were still soiling after the 14th week of treatment. The mean number of soils per week at the beginning of treatment was 17.14. Within the first week of treatment, the mean number of soils per week dropped to 2.16. All subjects were free of soiling at the end of the treatment program. Only one subject regressed to a pattern of soiling during the six months' follow-up period. This subject was placed on the program again and ceased soiling as a result of the follow-up treatment.

SUMMARY AND CONCLUSION

In concluding this chapter it seems fitting to note that there is a great deal of misinformation in the literature on the three topics discussed. Some of the confusion has resulted from authors expressing clinical impressions and personal biases as fact. Inadequately controlled research and abundant case studies add to the problem. It is indeed fortunate that most humans accomplish the tasks involved themselves with a minimal amount of help or interference from outsiders.

Toilet training is a matter of considerable concern to parents. However, relatively little real data are available, and there is much disagreement among the "experts." Training through the first four or five years of life should be gentle, employing patience and encouragement. Most children will learn quite readily when they are developmentally ready. For children who need extra help, the procedures outlined by Azrin and Foxx in their book *Toilet Training in Less Than a Day* are found to be helpful. However, most mothers appear to need professional guidance in addition to the book.

Organic and emotional problems are often thought to be causes of enuresis. However, the majority of cases are primarily instances in which the child has failed to learn to control and suppress the urination reflex. Behavioral methods, especially using the pad and bell apparatus, have been found to be the most efficient and effective treatment.

Encopresis may be caused by organic or emotional factors. However, the vast majority of the cases are caused by chronic constipation resulting in megacolon and overflow incontinence. Behavioral methods, particularly a procedure employing cathartics and reinforcement developed by Logan Wright at the University of Oklahoma Health Sciences Center, have been found to be highly effective.

REFERENCES

Alberti, R. E., and Emmons, M. L. 1974. Your Perfect Right. 2nd Ed. Impact, San Luis Obispo, Cal.

Anthony, E. J. 1957. An experimental approach to the psychopathology of childhood encopresis. Br. J. Med. Psychol. 30:146–175.

Atthowe, J. M. 1972. Controlling nocturnal enuresis in severely disabled and chronic patients. Behav. Ther. 3:232–239.

Ayllon, T., Simon, S. J., and Wildman, R. W. 1975. Instructions and reinforcement in the elimination of encopresis: A case study. J. Behav. Ther. Exp. Psychiatry 6:235–238.

Azrin, N. H., and Foxx, R. M. 1971. A rapid method of toilet training the institutionalized retarded. J. Appl. Behav. Anal. 4:89–99.

Azrin, N. H., and Foxx, R. M. 1976. Toilet Training in Less Than a Day. Pocket Books, New York.

Azrin, N. H., Sneed, T. J., and Foxx, R. M. 1973. Dry bed: A rapid method of eliminating bedwetting (enuresis) of the retarded. Behav. Res. Ther. 11:427–434.

Azrin, N. H., Sneed, T. J., and Foxx, R. M. 1974. Dry-bed training: Rapid elimination of childhood enuresis. Behav. Res. Ther. 12:147–156.

Bach, R., and Moylan, J. J. 1975. Parents administer behavior therapy for inappropriate urination and encopresis: A case study. J. Behav. Ther. Exp. Psychiatry 6:239–241.

Baer, R. F. 1961. Hypnosis applied to bowel and bladder control in multiple sclerosis, syringomyelia, and traumatic transverse myelitis. Am. J. Clin. Hypnosis 4:22–23.

Bakwin, H. 1973. The genetics of enuresis. In I. Kolvin, R. C. MacKeith, and S. R. Meadow (eds.), Bladder Control and Enuresis, pp. 73–77. J. B. Lippincott Co., Philadelphia.

Bakwin, H., and Bakwin, R. M. 1972. Behavior Disorders in Children. W. B. Saunders Co., Philadelphia.

Baller, W. R. 1975. Bed-wetting: Origins and Treatment. Pergamon, New York.

Bell, A. I., and Levine, M. I. 1954. Causes and treatment of chronic constipation. Pediatrics 14:259–266.

Bellman, M. 1966. Studies on encopresis. Acta Paediatr. Scand. (Suppl.) 170:1–137.

Bemporad, J. R., Pfeifer, C. M., Gibbs, L., Cortner, R. H., and Bloom, W. 1971. Characteristics of encopretic patients and their families. J. Am. Acad. Child Psychiatry 10:272–292.

Bernstein, D. A., and Borkovec, T. D. 1973. Progressive relaxation training. A manual for the helping professions. Research Press, Champaign, Ill.

Bjornsson, S. 1973. Enuresis in childhood. Scand. J. Educ. Res. 17:63–82.

Blackwell, B., and Currah, J. 1973. The psychopharmacology of nocturnal enuresis. In I. Kolvin, R. C. MacKeith, and S. R. Meadow (eds.), Bladder Control and Enuresis. J. B. Lippincott Co., Philadelphia.

Bostock, J. 1958. Exterior gestation, primitive sleep, enuresis and asthma: A study in aetiology. Med. J. Aust. ii:149, 185.

Boyd, M. M. 1960. The depth of sleep in enuretic school children and in non-enuretic controls. J. Psychosom. Res. 4:274–281.

Bransby, E. R., Blomfield, J. M., and Douglas, J. W. B. 1955. The prevalence of bed-wetting. Med. Officer 94:5–7.

Brazelton, T. B. 1969. Infants and Mothers: Differences in Development. Dell Publishing Co., New York.

Butler, J. F. 1976. The toilet training success of parents after reading "Toilet Training in Less Than a Day." Behav. Ther. 7:185–191.

Byrne, S. 1973. Hypnosis and the irritable bowel: Case histories, methods, and speculation. Am. J. Clin. Hypnosis 15:263–265.

Ciminero, A. R., and Doleys, D. M. 1976. Childhood enuresis: Considerations in assessment. J. Pediatr. Psychol. 4:17–20.

Cohen, S. I., and Reed, J. L. 1968. The treatment of nervous diarrhoea and other conditioned autonomic disorders by desensitization. Br. J. Psychiatry 114:1275–1280.

Collier, H. L. 1974. Enuresis and encopresis. In W. G. Klopfer and M. R. Reed (eds.), Problems in Psychotherapy: An Eclectic Approach, pp. 97–102. John Wiley & Sons, New York.

Collins, R. W. 1976. Applying the Mowrer conditioning device to nocturnal enuresis. J. Pediatr. Psychol. 4:27–30.

Collins, R. W., and Plaska, T. 1975. Mowrer's conditioning treatment for enuresis applied to geriatric residents of a nursing home. Behav. Ther. 6:632–638.

Collinson, D. R. 1970. Hypnotherapy in the management of nocturnal enuresis. Med. J. Aust. 1:52–54.

Conger, J. C. 1970. The treatment of encopresis by the management of social consequences. Behav. Ther. 1:386–390.

Cooper, C. E. 1973. Giggle micturition. In I. Kolvin, R. C. MacKeith, and S. R. Meadow (eds.), Bladder Control and Enuresis. J. B. Lippincott Co., Philadelphia.

Costello, C. G. 1970. Symptoms of Psychopathology: A Handbook. John Wiley & Sons, New York.

Creer, T. L., and Davis, M. H. 1975. Using a staggered-wakening procedure with enuretic children in an institutional setting. J. Behav. Ther. Exp. Psychiatry 6:23–25.

Crosby, N. D. 1950. Essential enuresis: Successful treatment based on physiological concept. Med. J. Aust. 2:533–543.

Cullen, K. J. 1966. Clinical observations concerning behavior disorders in children. Med. J. Aust. 1:712–715.

Davidson, M. 1973. Chronic nonspecific diarrhea syndrome. Irritable colon of childhood. In S. S. Gellis and B. M. Kagan (eds.), Current Pediatric Therapy, pp. 192–193. W. B. Saunders Co., Philadelphia.

deJonge, G. A. 1973. Epidemiology of enuresis: A survey of the literature. In I. Kolvin, R. C. MacKeith, and S. R. Meadow (eds.), Bladder Control and Enuresis, pp. 39–46. J. B. Lippincott Co., Philadelphia.

DeLeon, G., and Mandell, W. 1966. A comparison of conditioning and psychotherapy in the treatment of functional enuresis. J. Clin. Psychol. 22:326–330.

Dimson, S. B. 1959. Toilet training and enuresis. Br. Med. J. 2:666–670.

Dische, S. 1971. Management of enuresis. Br. Med. J. 2:33–36.

Dische, S. 1973. Treatment of enuresis with an enuresis alarm. In I. Kolvin, R. C. MacKeith, and S. R. Meadow (ed), Bladder Control and Enuresis. J. B. Lippincott Co., Philadelphia.

Doleys, D. M. 1977. Behavioral treatments for nocturnal enuresis in children: A review of the recent literature. Psychol. Bull. 84:30–54.

Doleys, D. M. Assessment and treatment of enuresis and encopresis in children. In M. Hersen, R. Ersler, P. Miller (eds.), Progress in Behavior Modification. Academic Press, New York. In press.

Doleys, D. M., and Arnold, S. 1975. Treatment of childhood encopresis: Full cleanliness training. Ment. Retard. 13:14–16.

Doleys, D. M., McWhorter, A. Q., Williams, S. C., and Gentry, W. R. 1977. Encopresis: Its treatment and relation to nocturnal enuresis. Behav. Ther. 8:77–82.

Douglas, J. W. B. 1973. Early disturbing events and later enuresis. In I. Kolvin,

R. C. MacKeith, and S. R. Meadow (eds.), **Bladder Control and Enuresis.** J. B. Lippincott Co., Philadelphia.

Easson, W. M. 1960. Encopresis—Psychogenic soiling. Can. Med. Assoc. J. 82:624–630.

Edelman, R. I. 1971. Operant conditioning treatment of encopresis. J. Behav. Ther. Exp. Psychiatry 2:71–73.

Engel, B. T., Nikoomanesh, P., and Schuster, M. M. 1974. Operant conditioning of rectosphincteric responses in the treatment of fecal incontinence. N. Engl. J. Med. 290:646–649.

Esperanca, M., and Gerrard, J. W. 1969. Nocturnal enuresis: Studies in bladder function in normal children and enuretics. Can. Med. Assoc. J. 101:324–327.

Fenichel, O. 1945. The Psychoanalytic Theory of Neurosis. W. W. Norton & Co., New York.

Fenichel, O. 1946. The Psychoanalytic Theory of Neurosis. Routledge & Kegan Paul, London.

Finley, W. W. 1971. An EEG study of the sleep of enuretics at three age levels. Clin. Electroencephalography 2:35–39.

Finley, W. W., Besserman, R. L., Bennett, L. F., Clapp, R. K., and Finley, P. M. 1973. The effect of continuous, intermittent, and placebo reinforcement on the effectiveness of the conditioning treatment for enuresis nocturna. Behav. Res. Ther. 11:289–297.

Finley, W. W., and Smith, H. A. 1975. A long-life, inexpensive urine-detection pad for conditioning of enuresis nocturna. Behav. Res. Meth. Instrum. 7:273–276.

Fitzgerald, J. F. 1975. Encopresis, soiling, constipation: What's to be done? Pediatrics 56:348–349.

Forsythe, W. I., and Merrett, J. D. 1969. A controlled trial of imipramine (Tofranil) and nortriplyline (Allegron) in the treatment of enuresis. Br. J. Clin. Prac. 23:210–215.

Foxx, R. M., and Azrin, N. H. 1973. Dry pants: A rapid method of toilet training children. Behav. Res. Ther. 11:435–442.

Fried, R. 1974. A device for enuresis control. Behav. Ther. 5:682–684.

Garrard, S. D., and Richmond, J. B. 1952. Psychogenic megacolon manifested by fecal soiling. Pediatrics 10:474–483.

Giles, D. K., and Wolf, M. M. 1966. Toilet training institutionalized severe retardates. Am. J. Ment. Defic. 70:766–780.

Glicklich, L. B. 1951. An historical account of enuresis. Pediatrics 8:859–876.

Goldsmith, H. 1962. Chronic loss of bowel control in a nine year old child. Am. J. Clin. Hypnosis 4:191–192.

Greaves, M. W. 1969. Scarring due to enuresis blankets. Br. J. Dermatol. 81:440–442.

Gruenberg, S. M. 1968. The New Encyclopedia of Child Care and Guidance. Doubleday & Co., Garden City, N.Y.

Hallgren, B. 1956. Enuresis I. A study with reference to the morbidity risk and symptomatology. II. A study with reference to certain physical, mental and social factors possibly associated with enuresis. Acta Psychiatr. 31:379–436.

Hallman, N. 1950. On the ability of enuretic children to hold urine. Acta Paediatr. 39:87–93.

Halverstadt, D. B. 1976. Enuresis. J. Pediatr. Psychol. 4:13–14.

Harper, P. A. 1962. Development of bowel and bladder control. In P. A. Harper (ed.), Preventive Pediatrics: Child Health and Development, pp. 27–35. Appleton-Century-Crofts, New York.

Harris, D. H., and Firestone, R. W. 1957. Are enuretics suitable for the armed services? J. Clin. Psychol. 13:91–93.

Hedberg, A. G. 1973. The treatment of chronic diarrhea by systematic desensitization: A case report. J. Behav. Ther. Exp. Psychiatry 4:67–68.

Henderson, W. 1976. A review of the current medical aspects of enuresis. J. Pediatr. Psychol. 4:15–16.

Hicks, W. R., and Barnes, E. H. 1964. A double-blind study of the effect of imipramine on enuresis in 100 Naval recruits. Am. J. Psychiatry 20:812–814.

Hilburn, W. B. 1968. Encopresis in childhood. J. Ky. Med. Assoc. 66:978–982.

Hoag, J. M., Norriss, N. G., Himeno, E. T., and Jacobs, J. 1971. The encopretic child and his family. J. Am. Acad. Child Psychiatry 10:242–256.

Homan, W. E. 1970. Child Sense. A Pediatrician's Guide for Today's Families. Bantam Books, New York. [New and expanded edition—Child Sense: A Guide to Loving, Level-Headed Parenthood, © 1969, 1977 by William E. Homan, Basic Books, Inc., Publishers, New York.]

Houle, T. A. 1974. The use of positive reinforcement and aversive conditioning in the treatment of encopresis: A case study. Devereaux Forum 9:7–14.

Hushka, M. 1942. The child's response to coercive toilet training. Psychosom. Med. 4:301–308.

Ilg, F. L., and Ames, L. B. 1962. Parents Ask. Harper & Brothers, New York.

Imhof, B. 1956. Bettnasser in der erziehingsberatung. Heilpaedagogische Werkblaetter 25:122–127.

Johnson, J. H., and Thompson, D. J. 1974. Modeling in the treatment of enuresis: A case study. J. Behav. Ther. Exp. Psychiatry 5:93–94.

Jones, H. G. 1960. The behavioral treatment of enuresis nocturna. In H. J. Eysenck (ed.), Behavior Therapy and the Neuroses, pp. 377–403. Pergamon, Oxford.

Kashinsky, W. 1974. Two low cost micturation alarms. Behav. Ther. 5:698–700.

Kelalis, P. P., King, L. R., and Belman, A. B. 1976. Clinical Pediatric Urology. Vol. 1. W. B. Saunders Co., Philadelphia.

Kimmel, H. D., and Kimmel, E. 1970. An instrumental conditioning method for the treatment of enuresis. J. Behav. Ther. Exp. Psychiatry 1:121–123.

Knobloch, H., and Pasamanick, B. 1974. Gessell & Amatruda's Developmental Diagnosis: The Evaluation and Management of Normal and Abnormal Neuropsychologic Development in Infancy and Early Childhood. 3rd Ed. Harper & Row, New York.

Kriegman, G., and Wright, H. B. 1947–48. Brief psychotherapy with enuretics in the Army. Am. J. Psychiatry 104:254–258.

Lehman, E. 1944. Psychogenic incontinence of feces (encopresis) in children. Report of recovery of four patients following psychotherapy. Am. J. Dis. Child. 68:190–199.

Levine, M. D. 1975. Children with encopresis: A descriptive analysis. Pediatrics 56:412–416.

Lifshitz, M., and Chovers, A. 1972. Encopresis among Israeli kibbutz children. Isr. Ann. Psychiatry 10:326–340.

Lovibond, S. H. 1964. Conditioning and Enuresis. The Macmillan Co., New York.

Lovibond, S. H., and Coote, M. A. 1970. Enuresis. In C. G. Costello (ed.), Symptoms of Psychopathology: A handbook. John Wiley & Sons, New York.

Macfarlane, J. W., Allen, L., and Honzik, M. P. 1954. A developmental study of the behavior problems of normal children between 21 months and 14 years. University of California Press, Berkeley.

MacKeith, R. C. 1972. Is maturation delay a frequent factor in the origins of primary nocturnal enuresis? Dev. Med. Child. Neurol. 14:217–223.

MacKeith, R., Meadow, R., and Turner, R. K. 1973. How children become dry. In I. Kolvin, R. C. MacKeith, and S. R. Meadow (eds.), Bladder Control and Enuresis, pp. 3–22. J. B. Lippincott Co., Philadelphia.

McKendry, J. B. J., and Stewart, D. A. 1974. Enuresis. Pediatr. Clin. North Am. 21:1019–1028.

McKendry, J. B. J., Stewart, D. A., Jeffs, R. D., and Mozes, A. 1972. Enuresis treated by an improved waking apparatus. Can. Med. Assoc. J. 106:27–29.

Matson, J. L., and Ollendick, T. H. 1977. Issues in toilet training normal children. Behav. Ther. 8:549–553.

Matthews, L. H. 1976. Toilet training: What do pediatricians know anyway? J. Pediatr. Psychol. 4:7–11.

Meadow, R. 1973. Practical aspects of the management of nocturnal enuresis. In I. Kolvin, R. C. MacKeith, and S. R. Meadow (eds.), Bladder Control and Enuresis, pp. 181–188. J. B. Lippincott Co., Philadelphia.

Mesibov, G. B., Schroeder, C. S., and Wesson, L. 1977. Parental concerns about their children. J. Pediatr. Psychol. 2:13–17.

Morgan, J. J. B., and Witmer, F. J. 1939. The treatment of enuresis by the conditioned reaction technique. J. Gen. Psychol. 55:59–65.

Morgan, R. T. T. 1974. Enuresis and the enuresis alarm. A clinical manual for the treatment of nocturnal enuresis. Department of Health and Social Security, Birmingham, Ala.

Morgan, R. T. T., and Young, G. C. 1972. The treatment of enuresis: Merits of conditioning methods. Community Med. 128:119–121.

Mowrer, O. H., and Mowrer, W. M. 1938. Enuresis—A method for its study and treatment. Am. J. Orthopsychiatry 8:436–459.

Muellner, S. R. 1960. Development of urinary control in children: A new concept in cause, prevention and treatment of primary enuresis. J. Urol. 84:714–716.

Neal, B. W., and Coote, M. A. 1969. Hazards of enuresis alarms. Arch. Dis. Child. 44:651.

Neale, D. H. 1963. Behavior therapy and encopresis in children. Behav. Res. Ther. 1:139–149.

Nilsson, D. E. 1976. Treatment of encopresis: A token economy. J. Pediatr. Psychol. 4:42–46.

Nisley, D. D. 1976. Medical overview of the management of encopresis. J. Pediatr. Psychol. 4:33–34.

Nixon, H. H. 1961. Participant on discussion on megacolon and megarectum with the emphasis on conditions other than Hirschprung's disease. Proc. R. Soc. Med. 54:1037–1040.

Nixon, H. H. 1975. The diagnosis and management of fecal incontinence in children. Arch. Chir. Neerl. 27:171–177.

Olatawura, M. O. 1973. Encopresis, a review of 32 cases. Acta Paediatr. Scand. 62:358–364.

Olness, K. 1975. The use of self-hypnosis in the treatment of childhood nocturnal enuresis. Clin. Pediatr. 14:273–279.

Olness, K. 1976. Autohypnosis in functional megacolon in children. Am. J. Clin. Hypnosis 19:28–32.

Oppel, W. C., Harper, P. A., and Rider, R. V. 1968. Social, psychological, and neurological factors associated with nocturnal enuresis. Pediatrics 42:627–641.

Paschalis, A. P., Kimmel, H. D., and Kimmel, E. 1972. Further study of diurnal instrumental conditioning in the treatment of enuresis nocturna. J. Behav. Ther. Exp. Psychiatry 3:253–256.

Pierce, C. M. 1972. Enuresis. In A. M. Freedman and H. I. Kaplan (eds.), The Child. Vol. I. Atheneum, New York.

Pinkerton, P. 1958. Psychogenic megacolon in children: The implications of bowel negativism. Arch. Dis. Child. 33:371–380.

Plag, J. A. 1964. The problem of enuresis in the naval service. U.S. Navy Medical Neuropsychiatric Research Unit, Report 64-3.

Poulton, E. M., and Hinden, E. 1953. The classification of enuresis. Arch. Dis. Child. 28:392–397.

Poussaint, A. F., and Greenfield, R. 1966. Epilepsy and enuresis. Am. J. Psychiatry 122:1426–1427.

Poussaint, A. F., Koegler, R. R., and Riehl, J. R. 1967. Enuresis, epilepsy, and the electroencephalogram. Am. J. Psychiatry 123:1294–1295.

Ravitch, M. M. 1958. Pseudo Hirschsprung's disease. Ann. Surg. 147:781–795.

Richmond, J. B., Eddy, E. J., and Garrard, S. D. 1954. The syndrome of fecal soiling and megacolon. Am. J. Orthopsychiatry 24:391–401.

Robertiello, R. C. 1956. Some psychiatric interrelations between the urinary and sexual systems with special reference to enuresis. Psychiatr. Q. 30:61–62.

Sacks, S., DeLeon, G., and Blackman, S. 1974. Psychological changes associated with conditioning functional enuresis. J. Clin. Psychol. 30:271–276.

Salk, L. 1972. What Every Child Would Like His Parents To Know. David McKay, New York.

Salmon, M. A., Taylor, D. C., and Lee, D. 1973. On the EEG in enuresis. In I. Kolvin, R. C. MacKeith, and S. R. Meadow (eds.), Bladder Control and Enuresis. J. B. Lippincott Co., Philadelphia.

Samaan, M. 1972. The control of nocturnal enuresis by operant conditioning. J. Behav. Ther. Exp. Psychiatry 3:103–105.

Schuster, M. M. 1974. Operant conditioning in gastrointestinal dysfunctions. Hosp. Pract. 9:135–143.

Seiger, H. W. 1952. Treatment of essential nocturnal enuresis. J. Pediatr. 40:738–749.

Shaffer, D. 1973. The association between enuresis and emotional disorder: A review of the literature. In I. Kolvin, R. C. MacKeith, and S. R. Meadow (eds.), Bladder Control and Enuresis. J. B. Lippincott Co., Philadelphia.

Shaffer, D., Costello, A. J., and Hill, I. D. 1968. Control of enuresis with imipramine. Arch. Dis. Child. 43:665–667.

Shane, M. 1967. Encopresis in a latency boy. An arrest along a developmental line. Psychoanal. Study Child 22:296–314.

Shaw, W. J. 1976. Enuresis: Survey articles. J. Pediatr. Psychol. 4:4–6.

Shirley, H. F. 1938. Encopresis in children. J. Pediatr. 12:367–380.

Silber, D. L. 1969. Encopresis. Discussion of etiology and management. Clin. Pediatr. 8:225–231.

Solomon, P., and Patch, V. D. 1969. Handbook of Psychiatry. Lange Medical Publications, Los Altos, Cal.

Spock, B. 1957. The Common Sense Book of Baby and Child Care. Duell, Sloan and Pearce, New York.

Starfield, B. 1967. Functional bladder capacity in enuretic and non-enuretic children. J. Pediatr. 70:777–781.

Starfield, B., and Mellits, E. D. 1968. Increase in functional bladder capacity and improvements in enuresis. J. Pediatr. 72:483–487.

Stedman, J. M. 1972. An extension of the Kimmell treatment method for enuresis to an adolescent: A case report. J. Behav. Ther. Exp. Psychiatry 3:307–309.

Stehbens, J. A., and Silber, D. L. 1971. Parental expectations in toilet training. Pediatrics 48:451–454.

Stehbens, J. A., and Silber, D. L. 1974. Experience and reason—Briefly recorded. Pediatrics 54:493–497.

Stewart, M. A. 1975. Treatment of bedwetting. JAMA 232:281–283.

Tapia, F., Jekel, K., and Domke, H. R. 1960. Enuresis: An emotional symptom. J. Nerv. Ment. Dis. 130:61–66.

Taylor, P. D., and Turner, R. K. 1975. A clinical trial of continuous, intermittent, and overlearning "bell and pad" treatments for nocturnal enuresis. Behav. Res. Ther. 13:281–293.

Torrey, E. F. 1972. What western psychotherapists can learn from witch doctors. Am. J. Orthopsychiatry 42:69–76.

Tough, J. H., Hawkins, R. P., McArthur, M. M., and Ravenswaay, S. V. 1971. Modification of enuretic behavior by punishment: A new use for an old device. Behav. Ther. 2:567–574.

Troup, C. W., and Hodgson, B. 1971. Nocturnal functional bladder capacity in enuretic children. J. Urol. 105:129–132.

Turner, R. K. 1973. Conditioning treatment of nocturnal enuresis: Present status. In I. Kolvin, R. C. MacKeith, and S. R. Meadow (eds.), Bladder Control and Enuresis. J. B. Lippincott Co., Philadelphia.

Turner, R. K., Young, G. C., and Rachman, S. 1970. Treatment of nocturnal enuresis by conditioning techniques. Behav. Res. Ther. 8:367–381.

Vaughan, G. F., and Cashmore, A. A. 1954. Encopresis in childhood. Guy's Hosp. Rep. 103:360–370.

Vaughan, V. C., McKay, R. J., and Nelson, W. E. 1975. Textbook of Pediatrics. 10th Ed. W. B. Saunders Co., Philadelphia.

Vincent, S. A. 1964. Treatment of enuresis with a perineal pressure apparatus: The irritable bladder syndrome. Dev. Med. Child Neurol. 6:23–31.

Walker, C. E., Hedberg, A. G., Clement, P. W., and Wright, L. Clinical Procedures for Behavior Therapy. Prentice-Hall Inc., New York. In press.

Werry, J., and Cohrssen, J. 1965. Enuresis: An etiologic and therapeutic study. J. Pediatr. 67:423–431.

Wolters, W. H. G. 1974. A comparative study of behavioural aspects in encopretic children. Psychother. Psychosom. 24:86–97.

Wolters, W. H. G., and Wauters, E. A. K. 1975. A study of somatopsychic vulnerability in encopretic children. Psychother. Psychosom. 26:27–34.

Wright, L. 1973. Handling the encopretic child. Prof. Psychol. 4:137–144.

Wright, L. 1975. Outcome of a standardized program for treating psychogenic encopresis. Prof. Psychol. 6:453–456.

Wright, L., and Craig, S. 1974. A comparative study of amphetamine, ephedrine-atrophine mixture, placebo and behavioral conditioning in the treatment of nocturnal enuresis. Okla. State Med. Assoc. J. 67:430–433.

Wright, L., and Walker, C. E. 1977. Treating the encopretic child. Clin. Pediatr. 16:1042–1045.

Yates, A. J. 1970. Behavior Therapy. John Wiley & Sons, New York.

Yeates, W. K. 1973. Bladder function in normal micturation. In I. Kolvin, R. C. MacKeith, and S. R. Meadow (eds.), Bladder Control and Enuresis, pp. 28–38. W. B. Saunders Co., Philadelphia.

Young, G. C. 1963. The family history of enuresis. J. R. Inst. Pub. Health 26:197–201.

Young, G. C. 1964. A staggered-wakening procedure in the treatment of enuresis. Med. Officer 111:142–143.

Young, G. C. 1973. The treatment of childhood encopresis by conditioned gastro-ileal reflex training. Behav. Res. Ther. 11:499–503.

Young, G. C., and Morgan, R. T. T. 1972. Overlearning in the conditioning treatment of enuresis. Behav. Res. Ther. 10:419–420.

Young, G. C., and Turner, R. K. 1965. CNS stimulant drugs and conditioning of nocturnal enuresis. Behav. Res. Ther. 3:93–101.

Young, I. L., and Goldsmith, A. O. 1972. Treatment of encopresis in a day treatment program. Psychotherapy: Theory, Research and Practice 9:231–235.

7
Disturbances of Eating and Feeding

Thomas R. Linscheid

Problems in eating and feeding are of great importance in a pediatric population because of their high frequency, nutritional and developmental implications, and psychological impact on children and families.

Palmer (1977) defines feeding problems as "the inability or refusal to eat certain foods because of neuromuscular dysfunction, obstructive lesions or psychological factors which interfere with eating, or a combination of two or more of these."

The best estimates suggest that approximately 25% of the pediatric population presents with varying degrees of feeding problems (Bartlett, 1928; Tilson, 1929; Kanner, 1957). Palmer (1977) reports a higher incidence, 33%, in specialized centers treating developmentally disabled children. It should be kept in mind that these figures represent feeding problems for which help is sought from professionals. It is highly likely that many feeding problems are dealt with at home or are tolerated and that the true incidence is undoubtedly higher.

Because of the nature of this book, emphasis is placed on those problems for which behavioral intervention or psychological input is appropriate. The reader is encouraged to consult other sources concerning problems caused by neuromuscular dysfunction or mechanical obstruction (cf. Illingworth, 1969; Coffey and Crawford, 1971).

Included in this chapter are such problems as bizarre food habits, mealtime tantrums, delays in self-feeding, difficulty in accepting various food textures, and multiple food dislikes. In addition, other less common childhood feeding disorders that have significant behavioral components are discussed, including infant rumination, childhood obesity, and anorexia nervosa. The chapter outlines the behavioral model and shows through example and case presentation how it can be used to treat the various feeding problems.

CLASSIFICATION OF FEEDING PROBLEMS

The causes of feeding problems are extremely varied. They range from intolerance of certain foods, because of allergies, to neuromuscular or mechanical obstructions to purely behavioral or psychogenic factors. In an effort to classify the types of problems and their causes, Palmer, Thompson, and Linscheid (1975) have suggested the classification system presented in Table 1.

While the list of problems is not exhaustive, most of the common problems, allowing for individual variation in expression, fit into one of the seven categories. Behavioral mismanagement is seen as the sole cause or a contributing factor in six of the seven major problem areas. This suggests that most feeding problems can be eliminated or alleviated by proper behavioral or psychological intervention. Schwartz (1958) divides children with nonorganically based eating problems into two main groups: a larger group whose eating problems are related directly to mismanagement of the feeding situation itself, and a smaller group whose eating problems are secondary to emotional disturbance in the family or child. He further suggests that many of the patients in the larger group can be treated by the pediatrician with no assistance from other professionals, whereas children in the second group will need input from other disciplines, such as educators, psychologists, nutritionists, and psychiatrists.

ETIOLOGY OF BEHAVIORALLY BASED FEEDING PROBLEMS

The roots of behaviorally determined feeding problems can often be traced to *infancy*. Initially, an infant has no realization that his behavior can affect what happens to him, but he soon learns that crying can bring satisfaction of his needs and that fussing and resistance may result in extension of adult attention. Most parents learn quickly to differentiate the meanings of crying in their infant children and to respond to crying that is purely manipulative in appropriate ways (e.g., ignoring). This is the beginning of an important normal process in which the child learns to

Table 1.   Classification of feeding problems

Major problems	Behavioral mismanagement	Neuromotor dysfunction	Mechanical obstruction
Mealtime tantrum	X		
Bizarre food habits	X		
Multiple food dislikes	X		
Prolonged subsistence on pureed food	X	X	X
Delay or difficulty in sucking, swallowing, or chewing		X	X
Delay in self-feeding	X	X	X

From Palmer, Thompson, and Linscheid, 1975; reprinted by permission.

delay gratification and learns that not all his desires will be met. Many parents feel that crying indicates their child is not happy and therefore they are not good parents. These parents are willing to do almost anything to prevent crying or to stop crying once it has begun. Because feeding often serves to pacify the child, overfeeding in infancy often occurs and can result in childhood obesity or bizarre food habits later in life (Illingworth and Lister, 1964; Hirsch, 1975). In addition, the subtle but significant emphasis placed on weight gain during the first year of life leads parents to believe "the more the better." Because a major component of the normal pediatric infant visit is the weighing and measuring, some mothers come to believe that the index of health is weight gain and growth. The pediatrician can reinforce this idea unknowingly by stressing questions about quantity eaten and types of food consumed. A pediatrician can prevent many later feeding problems by the information conveyed in the first few months of life. Emphasis should be placed on the extensive normal variability in growth and appetite. While educating parents in the normal patterns of weight gain and food intake, the pediatrician needs to remember that the statistical average is not necessarily the theoretical ideal. Within limits each child has his own ideal growth rate.

Problems with *food texture* often begin in the latter half of the first year of life. Illingworth and Lister (1964) suggest that there is a critical or sensitive period for the introduction of solid foods, age six to seven months. If this critical period is missed, the child is less likely to accept solid foods and the likelihood of behavioral feeding problems increases. Palmer, Thompson, and Linscheid (1975) describe a six-year-old child who was maintained on pureed foods. Because of medical complications and developmental delays, solids had not been introduced until much later than the normal time. The child's reluctance to accept the solid food had led to forced feeding and excessive mealtime tensions, resulting in a food phobia or solid food aversion. In addition, the child had developed several behaviors that effectively served to avoid eating all but pureed food.

It is common for feeding problems to develop in *children who are handicapped* or *who have a history of serious illness* (Palmer, Thompson, and Linscheid, 1975). Because of the illness or handicap, it is felt that the child deserves special consideration, and behaviors that would not be allowed in a nonhandicapped or well child are tolerated. Often these children are allowed to eat only a limited variety of food or an excess of food low in nutritional value. An interesting example of such a case treated at a child development center involved a six-year-old handicapped girl who ate only peanut butter and bread and drank only chocolate milk. Two years before referral she had been hospitalized for an extended period during which she was in a full body cast. Secondary to a reduced appetite she was allowed to eat whatever she wanted so that an adequate intake would be maintained. After removal of the cast and discharge from the hospital the girl refused to eat anything but her preferred foods. Efforts by her family to reinstitute a normal diet were met with refusals and tantrums and the girl was allowed to remain on her limited diet. Mealtimes became a source of tension, and medical problems such as constipation and limited weight gain developed and led to referrals for a behaviorally based treatment procedure.

Other problems such as bizarre food habits, multiple food dislikes, and delays in self-feeding often have their *origin between one and three years of age.* The rapid rate of growth seen during the first year of life diminishes dramatically, bringing with it a reduced need for calories and a relative decrease in appetite. Accompanying the reduced appetite is a change in feeding patterns. Children may be interested in food only once a day in contrast to the three or four regularly scheduled feedings characteristic of the first year of life (Bakwin and Bakwin, 1972). Also, they may refuse a food one day and then accept it the next. If parents are not made aware of the normality of this pattern, they may become overly concerned and resort to practices such as forced feeding or the placing of undue pressures on the child by threats of punishments or promises of excessive rewards. This is also an age when children begin to assert their independence, and the feeding situation often becomes the focus for this new expression. Children may refuse foods that they enjoy because the increased attention from their parents may be more rewarding than the actual consumption of the food (Schwartz, 1958). If mealtime tantrums and refusals are successful for the child, they will continue and "picki-ness" will become a characteristic of the child's feeding patterns. It is important during this stage to be aware that a child's adamant demands for a particular food may be founded more in a desire to know that he can in some way control his parent's behavior than in an actual preference for that food. Parents who resist these demands for a time and then submit to them are rewarding their child for persistent (stubborn?) behavior and are setting the stage for similar behaviors in other situations. There are those parents who, while they may not give in to a child's demands, encourage food refusals by extended periods of coaxing or offers of some artificial reward (e.g., a new toy) for eating. In this situation the child learns that his behavior can result in an extension of his parents' attention so that even for foods that he enjoys he can "have his cake and eat it too" by initially refusing these foods. In this situation, parents are rewarded as well because the child eventually does eat the food; thus, they persist in their efforts to talk their child into eating. It is important to stress to parents that how food is consumed is perhaps as important as what is consumed during this period. Bad mealtime behaviors learned during this period of naturally reduced interest in food can carry over and prevent the child from experiencing the variety and consuming the quantity of foods characteristic of later stages of development.

During the preschool years, a child encounters many *situations that can affect his feeding.* The birth of a sibling can have a significant effect on his eating patterns. It is common for children who have been drinking from a cup exclusively to demand a bottle again after the birth of a new sibling. Children are well aware of the amount of attention given a new baby by the parents and will engage in more infantile behaviors, feeling that this will bring to them the same attention lavished on the newborn. If parents reward these behaviors with their attention, the child will continue to elicit them and will be resistant to change when the novelty of the new baby has worn off for the parents. ·

Schwartz (1958) feels that *punitive toilet-training methods* can also lead to the development of feeding difficulty. He describes how an overly compulsive mother (or father) can communicate to her child an abhorrence of the messiness of toileting, which can lead to rejection of foods that are stool-like or excessively messy and may result in these foods being vomited if eaten.

Changes in a child's routine often cause short-lived variations in the child's eating habits. A family vacation or a visit from grandmother are high-risk times for the development of feeding problems if the parents do not handle these situations properly.

A child's appetite and willingness to eat can also be affected by the *nature of the family interaction during meals.* Hurried meals with unpleasant interactions serve to dissuade children and adults alike from viewing feeding as a pleasurable experience. Some families use the evening meal as a forum for discussion of the child's behavior during the day. A harried mother may recount a child's bad behavior to the father during mealtime while she has a captive audience. These factors all contribute to an anxiety-filled feeding situation for the child and may result in the child's avoidance of family mealtimes as he grows older. Most importantly, the carry-over from an emotionally charged encounter at mealtime reaches into all phases of family functioning.

Family interaction patterns not directly related to the consumption of food also play a role in the development of feeding problems. The expectation that a child be adult-like in table manners often places great pressures on the preschool child and results in undue tension in the feeding situation. Demanding that a preschool child come to the table sparkling clean, use perfect manners, empty his plate, and sit for long periods may result in a reduction in the child's appetite and escalate the conflict over eating (Schwartz, 1958). Those parents who use snacks and treats as rewards and distractors during the day may be forced to deal with their child's reduced appetite at mealtimes. Because the type of food given as snacks is usually less nutritious and higher in sugar than foods offered at mealtime, the child learns to expect these foods and may resist more normal foods on the basis of sweetness and appearance.

The psychological impact on a family with a feeding-problem child can be tremendous and can affect the family's interaction well beyond the feeding situation. Parents feel that one of their roles is to teach their children to eat a variety and adequate quantity of food. If this does not occur, parents can become extremely frustrated, and the resultant tension and pressures can lead to increased feeding problems and to interaction problems in other areas of family functioning. In families in which the problem is ignored and the child is allowed to feed the way he chooses, parents can suffer intense feelings of guilt if nutritional or other health problems arise. A sense of powerlessness often develops in parents after unsuccessful attempts to change food or eating patterns, which may result in the child increasing oppositional behaviors outside of the feeding situation. The child who is continually badgered and ridiculed for his eating habits by his parents, sibling, or peers can develop a poor impression of himself, affecting his self-confidence in new and unrelated situations.

For these reasons there is a great need for early intervention with feeding difficulties. Helping parents of developmentally disabled and normal children to solve long-standing feeding problems usually results in a reported reduction in other problems within the home and an improved attitude toward the child. Often this comes about because the parents gain confidence in their ability to influence their child's behavior in the ways they feel are important.

BEHAVIORAL APPROACH TO FEEDING PROBLEMS

Because most feeding problems are either caused or exacerbated by behavioral mismanagement, a treatment approach that emphasizes the interaction of child, feeder, and environment is essential. The behavioral approach with its emphasis on the interaction of behavior and environment provides a useful model in which to analyze feeding problems and plan appropriate treatment strategies. By placing emphasis on the interaction of behavior and environment, the behavioral approach avoids trait explanations that attempt to ascribe bad behaviors to something within the child and thereby deemphasize environmental interactions. To say that a child is refusing to eat because he is stubborn (i.e., a trait) focuses the problem on the child and may cause a therapist or parent to overlook specific behaviors in a feeding situation that may be encouraging the "stubborn" behavior in the child. The behavioral approach looks for the cause of the behavior not within the individual but in the interaction of his behavior with the environment. This does not mean that past experience is not important; it merely asserts that current conditions must be considered.

Behavioral Principles and the Feeding Situation

Behavior is defined as "any observable or measurable change or activity in an organism" (Mann, 1977). When behavior occurs it has some effect upon the environment, and this effect serves to determine the probability that the behavior will occur again. More simply stated, behavior is a function of its consequences. While it may be possible to think of situations in which this might not be true, in almost all cases of emitted or voluntary behavior the relationship does hold true.

Because basic data in the behavioral approach are response rates or response probabilities, the measurement of specific behaviors (responses) is very important. To accomplish this, behavior must be defined objectively and in ways that are measurable. A first step in any behavioral assessment or treatment is the pinpointing or defining of these specific behaviors. To use an earlier example, it would not be adequate to define a child's behavior as stubborn. There are many behaviors that could be included in this category, and it is probable that there would be disagreement as to some of them. To ensure agreement and to permit measurement, specific behaviors need to be defined. For example, a child described as stubborn in a feeding situation may push a spoonful of food away each time it is offered. The percentage of time the spoon is pushed away when offered is measurable (stubbornness is not), and with this measure there likely would be agreement among observers. Often, indirect but highly objective measures of behavior can be used. For example, in a feeding situation the weight of food or liquid consumed can provide such a measure.

An extremely important consideration in behavioral analysis is the specification of the conditions under which the undesirable behavior (e.g., spoon throwings, tantrums) is occurring and the conditions under which the desirable behavior (e.g., self-feeding) should occur. The environmental situation that is in effect just before or concomitant with a behavior is called the *antecedent* or *antecedent event*. Antecedents are important because they tell the child (or adult) what behaviors are appropriate for him in the situation. This signaling property comes about because of the child's previous experience under the same or similar antecedent conditions. Those behaviors that have been met with unfavorable results will tend not to be repeated. An everyday example is provided by people's adherence to the signals of a traffic control light.

It is not uncommon in feeding-problem cases for parents to report that the child will eat his vegetables for his father but not for his mother or vice versa. This is an immediate signal that certain behaviors of the child are being treated differently by the parents and should clue the therapist to look specifically at the behavioral differences between the parents in the feeding situation.

It was stated earlier that behavior is a function of its consequences. *Consequences* are defined on the basis of their effect on the future probability of the behavior. Those consequences that result in an increase in the probability that the behavior will be repeated are called *reinforcing consequences* or *reinforcers*. Consequences that result in a reduction or elimination of the behavior are called *punishing consequences* or *punishers*. It is important to note that these definitions are operational in nature and do not define the consequences on dimensions such as good/bad or pleasant/unpleasant. While it is true that most reinforcers are good or pleasant and most punishers are bad or unpleasant, the true criterion for the definition of a consequence lies in its effect on the behavior.

Many parents report that a child's behavior continues even though they scold the child severely each time that behavior occurs. At first thought, it would seem that scolding would be unpleasant and would tend to be thought of as punishment. However, because scolding reliably follows the behavior and the behavior is continuing, then by definition scolding is a reinforcer and not a punisher. The behavior might better be treated by ignoring it and providing pleasant attention when more appropriate behavior occurs. Because of their strong need for parental attention, children often prefer negative or punitive interactions with their parents to no interaction at all. Parents who complain that their child is never good and that they are continually reprimanding him are probably giving limited attention when the child is behaving appropriately. In working with children it is of utmost importance to remember that what is likeable or disagreeable to adults may not be so for children.

A word about natural versus arbitrary reinforcers is appropriate at this point. Arbitrary reinforcers or punishers are those that normally would not occur as the result of a behavior (Ferster, 1967). With children it is easy to provide an arbitrary or artificial reinforcer rather than have them experience the natural consequences of their behavior because such consequences are often upsetting to the child. In the feeding situation many problems are created when the natural consequence of not eating food that is offered, namely hunger, is prevented by the child's parents when they substitute less nutritious but tastier (from the child's viewpoint) foods.

Another important process is called *extinction*. This is the name given to the reduction in the rate of a behavior when a reinforcing consequence no longer occurs as a result of the behavior. Take the example of a child who has been eating his vegetables because he is given ice cream when he finishes. If we no longer give him the ice cream, he will most probably stop eating his vegetables.

A characteristic of the extinction process is that it results in an initial increase in the rate of behavior before reduction occurs. It is important to be aware of this so that the initial increase in not interpreted as a sign that the procedure is not working (Drabman and Jarvie, 1977). When a parent attempts to reduce mealtime demands for special foods by ignoring the demands, initially the child will probably respond by increasing the intensity and frequency of his demands. If this initial increase can be tolerated, the behavior will diminish; however, if the parent gives in to the demands at the increased level, the child is reinforced for his increased intensity and frequency and learns to be more persistent or "stubborn."

Because both result in a reduction in the rate of behavior, extinction is often confused with punishment. Extinction occurs when a reinforcing consequence is discontinued, whereas punishment occurs when a specific consequence is introduced contingent upon the behavior.

Behavioral Techniques Useful in Feeding Situations

If the objective of a behavioral intervention is to teach a new behavior or to increase one that is occurring, but at a very low rate, it is best to reinforce every occurrence of the response. This will produce the fastest acquisition. Once a behavior has been acquired, it can be maintained at a desired level without the need for reinforcement of each occurrence of the response. Reinforcement that is not provided for each occurrence of the behavior is called *intermittent reinforcement,* and in a therapy situation is usually delivered in accordance with a predetermined schedule based on time or number of behaviors emitted. For example, the child who has learned to eat vegetables because he has been given a bite of ice cream each time he has taken a bite of vegetables may be moved to a reinforcement schedule on which he receives the ice cream after every other bite and then after every third, fourth, fifth—tenth. The goal might be to increase the ratio until the ice cream is given only when all the vegetables are eaten.

If a child is to be taught to eat a new food or to engage in a new feeding behavior (eating with a spoon), two behavioral techniques can be extremely helpful. These are *shaping* and *fading*.

Shaping, or the method of successive approximations, involves the breaking down of the goal behavior into its various components and then systematically and cumulatively reinforcing the acquisition of these components until the goal behavior is exhibited. If the goal behavior is self-feeding with a spoon, we could elect to wait until the child spontaneously picked up the spoon and took a bite and then reinforce him. If the child has never used a spoon before, this may mean a long wait and might never occur at all. Feeding with a spoon is made up of many less complex behaviors. If we define these and then set out to increase the probability of each by reinforcing its occurrence, we can build the final behavior. Steps must be established so that each new step contains behaviors that have already been reinforced and does not ask for any new behavior other than that specified. Table 2 provides a sample program for shaping self-feeding in a child who would self-feed with his fingers but not with a spoon. The components of the final behavior are defined and are built into the chain by reinforcing each sequentially. In a shaping procedure it is important not to move to the next step before the previous component is well established. One must also be careful not to provide an excess of reinforcements at any one level, making it more difficult to move the child on to the next step. It is often necessary to go back a step or two if difficulty is encountered. In Table 2 a suggested number of reinforcements is given for each level but these should not be adhered to too rigidly. Experience is very important here, and it is sometimes hard even for the more experienced to fight the temptation to move ahead faster than warranted. Bensberg and Slominski (1965) and Whitney and Barnard (1966) both used shaping to teach proper spoon use in retardates.

With cooperative children a *fading procedure* may be used. O'Brien, Bugle, and Azrin (1972) used fading to teach proper spoon use to a retarded girl. They divided the process of using a spoon into six steps. The first step was the placement of the spoon in the child's hand and the holding of that hand by the trainer. The last step was the introduction of the food into the child's mouth and its removal by the child's upper teeth or lips. At first, the trainer guided the child's hand through all six steps. If the sequence of steps was completed successfully on three consecutive trials, the child's hand was guided through one less step on the next assisted trial. This was continued until the child could initiate and complete spoon use by herself.

Fading can be a fast and efficient method if the child will allow you to manipulate his movements physically; however, for those children who resist, a shaping procedure may be more effective.

Modeling is another way to teaching new behaviors. Therapeutically, it has been used for such purposes as reducing fear in children (Bandura, Grusec, and Menlove, 1967) and teaching new social behaviors

Table 2.   Shaping program for teaching self-feeding with a spoon

Reinforce when	Move to next step after ___ reinforcements
1. Johnny looks at the spoon	5
2. Johnny has his hand within one foot of the spoon	5
3. Johnny has his hand within six inches of the spoon	5
4. Johnny has his hand within two inches of the spoon	5
5. Johnny touches his spoon	5
6. Johnny holds the spoon	5
7. Johnny is holding the spoon within one foot of the food	5
8. Johnny is holding the spoon within six inches of the food	5
9. Johnny is holding the spoon within two inches of the food	8
10. Johnny touches the food with spoon held in his hand	8
11. Spoon is removed from food with food on it	8
12. Johnny holds spoon with food within eight inches of his mouth	8
13. Spoon with food is held within four inches of his mouth	4
14. Spoon with food is held within two inches of his mouth	4
15. Spoon with food is held within one inch of his mouth	5
16. Spoon with food touches face	5
17. Spoon with food touches lips	10
18. Spoon with food is placed inside the lips	15
19. Some of food is removed and is swallowed	10
20. All food is removed from spoon and swallowed	

(O'Connor, 1969). In reality, it is a learning process that is occurring all the time in everyday life. If we enter a new situation in which there are many people, we tend to behave as they do. As humans we have the capability of observing a behavior and noting the consequence that is desirable for us. One good way to encourage appropriate mealtime behaviors in a child is to provide a model of the appropriate behavior and ensure that the appropriate behavior is rewarded. It is sometimes adequate, and in many ways better, to reward an older sibling with praise for eating his vegetables than to chastise a younger sibling for refusal to eat the vegetables. In the former case the younger child observes the correct behaviors of the older child and notes that parental praise is the result.

The effectiveness of modeling, however, has been shown to be dependent on the subject's intellectual level and the behavior to be learned (Nelson, Cone, and Hanson, 1975) and is therefore more limited in its usefulness than shaping and fading techniques.

TREATMENT OF BEHAVIORALLY BASED FEEDING PROBLEMS

The treatment of feeding problems is discussed below in relation to those problems that can be prevented or easily managed by front-line professionals, usually the family pediatrician, and those problems that are more involved and require direct intervention from specialized professionals.

Role of the Pediatrician

Because the development of feeding skills is a stepwise process, the prevention or immediate treatment at an early age serves to ensure steady progress through later stages. The family pediatrician is in an ideal position to play the leading role in prevention and early treatment. Parents look to the pediatrician in all matters of infant management, and time spent with new parents in discussion of feeding patterns and stages will pay off in a reduced number of phone calls from anxious mothers later on. Schwartz (1958) suggests seven areas to be covered in such a discussion:

1. In the first few months of life there should be permissive management of feeding schedules with a gradual move toward the institution of a more structured feeding schedule near the middle of the first year.
2. Discussions should include techniques for introducing solid foods and the move toward chopped and home-cooked foods. The normality of food preferences should also be related at this point.
3. Techniques of weaning and the child's needs to suck independent of the feeding situation should be reviewed.
4. The pediatrician should outline expected weight gain and its correlation to age and describe changing patterns of food intake, weight gain, and appetite.
5. The expected growth rate should be discussed in reference to body type and hereditary factors.
6. Children should be encouraged to self-feed as maturation and interest allow.
7. Parents need to hear that messiness is a part of feeding for a child and that premature emphasis on manners and neatness can lead to disturbances in intake.

Restatement of these points during well-baby visits in the first year of life will also help to avoid problems.

If problems in feeding are reported, the pediatrician can use the behavioral model described in the previous section as a guide to the analysis of the difficulty once organic factors have been ruled out.

The first step would be to elicit from the child's mother (parents) an objective description of the behavior in question and an estimate of its frequency. Is it refusal to accept any food or just certain foods? Has it been increasing or decreasing? The physician should not accept non-specific descriptions of the behavior such as "he gets upset at mealtime" but rather should attempt to elicit a more detailed description that specifies the exact observable behavior. Also, it is important to get an estimate of the frequency of a behavior. Parents of a two-year-old often report that the child never eats. If these same parents are asked to record the actual amount and type of food eaten by their child, it is often found that intake is entirely appropriate for the child's age and weight. The conflict and distress engendered by a child's reduced food consumption tend to overly influence the parents' perception of the child's eating. Comparison of the obtained food records with developmental expectations is very important in this early stage of assessment.

In many cases it may be appropriate for the pediatrician to suggest that the parents count the behavior in question (e.g., bites of meat) for some preset time period such as a week. Measurement has two important functions. First, it provides a baseline measure of the behavior so that the effectiveness of a suggested treatment can be assessed realistically. Second, counting focuses the parents' attention upon the specific behavior and may help them see solutions to the problem themselves. Frequently, asking parents to count or in some other way measure the behavior of their child has resulted in the parents solving the problem on their own. Parents become more aware of the exact behavior in question, when and where it occurs, and notice the results or consequences of the behavior. In one case, a mother reported that her hearing-impaired son would not stay in his seat during breakfast. She was asked to record the number of times he left his seat during breakfast over a one-week period. She returned at the end of a week with a data sheet showing that her child's frequency of "seat leaving" had gone from 22 on the first day she measured it to 0 by the end of the week. When questioned as to why she believed the frequency had dropped she related that in counting the out-of-seat behavior she had not attended to her child when he was out of his seat but instead had gone to the kitchen counter to make a tally mark on her data sheet. She spontaneously offered the explanation that she had previously been attending to her child while he was up by coaxing or ordering him to return to his seat and that the counting had forced her to ignore the undesirable behavior. She came to this realization after the second day and from that point had deliberately ignored the out-of-seat behavior and had made an effort to attend to her son only when he was seated. As much as it is gratifying to feel that as professionals we have all the answers, this mother, when given a chance, had instituted a treatment similar to, if not exactly the same as, one that might have been suggested by a professional.

Once an adequate description of the behavior has been obtained, questioning should be directed to the antecedent conditions. When, where, and with whom does the behavior occur? For feeding behaviors a description of the feeding situation should be elicited from the parent. What times are the meals served? Who feeds the child? What is offered and in what portions? What is the child doing just before the meal is served? These are a few of the many questions that should be asked in determining the specific situation under which the behavior is occurring. The solution to the problem may be as simple as telling parents to reduce portion size if they have been pressuring their child to consume unrealistically large quantities, or to restructure premeal activities so that the child is not asked to give up some highly desirable activity to come to the table.

The next step in the process is to determine the consequences of the behavior in question. This is done by asking the parents what they do when the behavior occurs or what happens to their child as a result of the behavior. The same specificity required in the description of the child's behavior should be asked for in the parents' description of their behavior. It would not be helpful to permit a parent to say that he punishes his child each time the child spits out his food. The exact actions that the parent calls punishment should be determined: Is it scolding, is it sending the child to his room, or is it discussing with the child the social unacceptability of spitting his food out?

Remembering that behavior is determined by its consequences the actions of the parents that occur immediately following the inappropriate behavior should be the main focus in planning a behavior-change program. If the behavior is continuing, then what the parents are doing is reinforcing the child for that behavior even though they see it as punishment. Whether a stimulus event (parents' reaction) is a reinforcer or a punisher is determined entirely by its effect on the behavior.

As an example of the application of this model to mealtime behavior-change, the case of a two-year-old spoon thrower is reviewed (Cunningham and Linscheid, 1974). The mother of a two-year-old male child was referred because of difficulty in dealing with his mealtime behaviors. Because preliminary information from the referral source suggested that the case was not extremely involved, it was decided to schedule two appointments for the mother. During the first appointment the mother related that the child threw things at mealtime. With further questioning it was determined that the child threw his spoon, and only his spoon, and that this occurred after each bite of food. Spoon throwing occurred at lunch and dinner only, and it was reported to occur regardless of who was present. The child's mother reported that the family's usual response was to pick up the spoon, return it, and scold the child after each toss. The mother was asked to count the number of times the spoon was thrown during lunch and dinner for the next week and then to return for another appointment. At the second visit frequency of spoon throwing during the two meals was examined (Figure 1). Because there was no reduction in the behavior during the baseline week, a discussion of a specific procedure was conducted with the mother. From this discussion evolved the idea that the natural consequence of throwing the spoon away should result in a delay or elimination of the opportunity to eat more, and that by returning the spoon to the child immediately and scolding him they were preventing the natural aversive consequence (delay in feeding) and introducing a consequence (scolding), which to them seemed aversive but which to the child could be desirable because it meant that the family's attention was directed to him. The treatment decided upon involved imposing a one-minute time-out from positive reinforcement. Specifically, each time the child threw his spoon all food

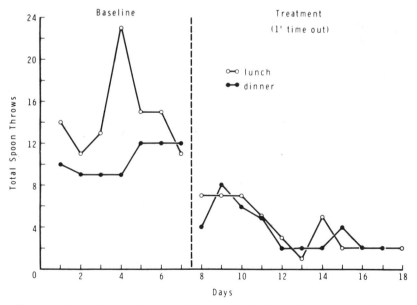

Figure 1.   Spoon throws at lunch and dinner during baseline and treatment conditions.

would be removed from his reach and the family would ignore him for a one-minute period. At the end of one minute, providing the child was not crying, his spoon and food would be returned to him, and, as long as he did not throw the spoon, the family would interact with him normally.

The results of the treatment are shown in Figure 1. Telephone contact was made with the family on the sixth and eleventh day of treatment. By the sixth day of treatment spoon throwing had decreased dramatically, and after the eleventh day of treatment it had stabilized at what to the family was an acceptably low level. The mother was not asked to take exact counts after the eleventh day but reported in later phone conversations that spoon throwing had disappeared.

This case was not presented to provide a universal treatment for spoon throwing but rather to present a model for treatment of feeding-behavior problems on a consultative basis using an applied behavior analysis model. In this case an effective treatment was conducted with minimal expenditure of professional time (total time was less than one hour). A strong but unmeasurable side benefit of this approach is the behavior analysis approach modeled for the parents by the professional. It is likely that this child's mother would look more toward the interaction of the child's behavior and her own in attempting to solve other conduct problems in the future.

TREATMENT OF COMPLEX FEEDING PROBLEMS

Many feeding problems are not amenable to the type of consultative treatment described in the previous section. When feeding problems are of long-standing duration or involve elements of fear or anxiety, a more specific approach involving behaviorally trained professionals may be required. Another reason for having the treatment conducted by professionals may be the parents' inability to comply with the procedures to be used. Some parents may be too busy with other children to impose the prescribed treatment consistently, or may be incapable of instituting some aspect of treatment that may be momentarily unpleasant for the child.

Most of the published reports of behavioral treatments by professionals are case studies. This is because of the great degree of variation in the specific expression of feeding problems, thus requiring highly individualized treatment procedures. Often cases requiring intense behavioral treatment involve children who have some type of mental or physical handicap or have suffered from a physical condition necessitating an interruption in the normal development of feeding skills and patterns.

Bernal (1972) describes the behavioral treatment of a four-year-old girl who would not feed herself and refused table foods. Two months before the first contact the child had undergone surgery to correct a congenital heart defect but was declared by her pediatrician to be in good health at the start of treatment. The child had begun to eat table foods at nine months of age, but when she choked on a piece of string bean her mother had reverted to baby foods. A few weeks later the mother attempted to reintroduce table foods; the child was resistant, and battles over food became a regular part of mealtimes, with the child winning most of the struggles. At 20 months of age the child's pediatrician recommended that all baby foods be removed and that the child not be fed unless she was willing to take regular foods. The parents were unable to tolerate the child's crying for her baby food, and after 36 hours of her not eating gave in to the child's requests. This is a common etiological description of the emergence of a feeding problem related to texture or bizarre food habits. The pediatrician's suggestion was appropriate had the parents been able to persevere. By not being able to follow the pediatrician's advice the parents in effect rewarded or reinforced their child's refusal and taught her that persistence in refusing regular foods would result in return of her preferred foods. The resources and capabilities of the parent must always be kept in mind when suggesting any extinction procedure.

Treatment of this case was conducted using several visits to the clinic in which video-taping of the feeding situation was done so that the mother-child interaction could be analyzed more easily. These tapes and other observation revealed that the child was receiving a great deal of social attention during the mealtime but that it was given contingent upon refusals and other behaviors not related to eating (i.e., chatting and playing with her food).

To reverse this pattern a treatment plan using a shaping procedure was instituted. Initially, the child was required to eat larger and larger quantities of strained foods, each bite of which was reinforced by social praise and smiles from the mother. When the present quantity was consumed she was allowed to eat her preferred foods. Table foods were introduced as the next step and were reinforced by social praise and brief access to a preferred food. The goal of the program was met when the child began to eat small portions of the family meal. Completion of the whole meal was reinforced with portions of preferred adult food and dessert. Within 20 weeks the child had added 50 foods to her diet that she had never eaten before.

This case illustrates the use of shaping to the desired diet through a series of steps, with each step in the process reinforced until it is well established. It is of interest that foods that were refused initially were used as reinforcers later in the program.

While Bernal used the mother as the primary therapist with the child, other researchers (Palmer, Thompson, and Linscheid, 1975; Thompson, Palmer, and Linscheid, 1977) have treated a number of cases in which a professional fed the child initially while the parents observed the techniques through a one-way mirror and then later in treatment moved into the feeding situation. Palmer, Thompson, and Linscheid (1975) outlined an interdisciplinary approach combining behavioral psychology and nutrition. In this way behavioral, nutritional, and developmental considerations are combined into a more effective program. The procedure involves an initial interview with the child's parents in which a nutritional and behavioral history is obtained. The nutritionist obtains a three-day food record as well and determines the child's current status in regard to caloric intake and recommended daily allowances of the various nutrients. The psychologist analyzes the reported behavioral interactions in objective terms and, through subsequent observations of feeding, formulates a treatment plan incorporating the most pressing nutritional needs of the child into the goals.

A common model involves treating the child at one meal per day at the clinic. During the rest of the day his food intake is limited in such a way as to ensure that he will be hungry during the treatment but will not suffer nutritionally. Before treatment begins a specific plan is evolved in which procedures and goals are stated in objective and behavioral terms. The treatment usually involves the reinforcement of a predetermined behavior by presentation of a preferred food and social approval. Noncompliance is treated by turning away from the child for short periods or until refusals or tantrums have ceased. This procedure is conducted daily, usually in 30–45-minute sessions.

Parents observe the treatment sessions and are instructed in the proper application of the techniques. When the child has made sufficient progress, the mother or father is brought into the room to actually feed the child. There is usually a slight regression when the parents begin feeding. However, this is short lived when the child realizes that the parent is imposing the same contingencies as the therapist. Often these sessions are video-taped and reviewed with the parents after the feeding session. Parents are reinforced by praise for correct applications of the techniques, and instances of incorrect applications are pointed out.

A specific program for extending the treatment to the other meals in the home is given to the parents, and follow-up is conducted by phone contact and periodic visits to the clinic for feedings. During the follow-up clinic visits, the behavioral interaction between the mother and child is observed and a nutritional analysis of the child's recent intake patterns is performed. Suggestions are made on the basis of these observations and a later follow-up visit is scheduled.

Not all cases can be treated on an outpatient basis, and occasionally a child has to be admitted to the hospital in order to conduct an in-depth program. In a recent case, a three-year-old, severely retarded child who also had cleft palate and visual and hearing losses was admitted for such a program. The child would refuse all food except formula offered in a bottle. As a result his nutritional status was always in question. In addition, his parents had been told that he would not be admitted to an appropriate school program unless he was trained to eat in a more normal manner. In the hospital four treatment sessions a day were conducted over a two-week period. Analysis of baseline sessions had revealed that the child became agitated and fearful when a spoon was brought anywhere near his mouth. A shaping procedure was used in which the child was initially reinforced with brief access to the bottle for sitting quietly with his fingers out of his mouth. When this was accomplished reinforcement was made contingent on quiet sitting while the spoon was brought progressively closer to the child's mouth. Eventually, access to the bottle was allowed only when food was actually taken from the spoon by the child.

It is doubtful that this case could have been treated successfully on an outpatient basis. Over 48 treatment sessions were needed to attain the goal for discharge. If this had been done on an outpatient basis it would have stretched over a two-month period and would have imposed an immense hardship on the family. It is unlikely that they would have continued for such an extended period had they been forced to live with the child's upset and whining because of reduced food intake. The child's mother took over the feeding before he left the hospital so that no problems in transfer to the home occurred.

Behavioral treatment for feeding problems also has been used extensively in institutions for the retarded. Nelson, Cone, and Hanson (1975) trained retarded males to use eating utensils using modeling and fading procedures, and Berkowitz, Sherry, and Davis (1971) used reinforcement and fading to teach self-feeding skills. Similarly, the specific inappropriate mealtime behaviors of retarded individuals were eliminated using time-out procedures by Barton et al. (1970).

APPLICATIONS OF BEHAVIORAL APPROACH TO FEEDING

Infant Rumination

Infant rumination is a rare but serious clinical entity characterized by the voluntary regurgitation of food or liquid. The food is usually ejected or allowed to run from the mouth but also is sometimes reswallowed. Rumination in adults was described as early as 1687 but was not reported in infants until 1907 (Kanner, 1957). To make the differential diagnosis one must rule out all other possible causes of vomiting, including brain stem lesions and gastrointestinal complications. A significant factor in the diagnosis is the lack of apparent distress experienced by the infant during rumination. The infant may be observed to be initiating the regurgitation deliberately, usually by arching, throwing his head back, and making deep chewing and swallowing movements with his mouth. In many instances children initiate the rumination by placing their fingers down their throats or by chewing on objects.

If the rumination continues and if enough food is lost, serious medical complications can result. These include severe malnutrition, electrolyte disturbances, developmental delays, and, in extreme cases, death (Bakwin and Bakwin, 1972). Kanner (1957) reports that, of 52 cases studied, "not less" than 11 died. Of this sample there was an equal number of each sex, all were between two-and-a-half and 12 months of age, and many had associated severe medical complications. Several recent studies report cases in this age range and do not reveal a higher incidence by sex or race (Lang and Melamed, 1969; Sajwaj, Libet, and Agras, 1974; Toister et al., 1975; Linscheid and Cunningham, 1977).

The etiology of the problem is not entirely understood. There are two seemingly divergent explanations, namely, psychoanalytic and behavioral. Richmond, Eddy, and Green (1958) suggest the psychoanalytic hypothesis that rumination is caused by an inadequacy in the mother, which does not allow her to provide a warm, relaxed, and physically intimate relationship for her infant. The infant, in an effort to create this missing gratification, regurgitates his food and rechews or retains it in his mouth.

The behavioral explanation defines rumination as a learned habit. Kanner's (1957) observations of infant rumination are supportive of this view. He states,

> Rumination is acquired incidentally and then taken up as a pleasurable habit practiced voluntarily. The complete abandon to the performance and the high degree of satisfaction derived from it are unmistakable. Whatever the primary occasion may have been, the habit nature of the act can hardly be questioned (p. 468).

But what is the source of reinforcement of ruminative behavior? Linscheid and Cunningham (1977) and Sheinbein (1975) have suggested that a combination of pleasurable self-stimulation and increased attention given to the infant during periods of rumination are the most probable causes for maintenance of the behavior. The normal occurrence of spitting up in infants may provide sufficient opportunity for the response to become reinforced given the right circumstances.

Upon close inspection the behavioral and psychoanalytic explanations are really not far apart. A mother who, because of her own problems, is unable to provide her infant with enough stimulation and who attends to the cleaning of the infant following vomiting is providing an ideal situation for rumination to develop. It is important to realize, however, that there may be many reasons why an infant receives reduced or inappropriate attention. For example, a mother who has several other children or who must work may not be able to give adequate attention to her infant. Also, infants in institutions are typically given less attention. In these cases the stage is set for establishment of habitual, self-stimulatory responses. While it is likely that rumination could occur because of psychopathology, its occurrence should not be seen as evidence of such. In the cases of rumination that we have treated (Cunningham and Linscheid, 1976; Linscheid and Cunningham, 1977), a clinical psychologist and a child psychiatrist found no evidence of family or mother-child psychopathology.

There are many approaches to the treatment of rumination. One approach involves prevention of the response by strapping the infant to a board that prevents arching or by placing tubes on his arms so that his fingers cannot be used to initiate vomiting. Feeding the infant very thick foods (e.g., thickened farina) would also fit in this preventive category, as would antiemetic medication. These approaches all have worked to an extent, but none seems to be totally reliable.

A treatment based on the psychodynamic view of rumination involves providing the infant with continual attention and stimulation. This is usually done in the hospital by assigning a nurse or volunteer to the infant exclusively (Richmond, Eddy, and Green, 1958). Berlin et al. (1957) reported success with this method with a four-year-old child who was hospitalized for eight months and whose parents received concomitant psychotherapy.

According to the behavioral explanation, rumination is learned or conditioned. Its treatment therefore can best be accomplished by counter-conditioning or relearning (Lang and Melamed, 1969). Using this approach with infants, a number of authors have eliminated rumination successfully by aversive conditioning procedures. These basic procedures, called punishment in behavioral terminology, involve the administration of an aversive or unpleasant stimulus contingent upon the response, in this case, rumination. Lang and Melamed (1969) were the first to use this procedure with an infant. After unsuccessful attempts to eliminate rumination by medication and posturing, a nine-month-old male infant was given brief electric shocks contingent upon vomiting. A dramatic reduction in rumination occurred in the first few days accompanied by a steady weight gain. Treatment was discontinued after six days but was reinstated three days later when a return of vomiting occurred.

This second treatment lasted three days and the patient was discharged. A one-year follow-up revealed that rumination had not returned and that the child was progressing normally.

There are at least three other case reports of the successful treatment of infant rumination by the contingent administration of electric shock (Toister et al., 1975; Cunningham and Linscheid, 1976; Linscheid and Cunningham, 1977). In all three cases infants were less than one year of age, and other treatment techniques had proved ineffective. Rumination was reduced to near zero within the first few days of treatment, and subsequent weight gain and development were normal. The effective shock level should be adjusted to a level that causes the infant to startle slightly. It is not necessary that the shock be excessively painful. In the cases treated at Georgetown University Hospital, an intensity level of 4.0 or 4.5 mA was used (Cunningham and Linscheid, 1976; Linscheid and Cunningham, 1977); this level caused the infants to suddenly orient and, on only a few occasions, to whimper briefly. Treatment should be conducted throughout the day and is most effective when delivery of the punisher is immediate. After an initial drop in the frequency, provision should be made for treating the infant in various locations and with the parents present to help ensure generalization of the suppressed response to the home (Cunningham and Linscheid, 1976).

Sajwaj, Libet, and Agras (1974) successfully employed an aversive conditioning procedure but used lemon juice squirted into the infant's mouth as the aversive stimulus rather than electric shock. Both methods seem to be successful in the rapid reduction of infant rumination. Because the intensity of the aversive stimuli used in these case reports is not extreme, it is not entirely clear whether the therapeutic effect is caused by the aversive property or by the distraction caused by its introduction. This needs further investigation because it would be unethical to use a painful stimulus if one were not needed. Sheinbein (1975) reports the successful treatment of a ruminator using contingent restraint, isolation, and social interaction. This method seems promising because it can be carried out at home as well as in the hospital. More research in this area is needed.

Childhood Obesity

The determinants of obesity in children as well as in adults are as yet not well understood. There is a theory that overfeeding in infancy produces either a greater number of adipose cells or cells that are larger than normal. This increase in size or volume remains with the child and serves to produce obesity in later childhood and adulthood (Hirsch, 1975). However, interactions between race, socioeconomic level, and age are inconsistent with this explanation (Garn, Clark, and Guire, 1975).

From a behavioral viewpoint obese adults show a characteristic eating pattern, typified by faster rates of biting, less chewing, and more extraneous responses during eating (Schacter, 1971). Recently, this pattern has been shown to exist in obese children between six and 14 years of age (Marston, London, and Cooper, 1976). This would suggest that behavioral feeding patterns characteristic of obesity begin early. The question of whether these patterns are causative of or merely secondary to an organic predisposition is certainly of interest.

Behavioral treatment of obesity has met with substantial success in adults (Bellack, 1977) and is just now being extended to children. The approach essentially teaches individuals to control intake by making them more aware of their eating patterns and introducing ways to modify these behaviors through self-monitoring.

Aside from the organic or behavioral explorations is the question of the fat personality. Is there a set of traits found in some people that somehow predisposes them to obesity? Certainly there exists the stereotype of the jolly fat person. Bruch (1973) reports on early studies that indicate that the obese child who characteristically is abnormally inactive has the greatest food intake and the greatest degree of emotional disturbance. These children typically have parents who are overprotective, indulgent, and overly apprehensive about the possible dangers of exercise. Children of these parents are extremely inactive and socially immature. The result of the parental overconcern is a home life in which gratification is obtained only from food.

The problem of understanding the determinants of childhood obesity is compounded by the emotional difficulties often produced by the obesity itself. In other words, are the emotional problems often seen in obese children the cause of or merely secondary to the social adjustment problems related to the condition?

For the purposes of this volume, suffice it to say that childhood obesity is a significant problem that can be many faceted in etiology and expression. Prevention may be possible through parent education and sensitive monitoring of weight gain early in life. Analysis of feeding patterns also plays a role in early intervention and treatment. Obese children are at risk for other problems, and referral for evaluation by medical, nutritional, and psychological specialists should be considered when extreme and persistent weight gain is seen in children. Many obese children do make a successful adjustment in later life (Bruch, 1973); however, many continue to have severe behavioral, emotional, and medical (e.g., hypertension, diabetes) problems throughout adulthood.

Anorexia Nervosa

Anorexia nervosa is a psychogenic disorder characterized by extensive weight loss. Onset often occurs between 10 and 15 years of age, and the condition is much more common in females than males. Despite its psychogenic origins, serious medical complications accompany the dramatic weight loss. Changes that are common include growth of lanugo hair, gastric hypoacidity, decreased sex drive, carotenemia, and hypoproteinimia. Usually menstruation ceases and in many cases does not resume until long after nutrition has improved (Bakwin and Bakwin, 1972).

It is felt that the condition is related to an unhealthy family relationship characterized by an ambivalent relationship with the mother and an increasingly anxious relationship with the father related to adolescent sexual development. The extreme weight loss serves to reduce some of the anxieties related to adolescent socialization. Adolescent anorexics remain active and energetic but usually do not date. This pattern continues until hospitalization is required (Bakwin and Bakwin, 1972).

Anorexia nervosa has been treated by a variety of approaches. In its early stages the family physician may be successful by prescribing a suitable diet and giving support and encouragement. Most often referral to other professionals for behavioral and psychotherapeutic treatment is required.

Behavioral treatment most commonly has involved the use of feedback of information about caloric intake and the reinforcement of weight gain by activities, privileges, and social interaction (Bachrach, Erwin, and Mohr, 1965; Blinder, Freeman, and Stunkard, 1970).

Agras et al. (1974) report weight gain in two cases using privileges granted based on weight gain. One of the subjects was a 17-year-old female whose weight had dropped from 63.5 kg to 43.2 kg over an 18-month period. Dieting had resulted in a cessation of menstruation, peroneal nerve paralysis, and loss of interest in food altogether. The second subject was a 10-year-old female who had lost weight steadily, from 26.0 kg to 17.5 kg over a six-month period. During an initial baseline phase, both patients were told that they should eat as much as possible and that the hospital staff was interested in them and expected improvement. Four 1,500-calorie meals were served each day. Each subject was to count the number of bites of food at each meal and was informed of the calories consumed following the meal. This information along with daily weight was plotted by the subjects.

During a reinforcement phase subjects were granted privileges such as television access or ward passes based on 0.1 kg increases in weight. The baseline conditions continued during this phase. A return to the baseline-only conditions followed the reinforcement phase.

Slight but steady weight gain for both subjects was observed during the initial baseline phase. Patient 1 increased her rate of gain fourfold during the reinforcement phase, while a rate of gain comparable to that during baseline occurred for Patient 2. During the second baseline phase both subjects continued to gain weight, Patient 2 at a rate about twice that of the reinforcement phase.

The authors identify three variables operating during behavioral treatment of anorexia nervosa. These are: 1) feedback of information about caloric intake and weight gain, 2) daily reinforcement for weight gain, and 3) the knowledge by the patient that weight gain will lead to discharge from the hospital. In subsequent experiments with adolescents and adults Agras et al. (1974) demonstrated the effects of these variables and suggested that the most effective treatment involves the active participation of the patient in data collection and reinforcement of weight gain. Linscheid, Malosky, and Zimmerman (1974) describe the successful treatment of a 21-year-old female in which discharge from the hospital was guaranteed contingent upon weight gain, reduction of inappropriate behaviors, and improvement in academics.

Despite the success of behavior modification in the treatment of anorexia nervosa, several criticisms of the approach have been advanced. Bruch (1974) criticizes behavior modification for treating only the symptom of the disturbance, namely, severe weight loss. She describes several cases in which weight gained during the treatment was rapidly lost following discharge and in which patients reported negative feelings about the procedure. In addition, inadequate follow-up and the lack of specific programs to be carried out at home have often characterized published reports of behavioral treatments.

These points are all well taken, and it should be stressed that the treatment of anorexia nervosa, especially in the child or adolescent, should involve an in-depth investigation of the physiological, emotional, and environmental factors operating in each case. Weight gain is important, however, and the behavioral approach has its place in the treatment of the problem both during hospitalization and during follow-up. An understanding of the environmental factors related to severe weight loss can be extremely beneficial, if not crucial, to the true understanding of the disease.

SUMMARY

In this chapter nonorganically based feeding problems are defined, and a behavioral model providing for the functional analysis and treatment of these problems is described.

Among the causes of childhood feeding problems are overfeeding in infancy, failure to introduce solid foods at the appropriate time, and mismanagement of undesirable mealtime behaviors. Suggestions are made for the prevention of these problems through parent education, and a consultative model for treatment by parents was described. Examples of the use of behavior modification in the treatment of more severe feeding problems are provided.

The applied behavioral approach presented in this chapter offers many advantages. It is flexible and can be used to treat a wide variety of problems from mealtime tantrums to solid food aversion. Even in cases in which the primary cause is not behavioral, the approach can be used to ensure that the child is performing to the best of his ability. The complexity of the treatment can be altered to fit the needs of the problem in question and can range from a single consultative session to an in-depth program lasting weeks or months.

Palmer, Thompson, and Linscheid (1975) have observed that, despite a growing interest in feeding problems, the literature contains little in regard to classification systems, discussion of incidence, diagnostic criteria, or appropriate treatment methods. They suggest that this may be because of the wide variety of disciplines involved in the treatment of feeding problems. Children may be treated by pediatricians (or pediatric specialties such as gastroenterology), as well as by nutritionists, dietitians, occupational therapists, psychologists, psychiatrists, and/or nurses. Each discipline has its own orientation, methods, and publications. What is needed is an interdisciplinary forum in which the various professionals interested in feeding problems can share their knowledge and experiences.

REFERENCES

Agras, W. S., Barlow, D. H., Chapin, H. N., Abel, G. G., and Leitenberg, H. 1974. Behavior modification of anorexia nervosa. Arch. Gen. Psychiatry 30:279–286.

Bachrach, A. J., Erwin, W. J., and Mohr, P. J. 1965. The control of eating behavior in an anorexic by operant conditioning techniques. In L. P. Ullman and L. Krasner (eds.), Case Studies in Behavior Modification, pp. 153–163. Holt, Rinehart and Winston, New York.

Bakwin, H., and Bakwin, R. M. 1972. Behavior Disorder in Children. W. B. Saunders Co., Philadelphia.

Bandura, A., Grusec, J. D., and Menlove, F. L. 1967. Vicarious extinction of avoidance behavior. J. Pers. Soc. Psychol. 5:16–23.

Bartlett, W. M. 1928. Problems of pre-school children. Teach Coll. Contrib. Educ. No. 536.

Barton, E. S., Guess, D., Garcia, E., and Baer, D. M. 1970. Improvement in retardates' meal time behaviors using multiple baseline techniques. J. Appl. Behav. Anal. 3:77–84.

Bellack, A. S. 1977. Behavioral treatment for obesity: Appraisal and recommendations. In R. M. Henson, R. M. Eisler, and P. M. Miller (eds.), Progress in Behavior Modification: Vol. 4, pp. 228–253. Academic Press, New York.

Bensberg, G. J., and Slominski, A. 1965. Helping the retarded learn self care. In G. J. Bensberg (ed.), Teaching the Mentally Retarded, pp. 46–62. Southern Regional Educational.Board, Atlanta, Georgia.

Berkowitz, S., Sherry, P. J., and Davis, B. A. 1971. Teaching self-feeding skills to profound retardates using reinforcement and fading procedures. Behav. Ther. 2:62–67.

Berlin, I. N., McCullough, G., Lisha, E. S., and Szurek, S. 1957. Intractible episodic vomiting in a three-year-old child. Psychiatr. Q. 31:228–249.

Bernal, M. E. 1972. Behavioral treatment of a child's eating problem. J. Behav. Ther. Exp. Psychiatry 3:43–52.

Blinder, B. J., Freeman, D. M. A., and Stunkard, A. J. 1970. Behavior therapy for anorexia nervosa: Effectiveness of activity as a reinforcer for weight gain. Am. J. Psychiatry 126:1093–1098.

Bruch, B. 1973. Eating disorders; obesity, anorexia nervosa, and the person within. Basic Books, New York.

Bruch, H. 1974. Perils of behavior modification in treatment of anorexia nervosa. JAMA 230:1419–1422.

Coffey, K. R., and Crawford, J. 1971. Nutritional problems commonly encountered in the developmentally handicapped. In M. A. Smith (ed.), Feeding the Handicapped Child. University of Tennessee Child Development Center, Memphis.

Cunningham, C. E., and Linscheid, T. R. 1974. Reduction of meal time spoon throwing in a retarded child using time out procedures. Unpublished manuscript.

Cunningham, C. E., and Linscheid, T. R. 1976. Elimination of chronic infant ruminating by electric shock. Behav. Ther. 7:231–234.

Drabman, R. S., and Jarvie, G. 1977. Counseling parents of children with behavior problems: The use of extinction and time out techniques. Pediatrics 59(1):78–85.

Ferster, C. B. 1967. Arbitrary and natural reinforcement. Psychol. Record 17(3):341–347.

Garn, S. M., Clark, D. C., and Guire, K. E. 1975. Growth, body composition, and development of obese and lean children. In M. Winick (ed.), Childhood Obesity, pp. 23–46. John Wiley & Sons, New York.

Hirsch, J. 1975. Cell number and size as a determinant of subsequent obesity. In M. Winick (ed.), Childhood Obesity, pp. 15–23. John Wiley & Sons, New York.

Illingworth, R. S. 1969. Sucking and swallowing difficulties in infancy: Diagnostic problem of dysphagia. Arch. Dis. Child. 44:655–667.

Illingworth, R. S., and Lister, J. 1964. The critical or sensitive period, with special reference to certain feeding problems in infants and children. J. Pediatr. 65:839–851.

Kanner, L. 1957. Child Psychiatry. 3rd Ed. Charles C Thomas, Springfield, Ill.

Lang, P. J., and Melamed, B. G. 1969. Avoidance conditioning therapy of an infant with chronic ruminative vomiting. J. Abnorm. Psychol. 74:139–142.

Linscheid, T. R., and Cunningham, C. E. 1977. A controlled demonstration of the effectiveness of electric shock in the elimination of chronic infant rumination. J. Appl. Behav. Anal. 10:500.

Linscheid, T. R., Malosky, P., and Zimmerman, J. 1974. Discharge as the major consequence in a hospitalized patient's behavior management program: A case study. Behav. Ther. 5:559–564.

Mann, R. A. 1977. Assessment of children's behavioral deficits. In M. Hersen and A. S. Bellack (eds.), Behavioral Assessment: A Practical Handbook, pp. 117–132. Pergamon, Oxford.

Marston, A. R., London, P., and Cooper, L. M. 1976. A note on the eating behavior of children varying in weight. J. Child Psychol. Psychiatry 17:221–224.

Nelson, G. L., Cone, J. D., and Hanson, C. R. 1975. Training correct utensil use in retarded children: Modeling vs. physical guidance. Am. J. Ment. Defic. 80(1):114–122.

O'Brien, F., Bugle, C., and Azrin, N. A. 1972. Training and maintaining a retarded child's proper eating. J. Appl. Behav. Anal. 5:67–72.

O'Connor, R. D. 1969. Modification of social withdrawal through symbolic modeling. J. Appl. Behav. Anal. 2:15–22.

Palmer, S., Thompson, R. J., Jr., and Linscheid, T. R. 1975. Applied behavior analysis in the treatment of childhood feeding problems. Dev. Med. Child Neurol. 17:333–339.

Palmer, S., and Horn, S. 1978. Feeding problems in children. In S. Palmer and S. Ekvall (eds.), Nutrition in Developmental Disorders, pp. 122–139. Charles C Thomas, Springfield, Ill.

Richmond, J. B., Eddy, E., and Green, M. 1958. Rumination: A psychosomatic syndrome of infancy. Pediatrics 22:49–55.

Sajwaj, T., Libet, J., and Agras, S. 1974. Lemon-juice therapy: The control of life-threatening rumination in a six-month old infant. J. Appl. Behav. Anal. 7(4):557–563.

Schacter, S. 1971. Some extraordinary facts about obese humans and rats. Am. Psychol. 26:129–144.

Schwartz, A. S. 1958. Eating problems. Pediatr. Clin. North Am. 5:595–611.

Sheinbein, M. 1975. Treatment for the hospitalized infantile ruminator. Clin. Pediatr. 14(8):719–724.

Thompson, R. J., Jr., and Linscheid, T. R. 1976. Adult-child interaction analysis: Methodology and case application. Child Psychiatry Hum. Dev. 7(1):31–42.

Thompson, R. J., Jr., Palmer, S., and Linscheid, T. R. 1977. Single subject design and interaction analysis in the behavioral treatment of a child with a feeding problem. Child Psychiatry Hum. Dev. 8:43–53.

Tilson, M. A. 1929. Problems of pre-school children. Teach. Coll. Contrib. Educ. No. 536.

Toister, R. P., Colin, J., Worley, L. M., and Arthur, D. 1975. Faradic therapy of chronic vomiting in infancy: A case study. J. Behav. Ther. Exp. Psychiatry 6(1):55–59.

Whitney, L. R., and Barnard, K. E. 1966. Implications of operant theory for nursing care of the retarded child. Ment. Retard. 4:26–28.

CHRONIC PHYSICAL CONDITIONS

The effects of a life-threatening illness on a child and his family are pervasive. Whether the disease is acute, progressive or chronic, the child and his family undergo substantial stress and change of daily life patterns.

When one considers diseases such as renal failure, diabetes, pulmonary disorders, and oncology, there is an emerging literature related to the psychosocial management of affected children that enhances and augments medical care practices. The following chapters summarize the body of knowledge that exists regarding psychological aspects of these diseases in the pediatric population.

8

Juvenile Diabetes

Ann M. Garner and Clare W. Thompson

There are few disorders of childhood that affect the child patient, the parents, siblings, peers, teacher, and physician as complexly as does juvenile diabetes mellitus. For one thing, diabetes is a chronic, lifelong condition, and may therefore interfere with the child's normal development in physical, emotional, and social spheres. For another thing, diabetes and its treatment involve the basic processes of feeding, urinating, and daily scheduling, which early acquire special meaning for the young child and parents alike. Control of the condition depends on dietary regulation, daily urine testing, insulin injections, and monitoring of exercise. First the parents and later the child assume responsibility for these significant aspects of the child's life.

Even under the best of circumstances, however, the degree of diabetic control fluctuates—sometimes with the strictness of regimen being followed, sometimes with emotional state, sometimes apparently capriciously. At these times, fear of later complications—vascular, retinal, neural—arises. Indeed, diabetic therapy itself, in the form of insulin injections, may prove threatening, as when the balance among insulin, food intake, and exercise is disturbed and a hypoglycemic reaction occurs.

Children, their families, and their physicians respond to this situation in a variety of ways. For example, in one study of the relative "comfort" of families with a diabetic child (Thompson, 1973; Garner and Thompson, 1974), two extreme reactions could be identified, as illustrated by the following cases:

> **Case 1** A nine-year-old boy, in preliminary interview, agreed reluctantly to participate with his family in the study but seemed frightened. His first comment to the experimenter was, "Well, anyhow, I have lots of friends." During his half-day visit with the research team, he declined to remove his heavy jacket although the laboratory rooms (in a hospital setting) were hot. His parents seemed tense, uneasy, and hasty in their responses to questions, frequently interrupting the interviewer. Insulin injections were handled exclusively by the mother, because the father reported he

This review was supported in part by Health Services and Mental Health Administration, Maternal and Child Health Services Project 920.

had a "phobia of blood" and so could not help, although no blood is involved in the injections. The parents described the child as "not spoiled," but they felt he got more attention than the other children in the family. After considering the history of their marriage and of their family, the parents agreed that the son's diabetes was "the worst thing that ever happened to us." The mother volunteered that she was already worried over what might happen to the boy's diabetic regimen when he reached adolescence and "rebelled." She also voiced the hope that she would never have any grandchildren lest they be afflicted with the diabetic condition. A variety of measures agreed in characterizing this family as "least comfortable" of all the families studied.

Case 2   Another little boy raced through the half-day of experimental procedures with a grin on his face. He was active in the local 4-H program, spent each summer in a regular camp, played trumpet in the school band, and was generally successful in a variety of school activities. Because of his special knowledge, he was greatly sought after in the school to give special talks on human physiology and on diabetes in particular; he always obliged willingly. The parents reported that they took turns administering the insulin but that the boy handled much of it himself, measuring the insulin and performing the injections efficiently. During the summer before the study, the entire family had gone on a camping trip through Mexico. They reported that they had been able to cope with urine testing, injections, and special diets with no difficulty. In fact, the parents reported they did not consider diabetes a particularly bad thing and that it had not, in their view, affected the family adversely. At the close of the interview, the mother volunteered, "I know what you mean; there are some families with diabetes that go into a tizzy over it. We aren't like that." A variety of measures agreed in characterizng this family as "most comfortable" of all the families studied.

The reasons for differences such as these lie in the complex interaction of many physiological, emotional, and environmental variables. It is the purpose of this chapter to discuss these variables and to show how professional persons can assist children and families in dealing with the chronic condition of juvenile diabetes mellitus.

NATURE OF JUVENILE DIABETES MELLITUS[1]

Definition

Juvenile diabetes mellitus is the most common endocrine abnormality of childhood. It is a chronic metabolic disorder of energy utilization, in which the ability to oxidize carbohydrates is decreased or completely lost as the result of inadequate pancreatic function. The immediate effect is increased sugar in the blood (hyperglycemia) and urine (glycosuria).

---

[1] For general discussions of the nature of juvenile diabetes mellitus, the reader is referred to Ehrlich (1974), Ganda and Soeldner (1977), and Paulsen and Colle (1969).

Two major forms of diabetes are recognized: *juvenile* (also called "brittle", or "insulin-deficient"), and *adult-onset*. Juvenile type diabetes accounts for 30% of all cases, and is most common in childhood. All other cases are classified as adult-onset. Children with juvenile diabetes constitute 4–5% of all diabetics. One child in 2,500 under age 15 suffers from the condition (Knowles, 1971). Onset may occur at any time during childhood, although the clinical symptoms appear most frequently in children aged 10 through 16 years. There is no difference in incidence between boys and girls.

There are other types of diabetes that may occur, although rarely, in young children. An occasional overweight child develops a syndrome resembling the maturity-onset diabetes mellitus and may be helped through dietary regulation alone. Even rarer forms include a transient diabetes of the newborn, lipodystrophic diabetes (in which there is atrophy of adipose tissue), and the diabetes of children suffering from cystic fibrosis.

Etiology

In juvenile diabetes, the insulin-producing capacity of the pancreas is markedly decreased at the onset of the conditon because of the failure of the beta cells of the islets of Langerhans, where insulin is synthesized. After a period of time, ranging roughly from six months to two years, the capacity of the pancreas to produce insulin disappears completely. Once developed, failure of the beta cells is permanent, and the child is entirely dependent upon insulin from other sources for the rest of his life. The nature of the process that renders the beta cells of the islets of Langerhans ineffectual is not known. Various suggestions have been advanced, including inflammation, viral effects, trauma, emotional reactions, and infections. At present there is no persuasive evidence favoring any of these explanations.

Genetic Considerations

It has long been thought that a propensity toward the development of diabetes was determined genetically. The exact mode of transmission, however, remains controversial—a "geneticist's nightmare" (Ganda and Soeldner, 1977). For example, the clinical manifestations of the condition may appear at any time in the life-span. However, both juvenile and adult-onset diabetes may appear in the same pedigrees, suggesting that they may be different manifestations of the same genetic predisposition. On the other hand, some evidence is available suggesting different modes of inheritance for these two forms.

Two main theories of transmission are common today: 1) Most writers argue that predisposition toward diabetes is an autosomal recessive trait. However, a number of studies in this country and elsewhere (Ehrlich, 1974) indicate that the frequency of occurrence of diabetes in children of diabetic couples is smaller than expected. However, when the occurrence of chemical diabetes (so-called "prediabetes," without clinical symptoms) is studied, frequencies of appearance in children of diabetic couples are much higher, approaching the predicted incidence. On the other hand, the concordance rates for the condition in identical twins is only 70%. Such findings cast doubt on the simple operation of an autosomal recessive trait. 2) In view of these findings, some writers hold that a multifactorial mode of transmission should be considered. A few investigators have thought that diabetes might be a dominant disorder, with variable expression and/or incomplete penetrance. Probably the most important factor in retarding progress toward unraveling the puzzle of inheritance here is the lack of a genetic marker or heritability index.

Whatever the specific mechanism of transmission proves to be, the expression of the clinical manifestations of diabetes seems to require that the abnormal propensity be present in both parents. In view of the tendency of distressed parents to use such information in coping with their anxieties about their diabetic child, it is important that both parents understand that both sides of the family are implicated. Otherwise, that parent in whose family the clinical manifestations occurred would be alone in carrying the feelings of guilt and responsibility that inevitably develop.

The development of clinical diabetes depends not only upon the particular genetic patterns but also upon the amount and type of environmental influence on the genes. At present, the complexities of genetic and environmental interactions are leading some authorities to propose a new diabetic typology not based, as is the present classification, upon age of onset (Ganda and Soeldner, 1977). In this system, *Type A* diabetes would be the insulin-dependent, severe condition, best explained as resulting from gene-virus interaction. *Type B* diabetes would be the non-insulin-dependent, milder condition, occurring at all ages, although more frequently with increasing age. Genetic factors would be considered predominant in this type, unlike Type A. Much research remains to be done on this intricate problem.

Clinical Manifestations

Insulin deficiency may be present in a child for a relatively long period of time before the typical clinical symptoms appear. When they do occur, the onset is ordinarily abrupt, dramatic, and often frightening to both adult and child. Typically, the early manifestations of diabetes are weight loss, excessive thirst (*polydipsia*), excessive eating (*polyphagia*), the frequent passing of large amounts of urine (*polyuria*), and general weakness and fatigue. The signs and symptoms are accounted for by insulin deficiency. Often parents are confused by these symptoms and may attribute the child's repeated requests for foods and liquids, or his bedwetting, or his irritability, to emotional distress or behavior problems.

If these misinterpretations cause parents to delay seeking medical help, the child may proceed rapidly into a graver stage of the condition. Acidosis may develop, with increased dehydration leading to dry skin and mucous membranes, flushed cheeks, and sunken eyeballs. The child becomes progressively more drowsy and slips at length into coma. Thus, for some families, the onset of diabetes is marked by the dramatic arrival of a comatose child in the emergency room, with all the fear and anxiety that such an event provokes. As will be seen later, however, the emergence of the child from coma and his resumption of normal activity and appearance may be equally abrupt and dramatic once the diagnosis has been made and treatment begun.

Except for this acute phase, diabetes does not produce visible changes in the child. There may be minor variations in height and weight, with diabetic boys slightly underweight and diabetic girls showing a tendency toward being overweight in adolescence, but studies in this area are conflicting. In general, diabetic adolescents proceed through the stages of sexual maturation at normal times. Menarche is normal and fertility is not decreased, although fetal loss and increased incidence of neonatal deaths in diabetic women are well known.

Therapeutic Regimen

For most young patients, the first step in treatment of their diabetes is hospitalization. This is necessary, not only to reverse the initial symptoms of hyperglycemia, glycosuria, and acidosis, but also to develop—for both child and parents—a regimen that will prevent the future development of these symptoms. Once the diagnosis is confirmed, often by means of a simple blood test, the next steps involve the determination of the unique balance of insulin and diet that will maintain the normal growth and development of the child. This is rendered somewhat difficult by the well-documented tendency of the insulin requirement of the child to decrease four to eight weeks after the initial diagnosis. This stage, often referred to as the "honeymoon period," is more common in boys than in girls, in children who are overweight rather than undernourished, and in children for whom the age of onset is roughly between three and 12 years, as compared with younger or older patients.

The honeymoon period is a time when the hopes of child and parent are understandably raised and anticipations of injection-free years develop. Because it is almost certain that this period of partial remission will terminate gradually, over a six- to 24-month period, these hopes inevitably prove to be false. Consequently, most diabetologists consider it unwise to stop insulin injections altogether at this time. A shift to oral hypoglycemic agents is usually disappointing in its results. Very small insulin dosages are therefore continued so that the family can become accustomed to the necessity of incorporating this procedure into the regular family schedule throughout the patient's childhood.

Insulin is administered to the child by means of injection with hypodermic syringe. Most juvenile diabetics require two injections daily. Typically the injections are administered first by the parents, but the child is expected to assume responsibility for this aspect of his care as he grows older. The amount of insulin to be administered may vary with the results of the daily urinary tests described below. Also, insulin requirements increase with the child's age but decrease with exercise. As the seasons change, the child's patterns of activity change, and so do his insulin requirements. Here is a first example of the many judgments that must eventually be made by parent and child in managing the diabetes. A devoted but anxious father of a diabetic child referred wryly to the time of deciding upon and measuring the insulin as "the moment of truth."

One important indicator of changing insulin requirements is, of course, the measured amount of sugar in blood and urine. Blood sugar levels are evaluated only at times of visits to the doctor or, on his referral, to the laboratory. Urine appraisals, on the other hand, can be performed at home. Most diabetologists recommend that the urine be tested for sugar four times daily. The times of these evaluations are set rather rigidly: the second voiding of the day, samples before lunch and dinner, and a nighttime evaluation. Regular investigations of possible acetone in the urine are also made. Indications of unduly high sugar levels or of the presence of acetone mean changes either in diet or insulin or both. Persistent evidence of acetone alerts the family to impending acidosis and means a trip to the physician's office or emergency room. Not infrequently, a brief hospitalization is necessary for regulation.

For many children, weekly 24-hour collections of urine are required as part of the evaluation of glycosuria. This means that every urination during a 24-hour period must be collected, and an analysis made. Reports of daily and weekly urine tests are often sent regularly to the physician so that he may keep abreast of the development of the diabetic condition.

Dietary considerations constitute one of the most controversial aspects of the treatment of diabetes. The controversy over strict versus lenient dietary control has raged for years. Some authorities favor a relatively "free" diet, depending on growth records as indicators of the adequacy of intake. Such diabetologists may recommend the use of polyunsaturated fats, the avoidance of concentrated sweets, and a regular schedule of food intake, but little else. Signs of excess sugar in blood or urine are taken as indicators that increased insulin dosage is required.

At the other extreme are those who recommend a highly organized and restricted diet, with carefully calculated weights of carbohydrates, fat, and protein, together with measures of total calories, to serve as guidelines for food intake (Ehrlich, 1974). For such diabetologists, signs of excess sugar in blood or urine are often seen as indicators that the child has not adhered to his dietary regulations. Between these two extremes is an almost infinite number of gradations of recommendations. The effects that these various approaches might have on the child's growth and development are considered later in this chapter.

Whatever philosophy is accepted by a particular family, there are additional judgments to be made, often daily, regarding types and amounts of foods to be offered the child, as well as the schedule upon which the meals are organized. Because of the complexity of the therapy for diabetes, and the responsibility of parents and patient in conducting tests and administering insulin, there are formal classes that furnish instruction in these matters. Physicians, nurses, dietitians, and laboratory technicians join in training child patients and their parents.

Although the careful evaluation of sugar levels, adherence to dietary regulation, and the use of insulin can keep the majority of diabetic children in reasonably good control, there are some special problems inherent in this therapy. For one thing, juvenile diabetes is by its very nature difficult to control. Its characterization as "brittle" is all too accurate: often levels of blood and urine sugar rise without any obvious or subtle indicators of the reasons. This is particularly likely when the child reaches adolescence. It has been suggested that emotional stress, factors associated with maturational processes, changing exercise patterns, and rebellion against restrictions may contribute to this variability. In any case, it is well documented that even the most faithful adherence to dietary and exercise requirements may not be enough to ensure adequate control.

Two other problems stem from the use of insulin itself. There is the ever-present danger of an "insulin reaction," the use of more insulin than is necessary to handle the food intake. This results in abnormally low blood sugar (*hypoglycemia*) and has a variety of behavioral consequences. Headache, irritability, and hunger are early signs of an impending insulin reaction. Feelings of being "shaky inside" are next reported. If not interrupted, the reaction may lead to unconsciousness and seizures, with the possibility of resulting brain damage. Although an insulin reaction can be interrupted through the administration of sugar (orange juice, sugar cube, a variety of other products), the child may not be in a condition either to locate these aids or to get to another person for assistance.

The other special problem caused by insulin injections is less threatening to the child's physical integrity, but it is still important. This is the cosmetic problem that results in a small percentage of juvenile diabetic patients as the result of repeated injections. There may occur an atrophy of fatty tissue at the sites of the injections (*lipodystrophy*), which causes those areas to appear wasted. Such changes appear about six months after the beginning of insulin injections and ordinarily disappear in two to three years. There are some methods that have been suggested for the control of lipodystrophy. Rotating the sites of injection has been said to help, as have a particular technique of using the needle and the use of special varieties of insulin.

The life-saving insulin therapy, then, is a mixed blessing. For this reason, recent experiments on transplants have been hailed with increasing enthusiasm (Ehrlich, 1974). Transplanting an entire pancreas has the disadvantage of risking rejection of the heterologous tissue. In 1973, however, Lacy succeeded in transplanting the islets of Langerhans in inbred rats and thus in curing the diabetes (Kemp et al., 1973). Subsequent research confirmed the initial finding. The generalization of such research to human diabetic subjects would revolutionize the entire field of diabetes.

Complications

It is not unexpected to discover that so basic a metabolic disorder as diabetes carries with it the possibility of later complications. Three systems of the body—the vascular, the retinal, and the neural—seem particularly susceptible to injury as the result of years of diabetes. *Vascular changes* have been found long before the clinical evidence of diabetes, suggesting that degenerative processes may be an integral part of the condition. In one study of the nailfold capillaries of 60 newly diagnosed diabetic children, for example, 75% of the subjects showed morphological vascular changes, as compared with 6% of a control group (Kohrman and Weil, 1971).

Related in part to the vascular changes are evidences of *retinopathy*. The time of occurrence of retinal changes, shown in hemorrhages, aneurysms, or neovascularizations, is unpredictable, as are the rates of progression and the severity of the condition. In general, the average time of appearance of retinopathy in juvenile diabetes is 10 years after the growth spurt. Incidence varies from 50 to 100%, depending on time of onset of the condition. The incidence is 70% in the twentieth year of the condition (Paulsen and Colle, 1969). A less common visual complication is the development of cataracts. The average time of appearance is in the tenth year of the diabetes; incidence ranges from 2 to 4% depending upon age at onset.

A third site for the development of complications is the nervous system (*neuropathy*). As in the other complications, there is evidence of changes—here electromyographic and electroencephalographic changes—in a small proportion of juvenile diabetic patients early in life. Clinical manifestations are evidenced after eight to 10 years of diabetes, and their prevalence ranges from 5 to 50% (Paulsen, 1969). This range seems correlated with age, duration, and adequacy of control. Some studies indicate a significant correlation between abnormal EEGs and frequency of hypoglycemic coma or seizures.

PSYCHOLOGICAL ISSUES

From the above discussion, it is clear that the complexities of juvenile diabetes and its treatment generate numerous problems for the diabetic child and for those who deal with him. Some of these problems arise largely because diabetes is a chronic, lifelong condition. Others develop from the unique characteristics of diabetes and its treatment. Whatever their source, however, the problems serve to put into focus at least five significant psychological issues: 1) the interdependence of metabolic disorder and emotional behavior, 2) the impact of this lifelong condition upon the usual stages of child development, 3) the ways in which the clinical characteristics of juvenile diabetes affect the behavior of child and family, 4) reactions to the therapeutic regimen, and 5) the methods that children and their parents develop for coping with this chronic condition. The present section deals with these points.

Interdependence of
Metabolic Disorder and Emotional Behavior[2]

Studies of the relationship between physiological states and emotional behavior have waxed and waned in frequency over the past decades. Indeed, one observation goes back as far as the seventeenth century, when Thomas Willis hypothesized that diabetes, with its "sweet urine," might be caused by a "long sorrow" (Koski, 1969). Perhaps the peak period, however, was in the 1950s, when many efforts were made to correlate personality traits or structure with predisposition to certain disorders. One example is the early work of Dunbar (Koski, 1969), in which an effort was made to identify a personality profile of the diabetic patient. This effort, along with many others during the same period, was not supported by further research, and the notion of a specific per-

---

[2] Koski (1969) presents a general review of this research.

sonality picture typical of diabetes has largely disappeared from the literature.

Similarly, attempts to relate a specific nuclear conflict to the development of metabolic disorder have decreased in recent years. Alexander and French (1948), following Freud in viewing certain bodily changes as neurotic symptoms, suggested that the basic conflict in diabetic patients was one between opposing wishes to be cared for and demands that they care for others. Reasonable as such hypotheses may seem on first reading, they do not find confirmation in subsequent studies.

If a typical personality structure or central conflict predisposing to the development of diabetes seems unlikely, there remain two other types of interrelationships between emotional reactions and metabolic disorder for which some evidence may be adduced. The *onset* of clinical manifestations of diabetes, for example, may be related to events in the patient's life. It is becoming increasingly clear that a relationship between stress and illness exists (Holmes and Rahe, 1967; Coddington, 1972a, 1972b). Diabetes is apparently no exception to this general finding. For example, a recent study (Stein and Charles, 1971) of 38 preadolescent and adolescent diabetic patients indicates a significantly higher incidence of parental loss and severe family disturbance than in a group of 38 nondiabetic, chronically ill children. The authors hypothesize that juvenile diabetes develops as a consequence of psychological stress in the physiologically susceptible individual. This emphasis upon the significance of loss in precipitating the clinical symptoms of diabetes echoes earlier findings with adult patients. Slawson, Flynn, and Koller (1963), for example, conducted psychiatric studies of newly diagnosed adult diabetic patients and reported that, in a few cases, there was direct or indirect evidence of object loss. Instances of unresolved grief and clinical depression were also cited.

The *course* of the diabetic condition, as indicated by the various indices of clinical control—blood and urine sugars, acidosis, insulin reactions, and hospitalization—has also been thought to be affected by life stresses. A recent study by Koski and Kumento (1975), reporting follow-up data on a large group of diabetic children, noted that a fair proportion of children whose level of diabetic control became poorer over time had suffered loss of parents by death, illness, or divorce.

The early studies of Hinkle and Wolf (1952) on adult patients were successful in correlating changes in blood sugar and blood ketones with stress. Goldner (1958) argued that nondiabetic persons may react to severe emotional disturbances with metabolic changes, including hyperglycemia, glycosuria, and ketonuria. Perhaps this reaction is exaggerated in the diabetic patient because of a predisposition to disordered carbohydrate metabolism. Weil (1967) varied the level of competition and cooperation over two weeks in a diabetic camp, and studied the corresponding glycosuria levels in two groups of diabetic children varying in age. The older children showed increased glycosuria with exercise and emotional stress under conditions of competition, while the younger boys showed reduced glycosuria at a time when an increase would have been expected.

Many of these findings fit in with the interpretation of Warnberg (1974), who, in a review of the experimental literature on these points, emphasizes the contradictory nature of the obtained results. When stressful stimuli are presented and blood glucose levels are measured, both lowered and elevated levels have been reported, as in the Weil study. Life stresses may therefore be associated with a general metabolic instability.

Impact of This Lifelong
Condition upon Developmental Stages

Like their healthy peers, children with juvenile diabetes follow a developmental sequence, confronting the same problems and tasks with which all children in their culture must deal. The presence of a chronic lifelong disorder, however, may distort or complicate these tasks. It is during the earliest years of life that patterns of interaction between child and parent are learned. Any chronic condition in the child may evoke reactions from the parent, which in turn affect the child's developing behavior. Such early dyadic interactions may lead to strains and disharmonies between parent and child. Evidence from studies of other chronic conditions suggests that "reading" the responses of a fretful, irritable child is difficult (Korner, 1974); meeting the needs of such a child becomes a trying task.

Along different lines, there is evidence that dealing over time with a child whose chronic handicap does not improve or change may lead to a decrease in warmth and an increase in psychological distance between child and mother (Kogan, Tyler, and Turner, 1974). Such children may also be subject to inconsistent or inappropriate disciplinary techniques (Barsch, 1968; Hewett, 1970), as a consequence of parents' uncertainty as to what measures might help and what might damage a vulnerable, chronically ill child.

Any chronic condition that, like diabetes, requires occasional hospitalization may intensify the usual anxiety that separation from parents brings. If hospitalization is necessary at a time when the child is also just mastering the task of control of bodily functions (Freud, 1952), the situation becomes further complicated. The early steps toward autonomy, including self-control and independence from the mother, may be reversed, and the child must deal all over again with these significant tasks.

Establishment of peer relationships and the forging of a position with one's peers may be made difficult because of the clinical manifestations of diabetes and its treatment. To be thought of as somehow "different"—either by oneself or by others—is particularly threatening in the later years of childhood and early adolescence. For the diabetic child the "difference" may be subtle but none the less important: the need to eat a special snack in mid-morning, the occasional spell of dizziness or outright hypoglycemic reactions, the monitoring of exercise, the foregoing of refreshments at parties—all these spell out the fact that the childhood diabetic patient is not like other children. It is hardly surprising that these children indicate (Richardson, Hastorf, and Dornbusch, 1964) that they feel isolated and somehow inferior to others.

It is during the period of adolescence, with its special physiological changes and social demands, however, that the impact of diabetes upon developmental progress is probably the strongest. Almost without exception, writers on the adolescent diabetic describe the tendency of the adolescent patient to experiment with his therapy, to reject his diet, his urine tests, even his insulin, in an effort to assume control over his own destiny. Such an attitude of experimentation, rebellion, or independence is a necessary part of the adolescent development of all young persons as they work toward a definition of their own identity. When this attitude finds expression in the rejection of the therapeutic program, however, the consequences are serious or even fatal.

The social tasks that confront the adolescent are many, and each of them may be affected by the fact that the teenager is diabetic. Preadolescent and early adolescent diabetic patients often have realistic, even rosy, plans for the future. In one study of patients at a diabetic camp, for example (Davis, Shipp, and Pattishall, 1965), 85% reported they planned to marry, and, of these, 98% planned to have children. All were counting upon college or professional school, and 53% specifically anticipated entering medicine or nursing. Despite the efforts of parents, teachers, and physicians to support such plans, optimism becomes tempered and may shift to frustration as the patient enters adolescence.

Heterosexual behavior in some cases becomes sexual acting out, as the young person seeks to demonstrate his bodily integrity in the face of chronic illness. Increased knowledge of the genetic aspects of the diabetic condition may limit or prevent plans for marriage and family. Adolescent diabetic girls are well aware of the special risks that pregnancy carries for them and for their infant. Vocational plans may be altered or even dropped as job opportunities are closed to diabetic teenagers, insurance may be refused, and driver's licenses may not be granted, or renewed only with frequent special examination. Although persons with diabetes may perform on the job at a level equal to the general population, prospective employers are reluctant to hire them

(Partridge, 1967). According to one study (Forsham, 1959), the most common reasons for refusing employment to diabetic persons are fear of insulin shock on the job, frequent absenteeism, and a variety of economic considerations, such as anticipated increased compensation costs, increased insurance costs, and the expense of disability caused by complications.

There is little if any justification for many of these social restrictions. The American Diabetes Association's recommendations on employment emphasized considerations of public and individual safety in hiring persons with diabetes but stated that cooperative diabetic persons under good control were satisfactory employment risks. One study of industrial employment indicated that the person with diabetes was comparable to the nondiabetic worker in performance and absentee record (American Diabetes Association, 1957). Nevertheless, the changing of social attitudes is a slow, discouraging process, and the diabetic teenager who is attempting to assume an adult role is easily frustrated or depressed.

Effects of Clinical Manifestations of Diabetes

Like any chronic condition, diabetes carries with it the threat of separation, of unwelcome dependence upon others, and of clinical characteristics unique to diabetes that inevitably affect the behavior of the children and their families. One obvious aspect is the genetic predisposition to the development of diabetes mellitus. Knowledge of the genetic factor cannot help but raise feelings of guilt and mutual reproach in parents, however unjustified. Such knowledge may also affect the adolescent's plans for marriage and family.

Other psychologically significant aspects of the condition are equally clear. Diabetes is an "invisible" condition: there is nothing that can be perceived by the child or by others as indicating a defect or disability, with the possible exception of areas of scarring or lipodystrophy secondary to the insulin injections. The child patient is not seen as physically different by the casual observer except at those rare but dramatic times when an insulin reaction occurs. The child is usually able to perceive certain warning signs that a hypoglycemic reaction is impending. Such reactions are unpleasant and frightening and are easily apparent to others: the child becomes pale, sweaty, and tremulous; he may become unconscious; or, in extreme cases, he may develop seizures. At best, such episodes are embarrassing; at worst, they may end in physical injury if the child falls, and in cerebral damage if they occur frequently.

The later complications of diabetes are pervasive and anxiety provoking. Parents are more likely to be aware of the possibility of complications than are their children, although parental anxiety is communicated to the child easily, especially during times when clinical control of the condition is poor. Concern over complications is particularly difficult to deal with because there is no clear cut evidence that even the most successful chemical control of the condition will prevent or allay later adverse systemic developments.

The whole question of control affects child, physician, and family in significant ways. Maintaining acceptably low levels of sugar in blood and urine is the central task given child and family. Regular monitoring of the urine provides regular, objective evidence of the success or failure of the child and of the parents in accomplishing this task. However, by its very nature, the juvenile type of diabetes mellitus eludes exact, consistent control. Periods of poor control seem to occur capriciously, without apparent antecedents in diet, insulin, or emotional events. During such periods, parents search anxiously for factors that may have contributed to the poor control and, in their haste and anxiety, may blame the child, the doctor, or one another unjustly.

One additional finding adds to the difficulty: the earlier the onset of the condition, and the longer its duration, the less adequate the control (Koski, 1969). This means that, in general, as diabetic children grow older, they may expect to have greater difficulty maintaining an acceptable level of control, regardless of their adherence to a therapeutic regime.

Two questions remain regarding the psychological aspects of the clinical manifestations of juvenile diabetes: 1) How do the young patients view their condition? 2) How do they look upon themselves? Some evidence is available on both these points.

1) How Young Patients View Their Condition   Young children have limited understanding of their bodily processes, and, like all patients, may distort what they hear when they are in a stressful situation. One small diabetic girl, for example, cried inconsolably during the first days of her initial hospitalization until it was discovered that she thought she was about to die. Sympathetic inquiry finally unearthed the fact that she had overheard a remark that she had diabetes, which the child perceived as "die-abetes," and which she therefore took to mean that she was about to die "of betes."

Systematic inquiry into the perceptions that young diabetic patients have of their condition provides some helpful information on this point. In one study of five diabetic teenagers, for example (Kaufman and Hersher, 1971), interview techniques and drawings were employed to identify the patients' views of their illness and of their internal bodily functioning. Although these adolescents had participated in the usual hospital educational program and had been given considerable instruction regarding the diabetic condition, their interviews and drawings were largely influenced by their own private thought systems. Images of a half-pancreas, of blockages within the pancreas, of dilatation of the stomach through overeating occurred. These teenagers saw external deprivation as related to the diabetes and felt that they themselves were somehow damaged.

In another study of younger diabetic children (Thompson, Garner, and Partridge, 1969b), the patients were asked to describe how they felt when their control was good or poor and what led to these conditions. These subjects gave almost textbook descriptions of symptoms, identifying "tiredness" and "weakness" as indicators of poor control and emphasizing dietary indiscretions as the common cause. They described feeling more energetic when in good control and again emphasized diet as leading to this desirable condition. In their answers to other questions, these children were able to distinguish the physiological indicators of diabetes from other bodily cues, especially those that occurred when they were "sick." Diabetes was seen as something different from sickness.

These same young children, together with a group of adolescent patients, were later asked to rate themselves on a five-point scale indicating how well controlled they thought their diabetic condition was. Both groups thought they were in "excellent" or "good" condition. Parents of the younger children also rated their offspring as in good control. These optimistic views did not, however, correlate with ratings obtained from each child's clinical record by means of objective scales, based upon blood and urine determinations, acidosis, coma, and other clinical indicators.

It is sometimes argued that the invisibility of juvenile diabetes, the "honeymoon" period just following diagnosis, and the extended times of good control all combine to cause the child to underestimate the seriousness of the condition. There are, indeed, some data that suggest that the diabetic child seems to prefer his own difficulties to those of others. When an experimental situation involves a choice between diabetes and a different handicapping condition, most children seem to prefer diabetes. This is particularly interesting in the study of Davis, Shipp, and Pattishall (1965), in which all the children stated a preference for diabetes over constipation, and a high proportion preferred diabetes to having pimples or six toes. It is possible, of course, that one determining factor in some of these choices is visibility. The findings do, however, fit in with the studies of Barsch (1968) and others (Wright, 1973), which suggest that persons typically prefer a familiar to an unknown handicap.

On the other hand, in the study of young children mentioned above (Thompson, Garner, and Partridge, 1969a), a series of choices was given the child, in which freedom from diabetes was compared with other presumably desirable things, such as having more money, being better looking, playing games better, being smarter, and having more friends. In these comparisons, the majority of the children chose freedom from their diabetes.

2) How Young Patients View Themselves   The stereotype of the handicapped or chronically ill child is that of a dependent individual with low self-esteem. The extent to which diabetic young people conform to this stereotype is not altogether clear. As we have seen (Kaufman and Hersher, 1971), some diabetic teenagers saw themselves as damaged and deprived. There is other suggestive evidence on the same point. Thus, Richardson, Hastorf, and Dornbusch (1964), using nondirective interviews with a group of handicapped children, including some with juvenile diabetes, found more negative self-references in the handicapped group than in a group of control children. The handicapped children also made fewer references to relationships with others and to group membership, suggesting some social impoverishment. These findings are supported in the detailed study of Swift, Seidman, and Stein (1967), in which diabetic subjects were characterized by impaired self-perception and a high dependency.

That this is not an uncomplicated situation, however, is indicated by a more recent study of 40 adolescent patients (Partridge et al., 1972). These teenagers were compared on a number of instruments with 200 nondiabetic adolescents. For present purposes, it is significant that, on a questionnaire tapping the degree of independence that the respondent feels he has achieved in a wide variety of areas, the diabetic and control subjects were similar in the ages at which they reported achieving independence. However, the diabetic adolescents reported that they wished to undertake responsibility in these areas earlier than the control subjects reported that they wished to, an indication of strivings for even greater autonomy. In the area of assuming independent responsibility for the treatment of their diabetes, these adolescents also reported close agreement between their age of independence and the "ideal" age of independence, again departing from the stereotype of the dependent handicapped child.

Reactions to the Therapeutic Regimen

Treatment for childhood diabetes requires a daily regimen that is comprehensive and emotion laden. Four general areas of the child's life are implicated: the daily food intake, urinary excretions, hypodermic administration of insulin, and daily exercise. Observation and daily monitoring of these aspects of the child's life go on in different ways in different families depending on the personal needs and sensitivities of those concerned. Inevitably, however, the therapeutic requirements occupy a significant place in the family's activities. There are a number of reasons for this.

For one, all these areas are laden with special meaning for child and family. For another, the therapeutic procedures focus daily attention upon the details of bodily reactions that, for most people, proceed unheeded. In some instances, as in urinary testing, there is immediate evidence of good or poor control. All procedures require repeated daily tasks, to be performed on a particular schedule. All are to some extent limiting of the activity or freedom of child and family. All identify the diabetic child to his family as "different."

Furthermore, the therapeutic procedures are unusual in that they are placed in the hands of the parents and eventually of the child patient. In a very real sense, they require parents and children to become their own physicians, nurses, laboratory technicians, dietitians, physiotherapists. How families respond to these requirements will depend on the individual, lifelong patterns of response to stress that have developed.

The *dietary regimen* ordinarily entails the calculation of food intake as well as limitation of certain sorts of foods, although the degree of rigidity will vary with the particular treatment philosophy. Inevitably, however, some desserts and other sweets will be forbidden altogether, so that the child is, in a sense, deprived of those foods that he may find most gratifying. The mother who must enforce this rule finds herself in the unaccustomed role of depriving her child of food rather than nurturing him. Indeed, mother and child may see this ambivalent situation as a punishing one, for withholding dessert is a much used form of punishment for a variety of transgressions in many families, and candy is a popular form of reward for good behavior. It is not surprising, therefore, that the diabetic condition has been said to produce more anxiety in mothers than any other child handicap.

If to the limitation on sweets is added the requirement that food intake be calculated carefully, additional strains occur at the family table. The diabetic child is again singled out, this time as the one for whom second helpings, spontaneous samplings of food, or unemptied plates are all forbidden. Again, the attention given the nature and amount of food may become almost ritualistic.

Urinary testing typically occurs four times daily on a definite schedule. Children are early taught both control of excretory functions and the fact that, in our culture, these functions are private. To share them even with a parent violates important early prohibitions. To test, analyze, and record urinary output—even when done privately by the older child— still focuses attention on functions that most people take for granted. An added source of tension is to be found in the necessity for following a particular schedule of testing. The combined requirements of breakfast time, urinary testing time, and insulin time mean that for most parents of young diabetic children, and for the children themselves, sleeping late on any day is no longer possible.

Most diabetic children find *insulin injections* painful, or at least uncomfortable. Here again, the parent is in a conflictual situation, for the inflicting of pain is contrary to the parental role. As in the case of dietary restriction, this therapeutic requirement takes on a punishing cast, and is therefore often distasteful to parents, even though they comprehend perfectly that the alternative—not to inject—is fatal.

Monitoring daily exercise adds one more requirement to the list of daily tasks, although this is neither onerous nor painful. The main hazard is forgetfulness; the child does not remember to report that the class is going on a hike, or the mother fails to note the start of the baseball season, or forgets on which day the gym classes meet. The extra snack required by the child to cover such contingencies presents no problem, except for the embarrassment felt by the occasional child who must eat while his friends wait and watch.

Methods for Coping with the Diabetic Condition

To the extent that diabetes mellitus is a stressful condition, it will call forth from those dealing with it their preferred techniques for coping with stress. If preexisting conflicts become involved in dealing with the diabetes, the means of coping with it may take a particular direction. The parents whose guilt is aroused easily by the stress of their child's condition may employ techniques of overprotection in their transactions with the child. Those who contain their anxiety by means of compulsive orderliness and ritual may make of the therapeutic requirements a more rigid, orderly procedure than even the most meticulous diabetologist would require. The handling of diabetes may become interwoven with marital problems, which have long antedated the diagnosis of diabetes in the child.

One of the most thoroughgoing studies of the development of coping techniques in diabetes has been conducted by Koski (1969) in Finland. The investigator raises these fundamental questions: How does the family react initially to the discovery of diabetes in the child? What more enduring attitudes ("coping processes") develop within the family? How does the child react individually to the discovery of diabetes? How well adjusted are the diabetic children after one year's duration of the condition?

The 60 children in Koski's study were divided into two groups according to the level of their diabetic control. Material was obtained by means of a series of parent interviews, child interviews, a variety of tests and observations, and teacher questionnaires. From these sources, it appeared that the *initial reaction of the family* was one of bewilderment and shock, with a variety of fears, anxieties, and depressive thoughts expressed. As usual, feelings of guilt were frequent in the parents, some of them related to realistic considerations, and others distorted into aggression or wishful thinking. The initial disorganization soon declined, however, and most parents were able to make a reasonable adjustment within a few weeks. It is noteworthy that, at this early stage, the mothers of children whose diabetes was in good control were more expressive and emotional in their initial reactions, while those of children in the poor-control group were less expressive and seemed to deny their strong emotions.

The *child's immediate reaction* to the discovery of diabetes appeared to be anxiety, but it is impossible to assign this behavior exclusively to the diabetes because the child was also hospitalized for regulation. The severity of the child's initial reaction of anxiety, however, did not appear to be related to the later rating of control of diabetes that was achieved.

The *later reaction of the parents* led Koski to postulate a classification of coping devices. External methods of adjustment were displayed as the diabetic regimen became part of the daily life of the family. At the same time, parental anxiety declined, particularly as the child took over some responsibility for diabetic management. Constructive external coping devices were evidenced as parents developed responsible acceptance of the situation and were able to emphasize the normal aspects of the child's life while respecting the limitations and requirements imposed by the condition. Some nonconstructive coping methods were observed, such as poor cooperation or helplessness in dietary matters, inability to give injections, and failure to participate in medical check-ups. The constructive methods were more frequent in good than in poor control cases.

Internal coping methods identified in this investigation included the control of feelings of anxiety and depression by finding the care of the child rewarding, as well as such less constructive approaches as denial, helplessness, depressive reactions, and mobilization of aggression.

The *later reaction of the children* suggested that the poorly controlled group had more additional symptomatic reactions than did the well-controlled group. Those children with poor control of the diabetic condition seemed particularly susceptible to difficulties in sleeping, bladder control, language development, and social behavior.

A five-year follow-up of the same 60 children (Koski and Kumento, 1975) indicated that there were nine cases in which the diabetic control improved, from poor to good. These nine families became able, over the five years, to overcome their early helplessness, and the nine children were able to recover from initial depressive reactions.

Although the Koski investigation is one of the few that focuses upon the details of coping techniques, it should be noted that there are limitations imposed by the design of the study. It is virtually impossible to determine, for example, which findings might be peculiar to diabetic children and their families because no control population, either normal or with nondiabetic handicaps, was employed. Also, as in most such studies, it is difficult to distinguish cause from result. The poor-control group, for example, may well have presented more realistic problems of management to the family than the good-control group; the difference in coping techniques might thus be the consequence rather than the antecedent of level of control.

The study of Swift, Seidman, and Stein (1967) employed 50 diabetic children and 50 matched normal controls and provides some further information on family methods of dealing with diabetes. Anxiety, hostility, and dysphoria distinguished the diabetic group. Discovery of the diabetes seemed to lead to the development of extreme attitudes of either protection or dominance in the parents. Acceptance of the condition by child and parents, as well as adjustment to the home, was associated with the child's self-concept. Swift and his associates are careful to point out that their results may represent the effects of chronic illness and not of diabetes alone. They also emphasize the point that no causal relationship between coping techniques and diabetic control can be demonstrated in their results.

Other studies touch upon the same points. Bruch (1948) early identified three ways in which mothers coped with the diabetic regimen: 1) a tolerant and relaxed acceptance, 2) a perfectionistic overcontrol, and 3) erratic or poor cooperation. Acceptance was least frequent in the Bruch study, and poor cooperation most frequent. Perfectionistic overcontrol was associated with the satisfactory regulation of the diabetes, but the child was susceptible to behavior difficulties in other areas, such as poor school work, sudden rebelliousness, or stealing. Frankel (1975), in an investigation of 68 diabetic children by means of the sentence-completion test, reported a high frequency of responses expressing denial, wishful thinking, and nonacceptance on the part of the children. He hypothesizes that it may be useful for the patient not to accept the finality of diabetes, so that he can stay hopeful about the future.

In the study of Garner and Thompson (1974), 40 triads of mother, father, and diabetic child participated together in a series of tasks and were rated by three observers on a number of variables, including "comfort." The coping techniques employed by the most comfortable families, as determined by this method, delineate a composite picture of a traditional family structure. The child occupies a low status as compared with his parents, and accepts it; he sees himself as like his siblings; he sees his mother as more forceful than he would like and himself less so. In the comfortable family, child and parents admit the fact of the child's diabetes. Such anxiety as this may arouse is mastered.

The relationship of diabetes in the child to the parents' marital adjustment was studied by Crain, Sussman, and Weil (1966). Parents of 54 diabetic children and their siblings were compared with parents of 76 nondiabetic control children on four measures of marital functioning. On all measures, the nondiabetic couples achieved higher marital integration scores, although only one difference reached statistical significance. Such findings could be interpreted as evidence of displacement of concerns about the child to the interaction between the spouses, as a form of coping with stress. At the most parsimonious level, they indicate the enmeshment of the child's condition within the pattern of marital functioning.

By now it is clear that juvenile diabetes presents child and family with numerous problems, opportunities, and challenges. How these are met is determined by the family history of dealing with frustration, as well as by the details of the individual child's condition. Some families eventually work out a comfortable pattern of living with the condition; a few do not. For both comfortable and uncomfortable families, and also for the vast majority who fall between these two extremes, there are forms of psychological intervention that may be beneficial. These are taken up in the next section.

PSYCHOLOGICAL INTERVENTION

As in other lifelong, chronic conditions, so in diabetes there are both immediate and more remote goals of treatment. A crucial immediate goal is to maintain the clinical control of the diabetic condition at a high level. Equally important is the goal of shifting the responsibility for care from the team of professional persons who initially assumed it to the parents and ultimately to the child. This goal, incidentally, reflects the contemporary emphasis upon patients' responsibility for their own health and care in general. It was an integral part of diabetic therapy long ago, however, when office instruction and diabetic classrooms were first used as means of intervention.

These two goals, significant as they may be, are not enough. A child whose diabetes is in excellent clinical control, who dependably and accurately performs the tasks necessary to the care of his condition, but whose life is made constricted and anxiety ridden by these requirements, is still a disabled child. If the balance among food, insulin, and exercise is crucial in diabetes, so also is the balance between ignoring a chronic condition on the one hand and making it the focal point of one's entire existence on the other. Consequently, a third goal of treatment is to assist child and family in developing and maintaining a comfortable attitude toward the condition so that the child may achieve normal social and emotional development.

These are ambitious goals. Their accomplishment depends on contributions from many different professions: pediatrics, dietetics, laboratory technology, nursing, psychology, social work, and the numerous specialties (cardiology, ophthalmology, neurology) that deal with diabetic complications. As important as access to the various specialists may be, however, it is of even greater importance for the family to have the support of a continuing relationship with some member of the helping professions. Many professional persons can fulfill this role; the main factor is that the relationship be a continuing one so that the inevitable questions, doubts, fears, and anxieties that arise in the course of a chronic condition in a developing child can be dealt with at once.

Psychological Considerations in Achievement of Clinical Control

Almost since the therapeutic use of insulin in diabetes began, there has been a controversy over the relative values of rigorous versus relaxed control. Proponents of tight control argue that low glucose levels are associated with delayed or decreased complications such as nephropathy and retinopathy. Opponents of tight control point to the complications that such control itself may induce, including increased frequency of hypoglycemic reactions. The controversy continues to the present time. Indeed, the American Diabetes Association has recently accepted and published as official policy a statement favoring relatively tight control (Cahill, Etzwiler, and Freinkel, 1976). Predictably, this led to replies from those who are skeptical of its value (Ingelfinger, 1977).

The controversy is by no means trivial or academic. The later complications of childhood diabetes are severe and life threatening. If tight chemical control is effective in preventing or mitigating these later developments, then perhaps its achievement should be accepted as a goal, no matter what the cost. The question is one of available evidence on both sides. And, as in most such cases, the evidence is conflicting.

To begin with, it appears that some types of changes that may eventuate in later complications are discernible even before the clinical manifestations of the diabetes. Particularly in the case of cardiovascular problems, we may be dealing with an inherent aspect of the diabetic process rather than with complications (Paulsen and Colle, 1969). When prospective studies are reviewed, as in the Knowles report of 300 studies (Kohrman and Weil, 1971; Cahill, Etzwiler, and Freinkel, 1976), no convincing evidence favoring or disconfirming a relationship between control and complications emerges. In the University Group Diabetes Project (Cahill et al., 1976), five different forms of therapy were studied; none demonstrated an unequivocal effect of treatment upon microvascular lesions. Such findings would argue against the recommendation of tight control as preventive of later complications.

On the other hand, recent studies on infrahuman animals have yielded evidence of a relationship between reduction of hyperglycemia in these animals and the prevention or mitigation of lesions that resemble retinopathy, nephropathy, and neuropathy. In one such study, of diabetic dogs (Bloodworth and Engerman, 1973), those animals kept under strict control showed a 10% incidence of vascular disease after five years; those under poor control showed an 80% incidence after the same time lapse.

Extension of such studies to human subjects seems to suggest that close control of hyperglycemia is associated with decreased retinopathy. It is this sort of evidence that supports the American Diabetes Association's policy that " . . . current clinical and experimental data clearly demonstrate that optimal regulation of glucose levels should be achieved in the treatment of diabetes, particularly in young and middle-aged persons . . ." (Cahill, Etzwiler, and Freinkel, 1976). The rejoinder to this argument has been to ask whether tight control does not carry with it an undue risk of hypoglycemic episodes, with their known relationship to cerebral deterioration (Ingelfinger, 1977).

The controversy over control is further complicated by a lack of standard criteria for control. By implication, "good" or "optimal" control involves levels of blood glucose that approximate those of healthy persons. But this would require continuous measurement of glucose concentration in the patient, together with multiple insulin injections—an achievement which seems remote at best. It is important to note, however, that no party to the controversy advocates loose control; and most diabetologists argue, in the last analysis, for individualization of treatment.

The psychological aspects of the tight versus loose control continuum are equally significant, and the evidence for them equally conflicting. The contribution of the child's emotional state to the level of control has been discussed earlier; if the enforcement of rigid requirements of management intensifies emotional reactions, the value of tight control may be offset. On the other hand, as indicated by Weil's results (1967), better control can be achieved when the child is free from crises; if the use of less stringent management requirements makes for relaxation, then the value of loose control is enhanced.

More specific consequences of rigid management were hinted at by Koski (1969), Bruch (1948), and others, where the mother's perfectionistic application of requirements was associated with the child's behavior difficulties in other fields. A similar finding is reported by Travis (Warnberg, 1974), who relates the degree of adolescent rebellion to the amount of rigidity in preadolescent diabetic management. Certainly compulsive orderliness is a not uncommon means of handling anxiety, and a rigid program of management encourages the further development of such a technique in those children and parents who may already be finding relief in its use. At present, however, neither research findings nor theoretical formulations provide a definitive answer to the relative value of the various levels of stringency of control.

Psychological Considerations in Achievement of Responsibility for Care

Eventually, all diabetic patients assume responsibility for the care of their own condition. They weigh, measure, or otherwise monitor their food intake. They perform their own urine testing at the required times and determine their insulin dosage. They measure and inject their own insulin. They learn the preliminary signs of hypoglycemia and acidosis and take appropriate preventive and therapeutic measures against these developments. They anticipate situations of increased exercise, emotional stress, or mild illness, and adjust food and insulin accordingly.

The initial responsibility for these details of management belongs to the parents. The effects of the management regimen, however, extend throughout the entire family. They are felt in the limitation of family activities, in a continuous vigilance toward the diabetic child's condition and an alertness to signs of adverse reactions, and in an emphasis upon daily scheduling. The processes involved in monitoring the child's condition are time consuming and, for some parents, unpleasant or even frightening. Like all lifelong, chronic conditions, juvenile diabetes may raise the general level of stress in the family, and require of family members additional effort and energy as they cope with management requirements.

It is always assumed that the child will take over the details of management eventually. This is a task that extends over many years and requires the patience and cooperation of parents and physician. It is primarily a learning task, complicated by the unique fears, anxieties, and attitudes developed around the condition by each individual child. Like all learning tasks, however, success in acquiring independence in self-care depends on 1) the child's *readiness* to undertake the responsibility, 2) the *methods of teaching* the necessary skills and information, and 3) the *consequences* of the learning. Each of these aspects of the learning process is considered separately below.

Readiness to Learn   The initial phase of diabetes, when parents and child have just been told the diagnosis and its implications, is at once the most convenient and least appropriate time to begin instruction. The shock and disorganization that characterize this early period make the process of learning and remembering difficult if not impossible.

However, the resources for teaching are available at this time, with hospital classrooms, dietitians, laboratory technicians, nurses, and physicians ready to demonstrate, instruct, and support. The opportunity to begin at the beginning, as it were, before misconceptions and adverse attitudes have become set, is one that is hard to forego. Consequently, most new patients begin their learning before they are emotionally ready.

Parents often report later that they remember very little of what was told them during the early days of instruction. Learning about diabetes is not restricted to content alone, however. Parents do recall the early classroom meetings as valuable opportunities to share with other patients and families the experiences of dealing with this new and disturbing event. And information itself can contribute to the alleviation of the initial anxiety. As one parent put it (Koski, 1969), "It is less frightening when you get to know the illness." More than that, the assumption during the first classroom sessions that something can be done about the condition also serves to allay feelings of helplessness and disorganization.

The child's readiness to learn to apply the information and skills required for self-care varies with a number of factors. *Chronological age* is an obvious criterion, although the different aspects of self-care might reasonably be undertaken at different times. Urine testing, for example, is more within the competence of a younger child than is insulin measuring and administration, or diet calculation. Writers in the field still differ in the recommended ages. One source (Paulsen and Colle, 1969), suggests that the child who is as young as six years can be taught to perform urine tests, and that a child of nine or ten years can give his own injections. Others set the ages somewhat later. Although the individual worker's experience may be a reasonable guide here, there are other, more objective indicators that can be used.

The child's measured *store of information* is one possibility. Many diabetic classrooms employ tests of one sort or another to evaluate the progress of their patient-students. More formal, standardized instruments have also been employed. Some years ago Etzwiler (1962) constructed a 34-item test of knowledge of diabetes and administered it to a group of diabetic children from six to 17 years of age. The patterns of increasing knowledge with increasing age varied with the particular area of information being tapped. The significance of such changes is considered below. For present purposes, however, it may be noted that Etzwiler's early results suggested the chronological age 12 to 13 as a reasonable average time for the child to assume responsibility for self-care.

In a more recent study (Garner, Thompson, and Partridge, 1969b; Partridge et al., 1972), a group of diabetic children and teenagers responded to a 25-item multiple-choice test of diabetic information, and scores were analyzed by age. The parents of 40 of the younger subjects also responded to the items. A fairly steady increase in mean score with age was obtained, up to the age of 15; there was no significant gain in score between the ages of 15 and 18. At age 12 the children scored as well as their fathers; by age 15 the teenagers approached the level of understanding of the mothers, whose scores were the highest of any of the groups and who typically carry most of the responsibility for the care of the diabetics. If information alone is used as a guide, therefore, it appears that young people between the ages of 12 and 15 are ready to assume responsibility for their own care.

Further analysis of the information test indicated that those diabetic children and adolescents who had developed diabetes when they were younger than 10 years old had a very poor understanding of the condition and its management. This is probably attributable to the fact that they were too young to comprehend the classroom materials when they were first hospitalized. Perhaps some had never attended class at all, because of their young age.

When the various areas of information are examined, further data emerge. The Kaufman and Hersher (1971) study suggested that teenagers' fantasies about diabetes revealed many misconceptions about the condition as it related to their own bodies, despite extensive instruction in the diabetic classroom. And in Frankel's (1975) study, confusion over or rejection of heredity as an etiological factor in diabetes occurred. Of his group of subjects, 42% had a family history of diabetes, but only 21% indicated that they might have developed the condition because of heredity. Forty-one percent specified a variety of extraneous causes, such as shock or fright.

Analysis of items frequently missed in an extension of the Etzwiler investigation (Collier and Etzwiler, 1971) revealed frequent misunderstandings in the areas of recognizing symptoms of acidosis, testing for acetone, differences among varieties of insulin, and in a number of items relating to dietary control. In the more recent investigations of Garner and Thompson (1974), items inquiring about genetics, diet calculation, and identification of symptoms relating to level of control were failed with significant frequency by children nine to 13 years of age. Of most concern to these authors, however, were two failures having to do with the philosophy of management. More than half of the respondents characterized a diabetic diet as made up of "special foods," rather than as a "well balanced diet that the whole family can use." Even more significantly, a majority of the respondents indicated that the preferred philosophy of care involved "rigidly following the rules for control, not engaging in unusual activities, and always asking the doctor before doing anything different." The relationship between such an implicit philosophy and the development of orderly, even compulsive behavior, together with dependence upon others, seems clear.

Another indicator of appropriate ages for self-care is provided by *reports of the patients* themselves. In the studies of young children and adolescents referred to above (Partridge et al., 1972; Garner and Thompson, 1974), the subjects were asked when they had assumed responsibility for insulin injections, urine testing, and diet control. They were also asked to indicate what they considered the "ideal" ages for assuming these responsibilities. The younger children reported that they undertook these tasks at the average age of 9.1 years, but they considered this too early. Their recommendation, as represented by the average "ideal" age, was 11.9 years. The teenagers, on the other hand, reported an average age of 12.6 years for assuming responsibility, and they considered this appropriate, as indicated by their average "ideal" age of 12.5 years.

The parents of the younger children in these studies also responded to the questionnaire regarding the age at which their children should assume responsibility for their care, and then all three together arrived at a consensus. Realistically, the higher the child's score on the information test, the younger was the age agreed upon. Once again, the necessity for individualizing the details of diabetic management to suit the particular needs and capacities of the child is apparent.

A final indicator relating to readiness to learn is to be found in the actual *performance* of the child as he attempts to carry out the tasks required for self-care. There is no substitute for direct observation of the behavior of parent and child. Indeed, such observation often exposes errors and difficulties not hinted at by interviews, tests, and questionnaires. In the familiar study of Watkins et al. (1967), observers visited adult diabetic patients in their homes and recorded the behavior of the patients as they administered their insulin or took their oral medication. Fifty-eight percent of the 115 patients on insulin made dosage errors, of which 35% were considered "potentially serious." A common error involved reading the wrong scale on a "convertible" syringe. Somewhat similar frequencies of errors in oral medication were reported. Follow-up observations on a sample of the patients 12 to 18 months later found 20% making fewer errors than before but 48% making more errors than before.

Comparable data for childhood diabetic patients are not available. However, a similar approach to the problem, involving testing in a practical situation, was made in the Partridge-Garner-Thompson studies (Garner, Thompson, and Partridge, 1969a; Garner and Thompson, 1974). After the instruction and day-to-day practice in diet calculation and food-weighing, which were part of the classroom offerings, were complete, the children and their parents participated in a weight-estimation experiment. Subjects were provided with samples of five common foods and were asked to demonstrate, without scales, the servings that represented a given weight in grams. The servings were then weighed, and instances of overestimation tabulated. Not only were there numerous examples of gross errors of estimation, but, more significantly, there was no relationship between the accuracy of estimation and score on the information test. This may be a situation analogous to the Watkins study, in which behavioral observations unearth errors not discovered through paper-and-pencil, or more casual, methods. Certainly the whole area of direct observational approaches to the details of self-care deserves more extensive and careful research.

Methods of Teaching Effective teaching in this field must begin with some effort at alleviating the shock and anxiety that prevent adequate learning in the initial period of diabetic onset. Some practical steps may speed the process of overcoming the initial anxiety. These include the assumption of an optimistic attitude on the part of those working with the family, a positive but not unduly demanding schedule of diet, urinary testing, and insulin injection, and an opportunity for the child and parents to verbalize and share their fears and misconceptions (Koski, 1969; Ehrlich, 1974). Perhaps most important is the willingness of professional personnel to proceed slowly and patiently during this early period, to repeat information and instructions as often as necessary, and to be easily available to listen to child and family and to offer support.

Once this initial period has passed, the usual introduction that diabetic children and their parents are given to information regarding the condition and its management occurs in the diabetic classroom during initial hospitalization. Because of the complexity of the condition and its management, many professional persons participate in these classes, including nurses, pediatricians, dietitians, technicians, psychologists, and social workers. The curriculum varies from one hospital to another, but all offer a combination of didactic material, often based on a textbook, and demonstrations of the various procedures involved.

Because of practical considerations, many hospital diabetic classes are made up of a heterogeneous group of patients, ranging widely in age and in duration and severity of diabetic symptoms. Classes organized for adults obviously will not appeal to small children. The problems that arise in the care of adult-onset diabetes are different in many ways from those that arise for young children. Special consideration of the role of the parents and siblings is necessary in the case of child patients but not in the case of independent adults. For these and many other reasons, it is desirable for classes to be grouped by age and for many young children and their parents to receive specially organized and selected types of instruction.

The formal imparting of information may begin very early in the child's life, depending on his age of onset. In one of Etzwiler's early studies (1962), children reported being read to about diabetes from the age of eight years on. When the initial hospitalization is over, and child and parents gradually become accustomed to the details of the condition, the sources of information widen. In the study by Collier and Etzwiler (1971), diabetic children and their parents were asked from what source most of their knowledge about diabetes came. Both the children and their parents regarded the family physician or pediatrician as the primary source of their information. Fewer children reported this than did their parents, however, which led the authors to speculate that the physician was not dealing with the child patient directly but rather focusing on the parents. The children reported obtaining more information from books and pamphlets, nurses, and American Diabetes Association meetings and materials than did their parents.

Although there have been many advances in teaching techniques over the past years, few of these have yet been adopted by those professional persons who instruct diabetic children and their parents. Some use of teaching machines has been reported (Collier and Etzwiler, 1971); extension of this method might well be useful. Warnberg (1974) suggests the application of an operant conditioning model in the training of children and adolescents to adhere to a program of control. He cites the work of Wright, Woodcock, and Scott (1969) on the use of conditioning techniques with preschool children who refused oral medication. Similar methods of shaping and reinforcement may well be appropriate to some aspects of diabetic self-care, but the research relevant to this point is not yet available.

One development that many writers agree would facilitate the details of diabetes management is the simplification of some of the equipment used. Confusions over scale reading in "convertible" syringes, for example, or between the varieties of slow- and fast-acting insulin, are known to lead to errors in medication (Watkins et al., 1967). Great strides have been made in other areas in specifying the sources of scale-reading errors and designing methods for overcoming them. Application of these data to the specific problems of insulin identification and use might well simplify instruction and decrease errors. Again, the actual research in this area remains to be done.

An integral part of effective teaching is regular review. The well-known tendency of complex learned information to fade with time, and particularly to become simplified through interaction of emotions and attitudes with the learned material, must certainly be involved in the information and techniques acquired by the diabetic child. Adaptation to the condition, while it brings relief of anxiety, may also lead to simplification and distortion. Such a relationship is suggested by Watkins' (1967) finding that the frequency of errors made in insulin administration increased with the duration of known diabetes, and also increased over the 12- to 18-month period studied. In addition, the period of adolescence is a time of particular susceptibility to careless and forgetful management, for a variety of developmental and individual reasons.

Systematic review and rechecking of information and practice are therefore essential. The provisions made for such review will vary with the particular diabetic practice. Most classrooms offer regular sessions to their patients. Most pediatricians reserve a portion of the regular follow-up visits of their patients for review and further instruction. In a number of diabetic practices, a bulletin or a newsletter, published regularly, calls the attention of patients and their families to various aspects of self-care and furnishes information regarding recent developments in the field (Holcomb, Partridge, and Belknap, 1928–). The well-known human tendency to postpone or to avoid visits to medical settings, however, makes it desirable to have special inducements or special sorts of review procedures to reach young patients. Some of these approaches are described below.

Consequences of the Learning   What happens immediately after the acquisition of new skills or new information is crucial in determining how well the material is integrated into the learner's behavior. Ideally, careful adherence to management requirements should provide immediate gratifying consequences to the child and parent. This is, in fact, often the case. Daily evidence of acceptably low urine glucose levels provides immediate evidence of the results of efficient management. The child profits from feeling more energetic, and the parents from temporary relief from stress. If chemical balance can be maintained, at least the unfortunate consequences of hyperglycemia, acidosis, and hospitalization can be avoided.

The difficulty comes from the observation that, for a sizeable proportion of children, juvenile diabetes is extremely difficult to control, so that the chemical indicators may vary without apparent relationship to management. In one study (Garner and Thompson, 1974), neither scores on information tests nor accuracy of food-weight estimation was related to the clinical control of the child as measured by a variety of tests. Furthermore, a positive relationship between the level of clinical control and the development of future complications has not been demonstrated unequivocally. Thus, neither the immediate nor the remote consequences of learning to assume management effectively are necessarily positive. Such a situation makes consistent learning over time unusually difficult.

Some serendipitous results of the successful learning of how to manage diabetes should be mentioned. Training the child in self-care before he is ready, or training in fairly rigid routines, may lead to greater adolescent rebellion, much as too early toilet training may lead to enuresis and encopresis later (Etzwiler, 1962). Thus, waiting for the indicators of readiness, and proceeding with respect for the child's capacities and attitudes, may reap the benefits of an easier adolescence. Also, encouraging the child to assume responsibility for his own care appropriately may eventuate in some lessening of maternal anxiety, an important goal in its own right if the entire family is to achieve a comfortable balance with regard to the diabetes. Still another advantage of adequate training in management is to be found in the child's own feelings of achievement. Swift and his associates (1967) point out, for example, that attention to self-care and successful assumption of responsibility lead to the development of feelings of competence and adequacy. Such developments are significant in the life of any child, but they assume special importance in the life of a handicapped child, whose self-esteem is unusually vulnerable to damage.

Special Approaches to Social and Emotional Problems

The nature of juvenile diabetes and its management occasionally produce problems that require specialized techniques of intervention. At various times, systematic psychotherapy has been recommended for most diabetic patients as supplementary to general medical care. The particular therapeutic approach favored has changed over the years, ranging from relaxation therapies, to extended psychiatric study of a more conventional type, to various techniques of confrontation. At present, however, it is more common to develop individualized approaches for those relatively few groups of young patients and families who seem to need special assistance.

Such needs arise most commonly when either the diabetic condition itself or aspects of the management regimen become involved with old problems that the patient or family faces. The father who hopes for a rugged, athletic son to compensate for his own physical shortcomings, the mother who is guilty over real or imagined neglect of the child, the adolescent who is already anxious and uneasy over his own competence—all may use the diabetic condition as a pathway for the handling of their prior problems. Some of the contemporary approaches to psychological entanglements of this sort are reviewed below.

Group Approaches with Adolescent Patients   The problems of testing, acting out, and rebelling, which become implicated in the diabetes of the teenager, are inherent parts of the adolescent's transactions with adults in authority. To be helpful to the teenager, then, the therapeutic approach should minimize involvement with authority figures. This can often be accomplished through the use of groups of diabetic adolescents, in which attitudes, problems, and solutions can be shared with peers. Medical and other specialists can be used as consultants to such groups, but group leaders are best recruited from young trained persons closer to the patients' age. Experience with such groups indicates that discussion ranges freely over the details of diabetic management and self-care, to the more compelling issues of job opportunities, dating, marriage, and parenthood. Available consultants might well include social workers and vocational counselors (Garner, Thompson, and Partridge, 1968; Thompson et al., 1968).

Young diabetic adults who have achieved success in their vocations, or have earned recognition as athletes or performers or independent world travelers, are often glad to participate in such adolescent groups. They may serve as helpful models to the diabetic teenagers who are unsure of their own competencies and limitations.

A special meeting place apart from adult and child patients has also been found valuable (Paulsen and Colle, 1969). When clinic visits are necessary, a special clinic for those between 14 and 21 years of age has been used, where both pediatricians and internists are available. The transition of care to the internist may then be accomplished slowly, in an orderly way.

Family Therapy   Juvenile diabetes is uniquely a family matter; thus, when special difficulties arise they are likely to involve all family members. Indeed, we have seen that families can be characterized by the differences in comfort with which they deal with the diabetes, and we have said that a comfortable adjustment of the family to the condition is an important goal of treatment. Moreover, some contemporary writers now argue that certain symptoms of chronic conditions such as diabetes are part and parcel of the family pattern of organization. Minuchin (1974), for example, relates the labile or brittle type of juvenile diabetes to family organization, the involvement of the child patient in parental conflicts, and to the physiological vulnerabilities of the child. He presents convincing evidence in the case of two diabetic sisters, one of whom was more deeply embedded in the conflict between her parents than was the other. Indicators of emotional arousal obtained from blood samples showed significantly greater and more prolonged stress in the "trapped" child than in her sister. The same indicators showed reduction of interspouse stress in the parents when they assumed their parental functions and interacted with their daughters in the parental rather than the marital role.

It is not surprising, therefore, to discover that family therapy is often suggested as a means of assisting troubled diabetic children and their parents (Thompson, 1973). The "structural family therapy" of Minuchin is one such approach. Another, based to some extent upon the Minuchin rationale, is under way at the University of Maryland School of Medicine (Bauer, Harper, and Kenny, 1974). This approach involves both individual and family therapy. Techniques of inducing relaxation and of learning to identify anxieties are employed in the individual sessions, where emphasis is placed on individual autonomy. The family sessions focus on two-person communications to facilitate conflict resolution. Because this therapeutic endeavor is part of a more general research on childhood diabetes, it is anticipated that systematic information concerning the place of family therapy in diabetes will be forthcoming. Still another approach, described by Haimowitz (1972), is to employ Berne's Transactional Analysis in dealing with the psychological problems of diabetic families. This group approach requires the individual to consider the present rather than the past and to develop new alternatives in the present situation.

Genetic Counseling   Misconceptions of parents regarding the genetic transmission of a predisposition to diabetes are common. The uncertainty still surrounding the exact pattern of transmission serves to increase the parental confusion. Consequently, many workers with diabetic children have found value in recommending, or themselves conducting, some sessions in which the genetic implications of the condition may be explained and discussed.

There are two times in the span of any diabetic child's life when genetic counseling is most appropriate. One is at onset of the condition, when the parents' anxiety and bewilderment provide a fertile field for the development of guilt and misconception. The parent who has diabetic relatives may assume exclusive responsibility for the child's condition, and, without intervention, may suffer needlessly from guilt and self-recrimination. At this time it is particularly important to counsel the parents regarding the probability that the abnormal potential is present in both parents if it finds expression in the child.

The other time for genetic counseling is at the patient's adolescence, when questions of marriage and parenthood arise. Often, discussion of genetic factors occurs in the adolescent groups. Here again, however, the lack of unequivocal information limits the counseling.

Resources in the Wider Community   Like other children, the diabetic child is a member not only of his own family but also of many other more remote but still important groups. He goes to *school,* and does not, according to a wide range of studies (Kubany, Danowski, and Moses, 1956; Ack and Weil, 1961), differ from his classmates in level of intellectual functioning or in school achievement. He may, however, be perceived by them as different, despite his desires to conceal some of the obvious aspects of his regimen. He may have to have a snack regularly at mid-morning; or he may need sugar cubes or fruit juice to offset impending hypoglycemic reactions. He may need frequent drinks of water, or he may make frequent trips to the bathroom. These departures from the usual behavior of a school child will not go unnoticed by his peers. Some diabetic children, fearing ridicule, ignore warning signals or regimens and put themselves in jeopardy. One child, for example, ran away and hid whenever an insulin reaction seemed imminent, and on occasion was found only after he had slipped into unconsciousness.

Given adequate information, the diabetic child's teacher may provide significant support in the school situation. The teacher needs information not only about diabetes in general, but also about the condition and reactions of the particular child. Knowledge of what sorts of emergencies may arise and what is to be done if they do serves to allay the teacher's anxiety. The American Diabetes Association publishes a succinct, practical sheet of informational material for school personnel that many school systems use regularly. A calm, understanding teacher can serve as a helpful model to the class in demonstrating acceptance of the juvenile diabetic patient as an essentially normal child.

Another valuable resource in many communities is the *diabetic camp*. Special camps organized around the medical and social needs of diabetic children are available both in the United States and in Canada. Association with other childhood diabetic patients, good medical and dietary supervision, and opportunities to extend further the responsibility for self-care are among the advantages of the special camp. A period at camp for the child also provides a brief respite from the heavy responsibility that parents of diabetic children assume.

Although there are undoubted benefits from the diabetic camp, there are those who argue against them, on the grounds that segregation of any handicapped group from the general population is undesirable. Some diabetic children refuse to attend special camps, feeling that their "difference" from others would thereby be emphasized. Whether or not a child should attend diabetic camp is an individual decision. The decision will be colored, however, by the knowledge that many ordinary camps for children hesitate to accept the responsibility for children with diabetes.

The *American Diabetes Association, Inc.* is another community resource that many families find useful. It provides a wide variety of information to diabetic patients and to those who work with them. The association supports and stimulates research, publishes a journal, and may adopt and disseminate policy regarding various aspects of diabetic treatment. State branches of the association furnish local contacts for diabetic patients and their families. There is also a recently organized group called the Juvenile Diabetes Foundation, which has many chapters and which specializes in offering assistance to those with the juvenile form of the condition.

In 1974, the Congress passed the Diabetes Mellitus Research and Education Act, which established a National Commission on Diabetes. That commission's final report to the Congress characterized diabetes as a major health problem and outlined a long-range plan to combat the condition. The plan calls for basic research into the causes, cure, and prevention of diabetes, and into the improvement of treatment methods. It calls also for the development of manpower for diabetes research and care, and of activities to bring health care to the diabetic population.

SUMMARY

Juvenile diabetes is a condition whose unpredictable clinical manifestations, demanding treatment, and involvement with social and emotional behavior exert pressure and make heavy demands on children and their parents. For the occasional family, the demands are too great. For other families, they are met relatively easily. It is the goal of those who work in the field of juvenile diabetes to facilitate normal growth and development of the children, within a context of comfortable family interaction. To achieve this goal requires the cooperative effort of many professionals.

If juvenile diabetes is one of the most complex and demanding of chronic childhood conditions, it is also one of the most challenging. The opportunities for research are almost limitless. Much remains to be learned about etiology, genetic transmission, regimens, teaching methods, and techniques of coping with stress. But the opportunities for service are also almost limitless, as research points the way toward more effective intervention. Only an interdisciplinary team committed to this dual task can hope to unravel, eventually, the intricacies of juvenile diabetes.

REFERENCES

Ack, M. I., and Weil, W. B., Jr. 1961. Intelligence of children with diabetes mellitus. Pediatrics 28:764–770.

Alexander, F., and French, T. M. (eds.). 1948. Studies in Psychosomatic Medicine. Ronald Press, New York.

American Diabetes Association. 1957. Analysis of a survey concerning employment of diabetics in some major industries. Diabetes 6:550–553.

Anderson, K. A. 1971. The "shopping" behavior of parents of mentally retarded children: The professional person's role. Ment. Retard. 9:3–5.

Anderson, K. A. 1974. Mothers of retarded children who shop for professional help. Clin. Pediatr. 13:159–161.

Barsch, R. H. 1968. The Parent of the Handicapped Child. Charles C Thomas, Springfield, Ill.

Bauer, R., Harper, R., and Kenny, T. 1974. Treatment for uncontrolled juvenile diabetes. Pediatr. Psychol. 2:2–3.

Bloodworth, J. M. B., Jr., and Engerman, R. L. 1973. Diabetic microangiopathy in the experimentally diabetic dog and its prevention by careful control with insulin. Diabetes 22(Suppl. 1):290.

Bruch, H. 1948. Physiologic and psychologic interrelationships in diabetes in children. Psychosom. Med. 11:200–210.

Cahill, G. F., Jr., Etzwiler, D. D., and Freinkel, N. 1976. "Control" and diabetes. N. Engl. J. Med. 294:1004.

Cherry, T. J., Thompson, C. W., Partridge, J. W., and Garner, A. M. 1968. The happening. Diabetes Bull. 44:2.

Coddington, R. D. 1972a. The significance of life events as etiologic factors in the diseases of children: I. A survey of professional workers. J. Psychosom. Res. 16:7–18.

Coddington, R. D. 1972b. The significance of life events as etiologic factors in the diseases of children: II. A study of a normal population. J. Psychosom. Res. 16:205–213.

Collier, B. N., and Etzwiler, D. D. 1971. Comparative study of diabetes knowledge among juvenile diabetics and their parents. Diabetes 20:51–57.

Crain, A. R., Sussman, M. B., and Weil, W. B., Jr. 1966. Effects of a diabetic child on marital integration and related measures of family functioning. J. Health Hum. Behav. 7:122–127.

Davis, D. M., Shipp, J. C., and Pattishall, E. G. 1965. Attitudes of diabetic boys and girls toward diabetes. Diabetes 14:106–109.

Ehrlich, R. M. 1974. Diabetes mellitus in childhood. In H. W. Bain (ed.), Pediatric Clinics of North America, 21:871–884. Symposium on Chronic Disease in Children. W. B. Saunders Co., Philadelphia.

Etzwiler, D. D. 1962. What the juvenile diabetic knows about his disease. Pediatrics 29:135–141.

Forsham, P. H. (ed.). 1959. Current trends in research and clinical management of diabetes. Ann. N. Y. Acad. Sci. 82:229–235.

Frankel, J. J. 1975. Juvenile diabetes—the look from within. In Z. Laron (ed.), Diabetes in Juveniles: Medical and Rehabilitation Aspects. Modern Problems in Paediatrics. Vol. 12, pp. 358–360. S. Karger, Basel.

Freud, A. 1952. The role of bodily illness in the mental life of children. In R. S. Eissler, A. Freud, H. Hartmann, and E. Kris (eds.), The Psychoanalytic Study of the Child 7:69–81. International Universities Press, New York.

Ganda, O. P., and Soeldner, S. S. 1977. Genetic, acquired and related factors in the etiology of diabetes mellitus. Arch. Int. Med. 137:461–469.

Garner, A. M., and Thompson, C. W. 1974. Factors in the management of juvenile diabetes. Pediatr. Psychol. 2:6–7.

Garner, A. M., Thompson, C. W., and Partridge, J. W. 1968. Adolescent group discussion. Diabetes Bull. 41:2.

Garner, A. M., Thompson, C. W., and Partridge, J. W. 1969a. Check your guesses: A research report. Diabetes Bull. 45:2.

Garner, A. M., Thompson, C. W., and Partridge, J. W. 1969b. Who knows best? Diabetes Bull. 45:3–4.

Garner. A. M., Thompson, C. W., Cherry, T. J., and Partridge, J. W. Teen age discussion groups. 1969. Diabetes Bull. 45:3-4.

Goldner, M. C. 1958. Stress, corticoids, and diabetes. Diabetes 7:410-413.

Haimowitz, M. L. 1972. Thoughts on helping the patient with diabetes. J. Am. Diet. Assoc. 61:425-428.

Hewett, S. (with John and Elizabeth Newson). 1970. The Family and the Handicapped Child. Aldine Publishing Co., New York.

Hinkle, L. E., Jr., and Wolf, S. 1952. The effect of stressful life situations on the concentration of blood glucose in diabetic and nondiabetic humans. Diabetes 1:383-392.

Holcomb, B., Partridge, J. W., and Belknap, C. S. (eds.). 1928-. Diabetes Bulletin. Published at 2222 N.W. Lovejoy St., Portland, Oregon.

Holmes, T. H., and Rahe, R. H. 1967. The social readjustment rating scale. J. Psychosom. Res. 11:213-217.

Ingelfinger, F. J. 1977. Debates on diabetes. N. Engl. J. Med. 296:1228-1230.

Kaufman, R. B., and Hersher, B. 1971. Body-image changes in teenage diabetes. Pediatrics 48:123-128.

Kemp. C. B., Knight, M. J., Scharp, D. W., Lacy, P. E., and Ballinger, W. F. 1973. Transplantation of isolated pancreatic islets into the portal vein of diabetic rats. Nature 244:447.

Knowles, H. C., Jr. 1971. Diabetes mellitus in childhood and adolescence. In P. Felig and P. K. Bondy (eds.), Symposium on Diabetes Mellitus. The Medical Clinics of North America 55:975-987. W. B. Saunders Co., Philadelphia.

Kogan, K. L., Tyler, N., and Turner, P. 1974. The process of interpersonal adaptation between mothers and their cerebral palsied children. Dev. Med. Child Neurol. 16:518-527.

Kohrman, A. F., and Weil, W. B. 1971. Juvenile diabetes mellitus. Adv. Pediatr. 18:123-149.

Korner, A. F. 1974. The effect of the infant's state, level of arousal, sex, and ontogenetic stage on the caregiver. In M. Lewis and L. A. Rosenblum (eds.), The Effect of the Infant on its Caregiver, pp. 105-122. John Wiley & Sons, New York.

Koski, M.-L. 1969. The coping processes in childhood diabetes. Acta Paediatr. Scand. 198(suppl.):7-56.

Koski, M.-L., and Kumento, A. 1975. Adolescent development and behavior: A psychosomatic follow-up study of childhood diabetes. In Z. Laron (ed.), Diabetes in Juveniles: Medical and Rehabilitation Aspects. Modern Problems in Paediatrics. Vol. 12, pp. 348-353. S. Karger, Basel.

Kubany, A. J., Danowski, T. S., and Moses, C. 1956. The personality and intelligence of diabetics. Diabetes 5:462-467.

Minuchin, S. 1974. Families & Family Therapy. Harvard University Press, Cambridge, Mass.

Partridge, J. W. 1967. Employment of patients with diabetes. Diabetes Bull. 43:1, 3.

Partridge, J. W., Garner, A. M., Thompson, C. W., and Cherry, T. 1972. Attitudes of adolescents toward their diabetes. Am. J. Dis. Child. 124:226-229.

Paulsen, E. P., and Colle, E. 1969. Diabetes Mellitus. In L. E. Gardner (ed.), Endocrine and Genetic Diseases of Childhood, pp. 808-823. W. B. Saunders Co., Philadelphia.

Rahe, R. H., Meyer, M., Smith, M., Kjaer, G., and Holmes, T. H. 1964. Social stress and illness onset. J. Psychosom. Res. 8:35-44.

Richardson, S. A., Hastorf, A. H., and Dornbusch, S. M. 1964. Effects of physical disability on a child's description of himself. Child. Dev. 35:893–907.

Slawson, F., Flynn, W. R., and Koller, E. J. 1963. Psychological factors associated with the onset of diabetes mellitus. J. Am. Med. Assoc. 185: 166–170.

Stein, S. P., and Charles, E. 1971. Emotional factors in juvenile diabetes mellitus: A study of early life experiences of adolescent diabetics. Am. J. Psychiatry 128:700–704.

Swift, C. R., Seidman, F., and Stein, H. 1967. Adjustment problems in juvenile diabetes. Psychosom. Med. 29:555–571.

Thompson, C. W. 1973. Bridging the gap between psychotherapy and rehabilitation psychology: Report on work with diabetic children and their parents. Presented at the 81st annual convention, American Psychological Association, August 27–31, Montreal.

Thompson, C. W., Garner, A. M., and Partridge, J. W. 1969a. Fantasticks: A research report. Diabetes Bull. 45:2.

Thompson, C. W., Garner, A. M., and Partridge, J. W. 1969b. Sick? or diabetic? A research report. Diabetes Bull. 45:2–3.

Thompson, C. W., Garner, A. M., Cherry, T. J., and Partridge, J. W. 1968. Adolescent group discussion. Diabetes Bull. 44:2.

Warnberg, L. 1974. Psychological aspects of juvenile diabetes. Pediatr. Psychol. 2:10–11.

Watkins, J. D., Roberts, D. E., Williams, T. F., Martin, D. A., and Coyle, V. 1967. Observation of medication errors made by diabetic patients in the home. Diabetes 16:882–885.

Weil, W. B., Jr. 1967. Social patterns and diabetic glucosuria: A study of group behavior and diabetic management in summer camp. Am. J. Dis. Child. 113:454–460.

Wright, B. A. 1973. Suffering as seen by the experiencer and the observer. Presented at the 14th Inter-American Congress of Psychology, April, 1973, Sao Paulo, Brazil.

Wright, L., Woodcock, J. M., and Scott, R. 1969. Conditioning children when refusal of oral medication is life-threatening. Pediatrics 44:969–972.

Wyler, A. R., Masuda, M., and Holmes, T. H. 1971. Magnitude of life events and seriousness of illness. Psychosom. Med. 33:115–122.

9
Renal Disease

Phyllis R. Magrab and Zoe L. Papadopoulou

During the past two decades substantial accomplishments have been achieved in the field of pediatric nephrology. Greater insight into understanding the pathophysiology and immunological basis of renal disease has been gained, accompanied by a greater sophistication in diagnosis and treatment. For many children with renal disease, early detection of the underlying renal pathology points to medical or surgical therapeutic modalities that may correct or arrest the progression of the disease. Yet, in spite of these measures, the incidence of chronic kidney failure in children is 3.0 to 3.5 per million total population per year (MacGregor et al., 1969; Meadow, Cameron, and Ogg, 1970). Fortunately today we have the ability to prolong the lives of many of these children through the life-saving techniques of hemodialysis and renal transplantation. In a 1973 amendment to the Social Security Act end-stage renal failure was established in the United States as a prototype of a catastrophic illness for which the cost of extending life is assumed in part by the government because of the inordinate financial resources required. But having enhanced our ability to preserve life through medical advances and social reform, we in the health profession must dedicate ourselves to the quality of life we preserve. Children with chronic renal disease and their families face multiple stresses. Ongoing attention to their emotional adjustments must be incorporated in comprehensive health care plans.

KIDNEY DISEASE

There are many diseases that may affect the kidney, but fortunately renal disease does not necessarily mean renal failure, because the child, as well as the adult, has more renal function than is necessary for the maintenance of life (Wenzl, 1975). The types of kidney disease that lead to renal failure are unique in the pediatric age group as compared to adults. Review of the reported cases in the literature (Fine et al., 1970; Fine, 1972; Grushkin, Korsch, and Fine, 1972, 1973) discloses that renal diseases leading to renal failure are characteristically associated with three distinct age groups: infants and toddlers, school-age children between the ages of five and 11 years, and adolescents (see Table 1). The

259

Table 1.   Renal disease leading to chronic renal failure in children

---

  I. Infants and toddlers
    A. Congenital (50%)
        1. Hydronephrosis (2° to obstruction)
        2. Dysplastic or hypoplastic kidneys
        3. Infantile nephrotic syndrome
        4. Infantile polycystic kidneys
    B. Acquired (50%)
        1. Hemolytic uremic syndrome (80–90%)
        2. Renal cortical necrosis (10–20%)
        3. Other
 II. Young children (ages five to 11 years)
    A. Congenital (44%)
        1. Hydronephrosis (2° to obstruction)
        2. Chronic pyelonephritis
        3. Dysplastic or hypoplastic kidneys
        4. Oligomeganephron
        5. Other (cystinosis, polycystic kidneys)
    B. Acquired (56%)
        1. Chronic glomerulonephritis (80%)
        2. Cortical necrosis (20%)
III. Adolescents
    A. Congenital (34%)
        1. Hydronephrosis (2° to obstruction)
        2. Chronic pyelonephritis
        3. Hypoplastic kidneys
        4. Hereditary (familial) nephritis
        5. Medullary cystic disease
    B. Acquired (66%)
        1. Chronic glomerulonephritis (90%)
        2. Miscellaneous (10%)
            a. Shunt nephritis
            b. Goodpasture syndrome

---

frequency of congenital and acquired conditions varies based on the age of onset of the disease.

Congenital and Structural Abnormalities

For about 50% of the children in the infant and toddler-age group as well as in the school-age group, chronic renal disease is the result *of congenital and structural abnormalities of the kidneys and urinary tract or of hereditary disorders.* These children become symptomatic early in life and are exposed to multiple medical and surgical diagnostic and therapeutic modalities. Congenital obstruction, leading to *hydronephrosis* (backing up of urine into the kidney resulting in marked distention and, finally, atrophy of kidney tissue), may be infravesical (below the bladder or lower urinary tract) or supravesical (above the bladder or upper urinary tract). Infravesical causes include bladder neck obstruction, posterior urethral valves or urethral stenosis. Supravesical obstruction usually occurs at the junction of the ureter with the bladder (ureterovesical) or at the junction of the ureter with the pelvis of the kidney (ureteropelvic). In each of these areas, the obstruction may be caused by either congenital stenosis or an extrinsic compression by blood vessels or fibrotic bands. If the obstruction is severe, it will then lead to marked dilatation of the kidneys and hydronephrosis with progressive loss of renal function.

The diagnosis of these conditions is based on clinical observation and various radiological and urological studies including intravenous pyelogram (IVP), cystourethogram, renal scan, and cystoscopy. The intravenous pyelogram and the renal scan involve injecting a substance into a small vein and thereafter obtaining a series of pictures. Both of these procedures are relatively nontraumatic. The cystourethogram is usually more traumatic because a catheter is inserted into the bladder while the child is awake. Cystoscopy requires hospitalization; under general anesthesia several instruments are introduced into the bladder in order to identify abnormalities.

If an obstruction is found, various surgical procedures may follow but may not be successful in preventing progressive loss of renal function. The overall prognosis often depends on the degree of normal kidney tissue that is present at the time of the initial diagnosis as well as on the frequency of associated urinary tract infections, because the latter can further damage the kidneys and cause further reduction of kidney function.

Other congenital renal anomalies that lead to chronic renal disease include maldevelopment of the kidney tissue during the early fetal life, leading to malformed kidneys, *renal dysplasia,* and the formation of numerous large cysts in the kidney leading to various hereditary *cystic disorders of the kidney.* The latter include polycystic kidney disease (infantile and adult polycystic disease), cortical cysts present primarily in the cortex or outer part of the kidney (seen often in syndromes of multiple congenital malformations), medullary cysts seen primarily in the medulla or inner portion of the kidney (e.g., medullary cystic disease), and congenital nephrosis (microcystic disease). In congenital nephrosis the infant develops the nephrotic syndrome soon after birth and has a poor prognosis because kidney failure usually develops during the first few months of life.

Structural and anatomical developmental defects of the kidneys lead to various degrees of renal malfunction, which become manifest early in life depending on the severity of the anomaly. For this reason congenital malformations constitute the major etiology of chronic renal failure in

infancy and early childhood. The incidence of congenital renal malformations as the etiology of chronic renal failure decreases during
adolescence. In this age group, acquired renal disease constitutes the
major etiological factor of chronic renal failure.

Acquired Renal Disease

In general, various types of acquired renal disease that are severe enough
to result in kidney failure characteristically present in the three age
groups. In infants and toddlers, the kidneys are more susceptible to acute
vascular injury and circulatory collapse than in older children and
adolescents. In this age group *hemolytic uremic syndrome and renal
cortical necrosis* are the two main causes of severe renal injury.

The *hemolytic uremic syndrome* is primarily a disease of early childhood. Ninety percent of the cases occur before the fourth year of life,
and the average age of onset is at or below one year of age (Herdman
and Urizar, 1975). These children present acutely sick with anemia,
bleeding tendencies, hemolysis, or fragmentation of their red blood cells.
The bleeding occurs primarily in the kidney. The clots that form block
the blood vessels, thus cutting off the blood supply to the kidney. This
results in necrosis or death of the kidney tissue and subsequent kidney
failure. Long-term follow-up has shown that 42% of these children
recover completely, 26% continue to recover slowly, 21% demonstrate
progressive renal lesions, and 13% progress to uremia and chronic renal
failure (Gianantonio, Vitacco, and Mendilaharzu, 1967; Gianantonio et
al., 1968).

Renal cortical necrosis (i.e., necrosis of the cortex of the kidney)
may occur in infants and young children where there is reduction of
normal blood flow to the kidneys, which may result following acute
depletion of blood volume secondary to blood or fluid loss, or hypotension (low blood pressure) following anoxia or sepsis. The kidney tissue is
then deprived of its normal blood supply (ischemia), and necrosis will
occur because oxygen cannot be delivered to keep the cells in the kidney
cortex alive. Ischemic damage to the kidneys after various insults occurs
more frequently in infants and young children whose kidneys are
somewhat immature in structure and function.

For older children and adolescents, the most commonly acquired
renal disease leading to chronic renal failure is chronic *glomerulonephritis.* Chronic glomerulonephritis is not a specific diagnosis of a
single entity but instead is a clinical and pathological condition that
arises from a variety of clinical disease entities. The types of disease
entities that result in chronic glomerulonephritis in children primarily
include severe forms of the nephrotic syndrome such as focal segment-
al glomerulosclerosis, membrane proliterative glomerulonephritis, and
renal basement membrane dense deposit disease. In these conditions,

damage occurs in the kidney, the etiology of which is unknown, resulting in chronic disease that is progressive, causing complete destruction of kidney tissue and hence kidney failure. Clinically, most of these children present with the nephrotic syndrome manifested by protein loss in the urine and swelling of the face, abdomen, and extremities (Arneil, 1971). Most of these forms of the nephrotic syndrome do not respond to corticosteroid therapy and progress to renal failure within an average span of two to 10 years from the onset of the disease. It is precisely because of lack of definitive therapy that these children continue to have varying degrees of edema over the face and other parts of the body, which may have profound physical and psychosocial implications.

It must be remembered, however, that children with the severe forms of the nephrotic syndrome who do not respond to therapy and eventually progress to kidney failure comprise only 20%, or one-fifth, of the total number of children who develop the nephrotic syndrome in general. The other 80% of the children with nephrosis (called lipoid nephrosis or nil disease), respond to therapy, and their long-term prognosis is good because their disease does not progress to chronicity.

PSYCHOLOGICAL ASPECTS OF RENAL DISEASE

Most of the psychological studies of renal disease have focused on children with the nephrotic syndrome and on patients with end-stage renal disease. The type of nephrotic syndrome that does not respond to corticosteroid therapy is exemplary of a long-term chronic illness because of its protracted, usually progressive course, resulting in end-stage kidney failure. The problems encountered in pediatric patients with this condition are in many ways similar to those of children with any type of long-term physical illness. These children are subjected to numerous, recurring, emotionally stressful situations. The child's response to these situations and to his illness depends on his developmental age, the personalities of the child/patient and his parents, and the latent sources of tension within his family unit (Korsch and Barnett, 1961). As in any other chronic illness, anxiety and guilt are the predominant emotional feelings, which become exaggerated both in the child and his parents. The younger the child, the more distorted or magical the interpretation of his illness may be. For example, the preschool child who has little ability to understand the nature of his illness tends to interpret his symptoms as a punishment for misbehavior. Because young children believe that nothing happens by chance, they look for explanations of an event in actions such as disobedience in the immediate past (Mattson, 1972).

Feelings of anxiety and a tendency to self-blame occur in the parents as well as the child/patient. Korsch, Fraad, and Barnett (1954) have shown that in group discussions the parents of children with nephrosis showed a consistent tendency to assume the burden of blame for their child's illness. In some instances these feelings of anxiousness and self-blame were so exaggerated that they led to inappropriate behavior on the part of the parents, poor understanding of the disease, and, more importantly, poor cooperation with the attending physician. A major task of the physician emerged to relieve anxiety and approach the parents with greater empathy and understanding.

Various forms of family conflict may be brought into focus and may develop into major crises when a child develops nephrosis (Korsch and Barnett, 1961). In situations in which there have been difficulties and dissatisfaction in the marriage before the child's illness, the marriage may not be able to withstand the demands and strains brought about by handling a child with chronic disease; a breakdown in the relationship between the parents may occur, in some cases ending in divorce. On the other hand, the occurrence of nephrosis in a child may act as a unifying force, bringing a family closer together to combat a common enemy (Korsch and Barnett, 1961). In this case, any preexisting problems in interpersonal relationships appear to be put aside as the family focuses primarily on the child's illness.

Siblings are often deeply affected by the changes in the family resulting from the illness of the child/patient with nephrosis. They may manifest excessive jealousy and various types of disturbed behavior, even somatic symptoms, in an attempt to attract parental attention and maintain their position in the family. Occasionally, latent fears concerning illness and death may become exaggerated in the well sibling because of the family's preoccupation with the sick child and his frequent visits to doctors and hospitals.

Problems often develop around the sick child's interpersonal relationships with family members. The role of the mother is an especially difficult one: to maintain a safe life-style for the child as well as to provide him with opportunities for emotional growth. Often mothers of children with nephrosis become overprotective and tend to keep them closer and more dependent than is developmentally appropriate. The extent of the mother's overprotectiveness and overindulgence with the physical care of the child may be related to the magnitude of her feelings of guilt for her own shortcomings as a mother and for the illness itself. She may devote herself to the care of the child in order to prove by martyr-like devotion that she is really a good mother (Korsch and Barnett, 1961).

The nephrotic child thus can be deprived of the normal progression toward independence. Guilt feelings on the part of the parents for imposed discomforts, restrictions, and deprivations of the child may interfere with their ability to set limits in appropriate areas. Thus, the child may be deprived of learning and following rules and principles of conduct that govern social living, which he must learn to be accepted by his peers and other adults.

This is in contrast to the severe limits that may be imposed on the child's social contacts. Because children with nephrosis are susceptible to infections, which when they occur may precipitate a relapse of their disease, many parents prohibit their children from playing with their peers, especially in the winter months, and even may prevent them from attending school on very cold days. This deprivation of social contacts may become further accentuated by frequent hospitalizations, leaving the child with little opportunity to develop social skills.

For the nephrotic child himself his privacy is often intruded upon. In general he is subjected to many painful and frightening procedures, the importance of which he cannot fully understand. Urine and blood specimens are collected frequently to stage the progression of his disease. He has to comply with doctors' orders while, at the same time, his family may prevent any efforts on his part for self-rule and rebellion. As a result of the nature of his illness, at times of relapse of nephrosis he may feel tired, fatigued, and become cranky, irritable, and negativistic—acting more "spoiled" than usual. The adults and other members within his immediate environment may respond with anger and criticism, which will aggravate the sick child's feelings of guilt and will increase his depression.

In addition to these problems, the nephrotic child's sense of body image may be severely distorted. During periods of relapse he becomes edematous and at times may look almost grotesque; during the diuretic phase he loses substantial weight often to the point of looking thin and puny. His arms are stuck with needles for special biochemical determinations, his urine volume is closely monitored, his parents are constantly concerned about his bodily functions, and he is prevented from participating in normal activities. Depending on the age of the child, these factors may result in a greatly distorted concept of body image.

Role of the Physician

The physician responsible for the care of the child with nephrotic syndrome is confronted with the management of a sick child who is handicapped in some of the essential functions at a vulnerable time in his growth and development (Korsch and Barnett, 1961). He also has to deal with anxious parents who are aware of the chronicity of the disease and the poor prognosis. The physician who manages the nephrotic child must be a pediatrician with sound knowledge of normal growth and development and of the emotional needs of children. The parents must be encouraged to provide the child independence by allowing him to make decisions appropriate for his age level and to participate in motor activities within safe limits defined by the physician. Parents must learn to allow the child to have normal contacts with other children and to participate in as many normal activities as possible, as permitted by the physician and the child's feeling of well-being. The physician also must help parents understand the reason for the sick child's aggressive feelings, which are used almost in self-defense against all the unpleasant things that are done to him, and give them insight into proper ways to handle these feelings (Korsch and Barnett, 1961). When hospitalization becomes necessary, the child should be prepared in advance so that he will not feel threatened about situations he cannot control; parents must become partners with the physician in this preparation. If the child's fears and emotional disturbances are recognized early, they usually can be alleviated by proper management.

The physician must be able to display empathy toward the parents, who at times may become overanxious and irrational in trying to cope with their feelings about the chronicity and the poor prognosis of their child's illness on the one hand, and the financial burden that the illness imposes on the family on the other hand. These mixed emotions and stresses may give rise to feelings of resentment and hostility toward the medical personnel and, at times, toward the child (Korsch and Barnett, 1961). Understanding and empathy on the part of the physician may help relieve the tensions and restore the parents' faith in themselves and in their ability to handle these problems with appropriate help from the physician (Korsch and Barnett, 1961). At times the physician must use the resources of other mental health professionals. In difficult situations such as these, the role of the pediatric psychologist, psychiatrist, and social worker, can be significant in helping to alleviate these conflicts. Proper guidance may help the parents overcome their feelings of self-blame and may offer constructive measures for their need to be actively involved in the total care of the child. Every effort should be made to support them in their own ideas, acknowledge their competence, and show recognition of their efforts in the many difficult tasks they have to perform.

MEDICAL ASPECTS OF END-STAGE RENAL FAILURE

The onset of end-stage renal failure with all the associated medical complications of uremia comes as a shock to the child and his family despite any or all the previous psychological preparation. Up to this point, the child with chronic kidney disease and especially his family maintain some hope that, in spite of what they are told by the physicians about the long-term prognosis of the disease, the end will never come; somehow they will be spared. Once faced with the inevitable truth, the family's first reaction is usually one of guilt. What did they do wrong to cause this; could they have prevented it? For most adults, adolescents, and pre-adolescents, end-stage kidney failure is a continuing reminder of impending death; for very young children less able to understand, but aware of the increased anxiety around them, it is a source of unremitting fear.

When kidney failure develops, there are basically two choices: death, if definitive medical treatment is denied, or prolongation of life through hemodialysis and eventual kidney transplantation. This choice is almost always decided by the parents if the child is below 18 years of age.

Hemodialysis and renal homotransplantation, as successful therapeutic modalities for end-stage renal disease, did not become available to children until the late 1960s. Before that time, kidney failure in children resulted in death. Today hemodialysis is available to almost all children with kidney failure, and it provides the hope of life until renal transplantation can occur.

The onset of kidney failure and subsequent hemodialysis, as a means of prolonging life, is the beginning of a new scope of a variety of potential medical complications as well as restrictions and deprivations imposed on the child. With the loss of kidney function, many of the normal body functions fail and medical measures then must be taken to maintain them. The normal function of the kidneys is to excrete water, some electrolytes, and various end products of protein metabolism such as urea and creatinine. With failure of kidney function, urine output is decreased markedly, with subsequent retention of water, of various electrolytes such as sodium, potassium, and phosphorus, and of certain proteinaceous waste products, especially urea and nitrogen. This then results in retention of fluid which may cause hypertension, in retention of potassium which may be toxic to the heart causing various cardiac arrhythmias and/or death, in retention of phosphorus which upsets the normal calcium and phosphorus metabolism and may result in bone abnormalities, and in retention of waste products of metabolism which are toxic to the function of various organs of the body such as the brain, blood cells, etc. Correction of most of these abnormalities is attempted through hemodialysis.

A variety of growth problems occur with children who have chronic renal failure. Unique in young children is the failure of growth, and, in older children, the failure or delay of sexual maturation. Extreme dwarfism may occur, especially in those children who develop poor kidney function early in life. Although a high caloric intake may promote near-normal growth, many times this is not successful or even possible to achieve because of fluid and other dietary restrictions. As a result of the abnormalities in the calcium and phosphorus metabolism certain bone abnormalities may develop, the severity of which will depend on the age of the child at the time of onset of poor kidney function. Rickets is one of these abnormalities that is more commonly seen in very young children, often resulting in severe bowing deformities of the legs. It can be treated effectively with high doses of vitamin D, but if not treated early it may contribute to poor growth. Other bone abnormalities can occur secondary to high levels of phosphorus and concomitantly low levels of calcium in the blood. This derangement will result in excessive secretion of parathyroid hormone, which in turn will stimulate removal of calcium from the bones, thus rendering the bones weak and susceptible to fractures. This can be prevented by administering Amphogel with each meal, which prevents the absorption of phosphorus from the food in the stomach to the blood stream, which in turn keeps the blood levels of phosphorus within a normal range. However, many children often refuse to take the Amphogel with their meals, claiming that it leaves a bad taste in the mouth, thereby exposing themselves to the development of bone disease.

In addition, most children with chronic kidney failure will develop severe anemia necessitating frequent blood transfusions. In spite of the transfusions, however, the blood count remains low, thus contributing to the pale appearance of the child, easy fatigability, and feeling of inertia, which further limits the child's participation in normal physical activities.

Hemodialysis

Hemodialysis is a process of artificially replacing the functions of the kidney—a life-saving technique for children with chronic renal failure. During hemodialysis, blood is removed via an artery in one of the extremities, externally circulated by a tubing through an artificial kidney, and subsequently returned to the body via a vein in the same extremity.

For dialysis to occur, the blood slowly flows over a porous membrane, which substitutes for the kidney's glomeruli, or tufts of blood vessels, and filters out body wastes. The entire blood volume then circulates through the artificial kidney about two or three times each hour. Usually, each dialysis treatment lasts for five hours and is repeated three times a week. A good blood access to an artery and a vein of the body therefore is necessary on a chronic basis. This can be achieved by surgically creating either a shunt or fistula. With a *shunt,* a small piece of silastic tubing is inserted in an artery and a nearby vein of one of the extremities, joining them outside the skin with a small connecting piece of tubing, thus creating a loop through which blood is circulated. During the dialysis, the connecting piece is removed and the silastic tubing is connected with the larger tubes that carry the blood to and from the artificial kidney back to the body. Children with shunts must protect the extremity where the shunt is located from injury and from infection and must always keep it dry, so that they are forbidden to take showers or go swimming. Shunt complications consist of bleeding, infection, and clotting. A *fistula* is a direct surgical internal connection between an artery and a vein in one of the extremities followed by closure of the skin above it. This will cause engorgement of the blood vessels. During dialysis, a needle is inserted to one of the engorged vessels and through a connection on the other end of the needle to the blood tubing the patient's blood is pumped to the artificial kidney and then returned back into the body.

It must be noted that dialysis is only an intermittent measure because it is usually performed only three times a week with a total of 15 hours of treatment. Certain restrictions therefore must be imposed in between the dialysis treatments in order to avoid large amounts of retention of fluid, potassium, and the waste products of metabolism. The major restriction is dietary and consists of significant restrictions in the protein, fluid, and potassium intake. Because these are calculated on a weight basis, the younger the child, the more unpalatable is the diet. With these restrictions, eating hamburgers with ketchup, french fries, pizzas, chocolate, and drinking colas and milk shakes becomes a novelty—a treat that may be offered infrequently and with moderation of the total quantity.

PSYCHOLOGICAL REACTIONS OF CHILDREN AND FAMILIES TO END-STAGE RENAL FAILURE AND HEMODIALYSIS

Adjustment of Children

How do children respond to a parent's and doctor's decision to start hemodialysis, a situation that abruptly and suddenly changes life patterns? Different children, and families, handle the stress of chronic disease in a variety of ways and in sequential stages along the continuum marked at one end by withdrawal and denial and at the other by openness and acceptance. Studies by Korsch et al. (1971) and Sampson (1975) suggest that there are two predominant ongoing modes of response of children to end-stage renal failure: withdrawal behavior and coping behavior. The children who manifest depression and withdrawal under the impact of illness and painful treatment often sleep a great deal, eat poorly, refuse to play, and avoid interaction with others. Regression more frequently occurs in the younger patient (Sampson, 1975). After a few months on a dialysis program, as different complications occur and are dealt with, these children generally become more actively communicative and begin to accept the reality of their illness. The coping group of children appear to understand what is happening to them at the outset and accept help and caregiving while at the same time they may become increasingly dependent and often very demanding (Korsch et al., 1971). They use their illness to profit from secondary gains, such as attracting constant attention from their families and the medical and nursing personnel in the dialysis unit. Obviously, these two groups polarize the extremes; a number of children will fall somewhere between. The problems of withdrawal-depression cannot be minimized for any of these children. Khan, Herndon, and Ahmadian (1971) report continued depression in all of their dialysis patients. As in other chronic illnesses affecting children, one of the overriding emotional factors for the child is the uncertainty that will dominate the years ahead.

A major issue for dialysis patients is achieving a balance between dependence and independence (Korsch et al., 1971). However, this is often very difficult to achieve. Particularly for preadolescents and adolescents, there exists a fierce independence-dependence conflict. The preadolescent or adolescent is required to remain dependent on a machine (the artificial kidney) and to adhere to the restrictions imposed by his dialysis program, while at the same time he wishes to lead a normal life assuming normal responsibilities, such as attending school and participating in social activities (Abram, 1974). At the critical age when he begins to seek more independence, renal failure forces him to become more dependent upon his parents and the medical staff. If neurotic ambivalence exists in the areas of independence-dependence or activity-passivity, he responds by being "uncooperative," by becoming either excessively dependent or excessively independent, refusing in a rebellious way to accept the restrictions of the dialysis program (Abram, 1974). For others, attempts to break away from parents to achieve independence may be thwarted by the parents themselves whose oversolicitiousness may result in invalid-like behavior on the part of the patient (Salisbury, 1968).

The dialysis process itself—the machine, the procedures—is an unusual experience and may conjure up nightmarish fantasies. A child may or may not understand what is happening to him and why. Because his body image and self-concept are developing constantly, being attached to a machine can be devastating to his personality structure (Nordan, Ostendorf, and Naughton, 1971). Fear of the dialysis process because of lack of understanding can precipitate extreme responses at the outset. Schultz, McVicar, and Kemph (1974) described a nine-year-old girl who assumed a fetal position when hemodialysis was performed. She refused to change her position, stating that she would be hurt by the dialysis apparatus. She fantasized that parts of the "artificial kidney" would touch her body and injure her. The child improved once the functions of the different parts of the machine were described to her; thus, she was reassured that dialysis was used to help her rather than to hurt her.

In an extensive evaluation of children undergoing dialysis in Paris, Debre, Duhong, and Raimbault (1973) reported that in general the children's overall adaptation was good. However, projective tests showed that there were significant abnormalities in their personality structure characterized by diminution and narrowing. Their imaginary world was poor and most of them were functioning below their intellectual potential. They exhibited minimal emotional involvement; they felt isolated and had difficulty establishing good interpersonal relationships with others. They had almost no plans for the future, and their body image was profoundly disturbed in that it was mutilated and incomplete. For the majority of children school attendance and social activities were curtailed significantly, causing isolation of the child and of the family as a whole. Similar findings were reported by Khan, Herndon, and Ahmadian (1971) who studied nine children on chronic dialysis and found common problems in social isolation, depression, and dependency on parents. Such self-defeating behavior seems to be used as a defense against underlying feelings of fear and anxiety. Berger, Ginn, and Travis (1975) reported alteration of body images, illness-related anxiety, and emotional immaturity for the majority of their dialysis patients. When there are extreme psychopathological responses to dialysis, these must not be viewed as a result of treatment but rather as an accentuation of previous problems that burgeoned under stress.

From the psychological point of veiw, hemodialysis can be characterized as a process that stifles the child's ability to work through his personal problems and to develop his personality (Bouras et al., 1976). The usual arena for working through these issues is not readily available to these children; thus, the importance for developing supportive mechanisms, such as activity programs, tutors, liaison with the schools, is critical.

Adherence to dietary restrictions is a recurring problem for children on hemodialysis. Problems with dietary control can occur as a result of a variety of factors. Most children, and especially teenagers, have many psychosocial adjustments to make as they start hemodialysis, and severe restrictions or major changes in their eating style may become further barriers to normal social activity (Wilson, Potter, and Holliday, 1973). Often, family problems, lack of family support, low level of education, and rebellion against strong parental supervision may result in dietary abuse. For those children who fail to adhere to their prescribed diets, there is an increased risk for fluid overload and congestive heart failure, hypertension, hyperkalemia, azotemia, and bone disease. Often, in spite of careful and repeated instructions for adherence to the dietary restrictions and the consequences of dietary indiscretion, a number of children manifest their aggression and possible self-destruction by lack of dietary compliance and present with episodes of these problems.

Patient compliance is recognized as a major problem in clinical medicine, and few useful techniques beyond the quality of doctor-patient relationships have been developed (Zifferblatt, 1975). Zifferblatt supports an applied analysis of behavior, evaluating antecedent and consequent events in compliance situations, which is applicable to dialysis patients. The effect of behavior modification using a token economy in maintaining dietary control is reported by Magrab and Papadopoulou (1977) for patients ages 11–18 resulting in significant changes in the dietary pattern of problem children. The average weight gain between dialysis sessions for the subjects during treatment was reduced by 45%, and the degree of weight fluctuation was lessened. Potassium and blood, urea, and nitrogen (BUN) were controlled to their appropriate levels for subjects who initially exceeded the criterion levels.

Family Reaction

Most families do not acknowledge the seriousness of their child's illness until they are told of the imminence of dialysis. Khan et al. (1971) reported in their study of 14 families that the news seems to create a major crisis in families. Offered the choice of death or dialysis for their child, most families chose the latter but not without deliberating the long periods of suffering, the effect on the siblings and family unity, and the financial strains it would impose.

Like many other stressful situations, chronic kidney failure may accentuate potential problems in family adjustment and social relationships. As noted in kidney disease cases (Korsch and Barnett, 1961), preexisting problems in certain marriages may become heightened, resulting in divorce. Conversely, very close-knit families may become even more united when faced with the same painful experiences (Khan et al., 1971; Korsch et al., 1971). Sampson's (1975) subjects reported a general increase in closeness between patient and mother but not between patient and father. A feeling of role displacement expressed in resentment toward wife and job was predominant among fathers. Khan et al. (1971) and Morse (1974) describe the fearful and negativistic responses of siblings. Siblings worry about incurring the same disease and resent the time parents spend with the sick child. Acting-out behavior and school problems were often seen.

Special problems arise among extremely interdependent-child couples where the overidentified parent is unable to cope effectively with the child's illness and instead feels every pain along with the child (Korsch et al., 1971). Ultimately the child suffers and takes advantage of this situation. This causes problems in the relationship of the medical staff with the child and the overidentified parent. Problems may also arise at home where the siblings may feel neglected. Often the other parent has to carry the burden in dealing effectively with the needs of the sick child, the neglected siblings, and the disturbed parent.

Some parents appear on the surface to adjust to the demands made upon them in a controlled way but become extremely hostile with the medical staff and make unreasonable demands each time their child goes through a difficult period. This causes particular problems to the dialysis staff, who also have to deal with their own anxiety feelings concerning the child's welfare. In certain stressful situations they become less tolerant of parental interference, thus causing greater friction in their relationship with the overanxious parent.

PSYCHOLOGICAL MANAGEMENT AND RENAL DIALYSIS

Because of the complexity of the problem of chronic renal failure and the extent of need of the child on hemodialysis and of his family, an interdisciplinary team approach to care is most appropriate. The composition of a complete team will include the medical staff, the nursing staff, the dietician, the technicians, the social worker, and the pediatric psychologist or psychiatrist. The support of the total team is essential for the psychological management of the child, and this is accomplished only through developing an open communication system.

The role of the mental health professionals on the team is to serve as a primary advocate for the emotional adjustment of the child. Too often in hemodialysis a staff can become too preoccupied with medical and technical management. In part this relates to real necessities in medical care, but it also relates to the impact a chronically ill child will have on a staff, resulting in a type of staff withdrawal from the constant confrontation with potential death. DeNour and Czaczkes (1968) point to the feelings of guilt, possessiveness, and overprotectiveness and the withdrawal reactions that often develop among the dialysis care team members who may take on the role of a quasi-family. Critenden, Decker, and Levin (1975) report the feelings of uncertainty, helplessness, and dependency that arise out of the high level of ambiguity about the success of treatment. An important task for the psychologist and other mental health professionals on the team is to facilitate an understanding of these reactions as well as an understanding of the process of the group.

The need for a comprehensive psychosocial management program cannot be overstressed. The program should begin well before dialysis occurs. The first stage clearly relates to patient selection and some preassessment of the family dynamics and the emotional development of the child, so that families or children at "high emotional risk" can be identified and early psychosocial intervention can take place. Repeated evaluations should occur throughout dialysis and extend to posttransplantation so that specific problems can be identified early and appropriate therapeutic measures can be applied (Magrab, 1975).

An evaluation of the child should include intellectual as well as emotional assessment to document status and change. Of special importance is determining the child's social and educational activity level because withdrawal is such a frequent problem. Focusing on the child's adjustment to his illness and medical treatment, the Magrab-Bronheim Hospital Sentence Completion Technique (Table 2) and the Kinetic Hospital drawing can be useful. For example, the child whose primary defense is denial may respond on Sentence Completion, "My body is perfect," as compared to the child who is more accepting of the reality who responds, "My body has a kidney that doesn't work." In terms of body integrity on the Kinetic Hospital Test, one child who was particularly anxious about his body image drew a picture of himself with a kidney in the center of

Table 2. Magrab-Bronheim Hospital Sentence Completion

1.   Friends
2.   At home
3.   I am at my best when
4.   My family
5.   Most women
6.   It hurts when
7.   Most nurses
8.   I wish
9.   I feel down in the dumps when
10. My body
11. I like
12. I feel happiest when
13. My worst fault
14. My mother
15. I get angry when
16. The future
17. When I am on dialysis
18. My favorite person is
19. Most men
20. Lately, I think about
21. This place
22. Most doctors
23. My father
24. I get sad when
25. Being in the hospital

his body. The most depressed children drew themselves on the machine with no other person in the room.

Repeated psychosocial evaluations of the children and their families play an important role in the team approach to care. They serve as a vehicle for total team intervention when additional support is necessary and as a source of feedback for positive changes that have occurred as a result of team effort. The evaluations also become an integrated aspect of the supportive group treatment programs for parents and children.

Supportive therapy for the family members is an important part of a program for psychological management. To reduce crises, to facilitate identity changes, and to ameliorate depression and anxiety, parent groups and ongoing child-activity groups serve a continuing need. In these groups, members gain emotional support and learn alternate ways of viewing life. The overwhelming sense of isolation and uniqueness is reduced, and approaches to greater life normalcy can be learned. Along with supportive therapy, total staff involvement with patient and family members around adjustment issues must be encouraged. The families must be invited to come in for conferences on a regular basis while their children are on hemodialysis and during the immediate post-transplant period. These regular conferences are extremely important in maintaining the emotional adjustment of the child and his family, in providing adequately for social and educational needs, and in ensuring proper health care for the child (Korsch et al., 1971). When severe problems develop requiring actual therapeutic intervention, they can be detected early so that appropriate referrals can be made to the proper specialists. Open staff communication has the potential for being a crucial part of the team process and serves as an important foundation for developing more optimal psychological adjustment to dialysis.

RENAL TRANSPLANTATION

Hemodialysis in children is considered to be only a temporary measure in controlling kidney failure, the ultimate goal being renal transplantation. Both the child and the parents anticipate the time of transplantation with great hope, as the moment when the miracle will be achieved and the child will gain his good health with the acquisition of a functioning kidney. Subsequently, as they learn more about the necessity of certain surgical procedures that may be required before kidney transplantation, as well as about the ultimate success of transplantation, the picture becomes more complicated, causing new feelings of concern and anxiety.

For a large number of children, nephrectomy (removal of their own diseased kidneys) is a necessary surgical procedure that must take place several weeks before transplantation. This procedure is very difficult for the child and his family to accept. The child views nephrectomy as a loss of part of himself and the ultimate realization that his own kidneys have actually failed him and that now his life really must depend on the "kidney machine." From the parents' point of view it implies a negative verdict concerning the irreversibility of their child's kidney disease that they may be unwilling to accept, often questioning and arguing about the necessity of such a procedure.

With regard to transplantation itself, the initial enthusiasm and exuberance in its anticipation are dampened considerably as parents gain more information about the complications that may be encountered and the available statistics concerning survival of the transplanted kidney. Fine et al. (1973) and Fine and Gruskin (1973) showed that, in a five-year follow-up of 81 children who received a kidney transplant, 65 of them (80%) were alive with functioning kidneys (17 of these children had received a second kidney transplant because of previous rejection), nine children had died (11%), and seven children (3%) had rejected the kidney and were returned to hemodialysis awaiting a subsequent transplant. Kidney transplantation, therefore, is not always associated with 100% success. The greatest success is achieved in those children who receive a kidney from either a parent or sibling (living, related donor). Cadaver kidney transplants, i.e., kidneys obtained from a person who has died, show a lesser success. Furthermore, pediatric renal transplant recipients may experience several untoward side effects secondary to the immunosuppressive drugs that they must receive in order to avoid rejection of the transplanted kidney. The most common are obesity with typical "moonface" appearance secondary to steroid therapy, which can be quite devastating especially in adolescent girls. High blood pressure also may occur in a number of children, especially those receiving a cadaver transplant. Bone disease is another complication secondary to the steroid therapy and occurs in approximately 25% of the children. Resumption of a normal rate of growth can be hoped for in most young and preadolescent children. However, for those children over 12 years of age whose growth centers in the bones already have matured, the expectation for growth is much less favorable.

Preparation for Renal Transplantation

Preparation for transplantation is an educative process that begins even before the advent of renal failure. The key to a successful approach is the communication process between the physician, the renal team, and family members. Understanding the role of dialysis and transplantation, the options for donorship, and the potential outcomes must clearly be understood by the family if they are to participate meaningfully in the difficult decisions they will have to make. Because of the multiple stresses on these families, it is often a long process.

As the necessity for transplantation becomes imminent, frank discussions with the patient and his family must ensue around the medical alternatives and respective outcomes. A statistical comparison of the results of transplantation following cadaveric or living related donors must be given, along with the caution that family donors who initially wish to donate may not be medically acceptable (Wenzl, 1975). Donorship clearly must be voluntary with a full understanding of the risks involved. After blood typing, tissue typing, and assessment for general health and potential latent kidney disease, a bona fide family member donor still must be assured that he can withdraw.

The dilemmas of donorship can be exceedingly painful for families. To give or not to give, to be able to give or unable to give, to risk one's life, however small the risk, for the life of another are heavily emotionally charged issues and call forward numerous feelings of fear, guilt, anger, love, and a higher sense of humanity.

If a donor comes forward, the team must not only evaluate his medical appropriateness but also his emotional stability, freedom from coercion, and intellectual capacity to understand the ramifications of his decision (Wenzl, 1975). The family situation and the attitude of other family members are also of noted importance. When no donor comes forward in a family after several months' time and a repeated overture, it is important that blame and guilt not be assigned by the renal team and that a constructive approach to cadaver donorship be initiated.

Once the road to transplantation is taken, the waiting and the uncertainty of when it will take place become major stresses for the family. As the date nears, when it is known, tension and anxiety will increase (Sampson, 1975). Unlike adults, children do not manifest guilt for obtaining someone else's kidney—not even adolescents who have had previously hostile relationships with parents—but a variety of fears and fantasies about organ transplantation often ensue (Sampson, 1975). The donor-recipient relationship from the outset requires substantial insight on the part of the renal team. Receiving an organ from a relative or from a cadaver is a significant source of stress: the idea of having a foreign body inside oneself can be extremely disturbing to the child recipient (Malekzadeh et al., 1976). With cadaver donors, speculations arise regarding the source of the kidney; with living related donors, potential ambivalence about the source of the kidney. Sampson (1975) reports the potential for a quasi-symbiotic relationship emerging with attempts on the part of the donor to control aggressive behavior of the recipient.

Psychological Problems Associated with Transplantation

Transplantation cannot be viewed as an isolated phase because from the psychological point of view it is closely linked with the past experiences of the child. In order to understand some of the problems that may be encountered in children following transplantation, it is necessary to know their prior experiences, especially during the period on dialysis (Bouras et al., 1976). Debre, Duhong, and Raimbault (1973) have equated the period on dialysis with a still-life picture or a time spent in a waiting room, a time filled with a series of restrictions, anxieties, fears, and frustrations that will be removed miraculously at the time of transplantation. What each child expects from transplantation is a brand new life free of physical pain and restrictions, a chance to be his old self again, that is, a normal child.

One of the outstanding early sources of anxiety in the posttransplant period is the fear of rejection of the new kidney. The continuous underlying fear of rejection has been emphasized by Beard (1969, 1971), Fine et al. (1970), and Korsch et al. (1971).

During the immediate posttransplant period surgical complications, rejection crises, infections, and daily variations of the blood, urea, and nitrogen (BUN) and creatinine, which are used as indicators of kidney function, constantly torment the child patient, the family, and the medical staff. Once these initial problems are overcome, new complications may arise that are primarily caused by the immunsuppressive medications. At this point it must be emphasized that immunosuppressive therapy, consisting primarily of Prednisone (a steroid) and Immuran (an immunosuppressive drug), is absolutely necessary for the survival of the kidney graft. Failure to take these medications on a regular daily basis may result in rejection of the kidney.

Steroid therapy can represent a major psychological adjustment for the child. Steroids stimulate the appetite, which, when not carefully controlled, may result in excessive weight gain. The "moon facies" and acne that may occur as a result of steroid therapy, together with body disfigurement caused by excessive weight gain, are especially difficult for adolescent girls, who in desperation may resort to temporary noncompliance in therapy, thus endangering the function of the transplanted kidney (Malekzadeh et al., 1976). Korsch et al. (1973) reported that a number of children who exhibited problems of noncompliance to medications were found to have underlying personality disturbances that were not reactive to illness but a part of their preillness personality. Of additional note with respect to steroid therapy large doses of steroids occasionally may result in emotional and mental changes that can further complicate the posttransplant course.

Psychological problems stressed during the first year after transplant include: great anxiety and fear of graft rejection (Fine et al., 1970), difficulties linked with physical appearance and self-image (Fine et al., 1970; Khan, Herndon, and Ahmadian, 1971), and difficulties in adjusting to school (Beard, 1969; Sampson, 1975; Bernstein, 1971). Bouras et al.

(1976) reported that the immediate posttransplant period is characterized by great outbursts of vitality especially in children below 10 years of age. This buoyancy, almost hyperactive in quality, is in sharp contrast to the passive behavior exhibited during the period of chronic kidney disease. Increased anxiety may account, in part, for school problems that often occur. Adolescents were observed to give a superficial impression of adequate adjustment; yet, they evidenced underlying personality impoverishment, especially in the areas of creativity and sexuality.

The later period, one year and more after transplant, is generally described as a time when equilibrium is restored. Fear of rejection and feelings of depression persist (Beard, 1969, 1971), sometimes in the form of what Bernstein (1971) describes as "short-life syndrome," a fear of rejection and fear of death when signs of rejection are at a minimum. For adolescents, in particular, questions arise around the quality of this "new life." Attempts to enter the job market are among the most unsettling aspects of adjustment (Malekzadeh et al., 1976). Vocational rehabilitation and career opportunities become important considerations.

Studies of the families of posttransplant children (Korsch et al., 1973) show that, although the time period of treatment for end-stage renal disease, hemodialysis, and kidney transplant causes severe disturbances in family routines, relationships, education, and recreational patterns, usually family equilibrium is restored to normal within approximately one year after successful transplantation.

Typically there is a good potential for recovery and rehabilitation for the child and his family after hemodialysis and renal transplantation (Korsch et al., 1973). Usually the child's personality pattern returns to preillness balance if the kidney transplant is successful, and the child's physical health improves. Even severe disorganization in the personality of the child during the acute phases of treatment is reversible. Korsch et al. (1973) point out that experiences with treatment for end-stage kidney disease are not as traumatic, after all, as assumed by previous investigators, because the prognosis for graft survival is increasingly good with improvements in posttransplant surgical and medical care. The active participation of a comprehensive health care team in the management of the child and the family early in the onset of chronic kidney disease, providing constant attention to their needs and anticipatory guidance at times of great stress, is especially instrumental in observed successful recovery after kidney transplantation.

If a kidney transplant begins to fail, new issues emerge. When severe signs of kidney rejection develop and especially when the transplanted kidney is rejected completely, the resultant anxiety and deceit may become violent. Having to return to hemodialysis becomes nightmarish; dialysis sessions and physical pain are much harder to tolerate. Such children may undergo a period of deep depression and may exhibit symptoms of severe withdrawal (Bouras et al., 1976). In these instances the active participation of the comprehensive health care team in the rehabilitation of the child becomes extremely important.

SUMMARY

Renal disease, renal failure, hemodialysis, and transplantation—all have a strong psychological impact on the afflicted child and his family. The stress of a protracted, progressive illness such as the nephrotic syndrome gives rise to feelings of self-blame, as well as to problems with the development of interpersonal relationships, self-concept, and body image in the child patient. The onset of end-stage renal failure is the beginning of a new scope of medical issues and emotional problems. When kidney failure develops there are basically two choices: death or prolongation of life through hemodialysis and eventual kidney transplantation. Hemodialysis represents an abrupt and sudden change in life patterns that is often met with withdrawal and depression on the part of the child patient. A major issue becomes achieving a balance between dependence on the kidney machine and independence in social adjustment. From a psychological point of view, hemodialysis stifles a child's ability to develop his personality in the normal arenas such as school and social activities. Dietary restrictions become a source of frustration, and patient compliance is a recognized clinical problem. The need for comprehensive psychosocial management of the child/patient and his family by a team of professionals cannot be overemphasized. The preparation for transplantation is enhanced by good psychological management before the event. Transplantation cannot be viewed as an isolated phase because it is so closely linked with the past experiences of the child and the family. The problems surrounding kidney donorship, the anxiety waiting for the transplant to occur, and the fears of rejection that follow are pervasive issues. Encouragingly, most transplant patients return to normal psychological adjustment within a year after the transplantation, but continued problems persist around self-concept and future planning. If a kidney transplant fails, a new cycle of fears and anxieties begins; the hoped for chance for a normal life dissolves with increased uncertainty about the future.

The complex saga of the kidney patient is linked intimately with the saga of the health care team, the members of which are constantly confronting the potential failure of their life-saving efforts. The nature of hemodialysis—an almost daily process—brings together a new pseudo-family structure replete with its own organic issues. The questions of guilt, possessiveness, and overprotectiveness become critical components in the resolution of care. The shifting of care to a new team, the transplant unit, is a difficult event for all involved. It is through a good communication process and an understanding of each team's role in the psychodynamic triangle of child, parent, and team that optimal care can be provided.

REFERENCES

Abram, H. S. 1974. The uncooperative hemodialysis patient: A psychiatrist's viewpoint and a patient's commentary. In N. Levy (ed.), Living or Dying—Adaptation to Hemodialysis, pp. 50–61. Charles C Thomas, Springfield, Ill.

Arneil, G. C. 1971. The nephrotic syndrome. Pediatr. Clin. North Am. 18:547–559.

Beard, B. H. 1969. Fear of death and fear of life: The dilemma in chronic renal failure, hemodialysis and kidney transplantation. Arch. Gen. Psychiatry 21:373–380.

Beard, B. H. 1971. The quality of life before and after renal transplantation. Dis. Nerv. Syst. 32:24–29.

Berger, M., Ginn, R., and Travis, L. 1975. Pediatric dialysis and its psychosocial implications. Pediatr. Psychol. 3:17–19.

Bernstein, D. M. 1971. After transplantation—the child's emotional reactions. Am. J. Psychiatry 127:109–113.

Bouras, M., Silvestre, D., Broyer, M., and Raimbault, G. 1976. Renal transplantation in children: a psychological survey. Clin. Nephrol. 6:478–482.

Crittenden, M. R., Decker, B., and Levin, C. 1975. Pediatric renal team reactions to treatment of children by hemodialysis and transplantation. Pediat. Psychol. 3:6–10.

Debre, M., Duhong, O., and Raimbault, G. 1973. Etudes psychologiques d'enfants en hémodialyse. Arch. Fr. Pediatr. 30:163–167.

DeNour, A., and Czaczkes, J. 1976. The influence of patient's personality on adjustment to chronic dialysis. J. Nerv. Ment. Dis. 162:323–333.

DeNour, A., and Czaczkes, J. 1968. Emotional problems and reactions of the medical team in a chronic hemodialysis unit. Lancet 2:987–991.

Fine, R. N. 1972. Renal transplantation in children. In Proceedings of the Ninth Conference of European Dialysis and Transplantation Assoc. p. 200. Florence, Italy.

Fine, R. N., and Gruskin, C. M. 1973. Hemodialysis and renal transplantation in children. Clin. Nephrol. 1:243–256.

Fine, R. N., Korsch, B. M., Brennan, L. P., Edelbrock, H. H., Stiles, Q. R., Riddell, H. I., Weitzman, J. J., Mickelson, J. C., Tucker, B. L. and Grushkin, C. M. 1973. Renal transplantation in young children. Am. J. Surg. 125:559–569.

Fine, R. N., Korsch, B. M., Grushkin, C. M., and Lieberman, E. 1970. Hemodialysis in children. Am. J. Dis. Child. 119:498–504.

Gianantonio, C., Vitacco, M., Mendialaharzu, F., and Gallo, G. 1968. The hemolytic uremic syndrome. J. Pediatr. 72:757–765.

Gianantonio, C. A., Vitacco, M. and Mendilaharzu, F. 1967. The hemolytic uremic syndrome. In Proceedings, 3rd International Congress on Nephrology. Vol. III, p. 24. Karger, Basel.

Grushkin, C. M., Korsch, B. M., and Fine, R. N. 1973. The outlook for adolescents with chronic renal failure. Pediatr. Clin. North Am. 20:953–963.

Grushkin, C. M., Korsch, B., and Fine, R. N. 1972. Hemodialysis in small children. JAMA 221:869–973.

Herdman, R. C., and Urizar, R. E. 1975. Coagulopathy in renal disease, including hemolytic uremic syndrome. In M. I. Rubin and T. M. Barratt (eds.), Pediatric Nephrology, pp. 189–216. The Williams & Wilkins Co., Baltimore.

Khan, A. U., Herndon, M. A., and Ahmadian, S. Y. 1971. Social and emotional adaptations of children with transplanted kidneys and chronic hemodialysis. Am. J. Psychiatry 127:1194–1198.

Korsch, B., and Barnett, H. L. 1961. The physician, the family and the child with nephrosis. J. Pediatr. 58:707–715.

Korsch, B., Fraad, L. M., and Barnett, H. L. 1954. Pediatric dicussion with parent groups. J. Pediatr. 44:703–717.

Korsch, B. M., Fine, R. N., Grushkin, C. M., and Negrete, V. F. 1971. Experiences with children and their families during extended hemodialysis and kidney transplantation. Pediatr. Clin. North Am. 18:625–637.

Korsch, B. M., Negrete, V. F., Gardner, J. E., Weinstock, C, Mercer, A., Grushkin, C. M., and Fine R. N. 1973. Kidney transplantation in children: Psychosocial follow-up study on child and family. J. Pediatr. 83:399–408.

MacGregor, R. R., Sheagren, J. N., Lipsett, M. B., and Woff, S. M. 1969. Alternate-day prednisone therapy. New Engl. J. Med. 280:1427–1431.

Magrab, P. 1975. Psychological management and renal dialysis. J. Clin. Psychol. 4:38–41.

Magrab, P., and Papadopoulou, Z. 1977. The effect of a token economy on dietary compliance for children on hemodialysis. J. Appl. Behav. Anal. 10:573–579.

Malekzadeh, M., Pennisi, A., Uittenbogaart, C., Korsch, B. M., Fine, R. N., and Main, M. 1976. Current issues in pediatric renal transplantation. Pediatr. Clin. North Am. 23:857–872.

Mattson, A. 1972. Long-term physical illness in childhood: A challenge to psychosocial adaptation. Pediatrics 50:801–811.

Meadow, R., Cameron, J. S., and Ogg, C. 1970. Regional service for acute and chronic dialysis of children. Lancet 2:707–709.

Morse, J. 1974. Family involvement in pediatric dialysis and transplantation. Social Case Work, April, 216–223.

Nordan, R., Ostendorf, R., and Naughton, J. P. 1971. Return to the land of the living: An approach to the problem of chronic hemodialysis. Pediatrics 48:939–945.

Salisbury, R. E. 1968. Behavioral responses of a nine year old child on chronic dialysis. J. Am. Acad. Child Psychiatry 7:282–295.

Sampson, T. 1975. The child in renal failure—emotional impact of treatment on the child and his family. J. Am. Acad. Child Psychiatry 14:462–475.

Schultz, M. T., McVicar, M. I., and Kemph, J. P. 1974. Treatment of the emotional and cognitive deficits of the child receiving hemodialysis. In N. Levy (ed.), Living or Dying—Adaptation to Hemodialysis, pp. 62–73. Charles C Thomas, Springfield, Ill.

Wenzl, J. 1975. Preparation of the patient and family for renal transplantation. Pediatr. Psychol. 3:14–16.

Wilson, C., Potter, D., and Holliday, M. 1973. Treatment of the uremic child. In R.W. Winter (ed.), Body Fluids in Pediatrics, pp. 579–594. Little, Brown & Co., Boston.

Zifferblatt, S. 1975. Increased patient compliance through the applied analysis of behavior. Prev. Med. 4:173–182.

10
Pediatric Oncology

Gerald P. Koocher and Stephen E. Sallan

The treatment of childhood malignancies has changed dramatically over the past decade. Although cancer remains second only to accidents as a leading cause of death in children, great strides have been made in the treatment and control of these life-threatening diseases. Children who almost certainly would have died in the course of a few months 10 years ago have an even chance of surviving five years or more under current therapies. Medical science has essentially altered the natural history of many of these diseases, even though complete or permanent control may not be achieved. What were once acutely fatal illnesses have become chronic life-threatening ones.

The psychological impact of these events is rather complex. To begin with, there are probably more pediatric cancer patients alive today than ever before. Although these diseases are relatively rare, the children who have them are living much longer and fuller lives than in the past. As a result more families and people in our communities have the occasion to encounter pediatric cancer patients at home, in school, and on the playground. Families who might have once been told with a high degree of reliability that their child would die, are now met with guarded optimism by the oncologists who treat their child. For many families this is somewhat like sitting beneath the sword of Damocles. That is to say, they do not know whether they should prepare to mourn the loss of their child or whether they should dare to hope for a sustained remission or even the elusive "cure." Once "predictable" events in the course of the child's illness are in many ways less predictable, and families must learn to tolerate stressful periods of uncertainty.

Whereas therapeutic programs in the past were aimed at palliation, modern therapies are undertaken with curative intent. Such therapy is frequently aggressive to the point that patients and families are often uncertain as to whether the aggressor is the disease or the physician. Parents and children must accept and incorporate this "willing" capitulation to body (and, at times, spirit) destroying life-style in the service of

During the preparation of this chapter the first author was supported in part by National Cancer Institute Grant No. CA 18429 CCG.

a greater good—survival. Unfortunately, only about half of those who make this choice eventually succeed.

This is a rather grim field in which to work. In a nutshell, individuals involved in the care of children with malignancies must be able to form multiple, extraordinarily close interpersonal relationships and then to separate from half of these under the least desirable of circumstances, often finding themselves enmeshed in fundamental human tragedies. While the unacquainted observer ordinarily focuses on the tragic component, there are many personal rewards to be found in the fundamental human elements of these relationships. The potential for meaningful and helpful interventions in the lives of these families is quite significant, and much beneficial work can be accomplished in relatively brief periods of time. Only rarely in the work of the physician or mental health professional is the impact of one's day-to-day contact with a family so dramatically important and so much appreciated.

THE ILLNESSES

The majority of patients with childhood malignancies and their parents will quickly learn a multitude of facts and details about their individual disease and its treatment. Their knowledge and understanding will be communicated in "medicalese," a foreign language comprised of proper medical terminology and assorted malapropisms. The latter are often significant and readily interpreted by the sophisticated listener. Individuals who are not fluent with this language undoubtedly will suffer and lose a great deal from their communications. It is therefore quite important that the concerned caregiver without a medical background obtain a relatively detailed education regarding the various diseases, concepts of treatment, individual drugs, and the acute and chronic side effects of all these variables. The inability of the caregiver to interpret medicalese fluently will add a cumbersome barrier to ready communication.

The childhood malignancies (i.e., cancers) are a heterogeneous group of diseases characterized by a common bond: untreated, they are fatal. Each disease has its own natural history: a relatively predictable course from the time that it first becomes apparent, through a period of spreading, to death. The goal of treatment is to interrupt or alter the natural history of the disease. At the very least, pain can be allayed, bleeding controlled, and body functions stabilized as close to normal as possible. Usually, one can expect a great deal more of treatment. In addition to palliating disturbing symptoms, tumor masses can be controlled (using surgery and/or radiation therapy), and widespread disease can often be managed (using drugs).

Although each disease is different, childhood cancer can be divided generally into two broad categories: hematologic (i.e., blood) malignancies and solid tumors. Each category accounts for approximately one-half of all pediatric cancer.

The hematologic malignancies, leukemias and lymphomas, can be subdivided further into four diseases: acute lymphoblastic leukemia (ALL), acute nonlymphoblastic leukemia (ANLL), Hodgkin's lymphoma, and non-Hodgkin's lymphoma. Common solid tumors of childhood include brain tumors, neuroblastoma, Wilms' tumor, bone tumors, and soft tissue sarcomas (e.g., rhabdomyosarcoma, etc.). In the following pages the most common diseases in each of these two broad categories are discussed.

General Issues in Hematologic Malignancies

In general hematologic cancer involves rapid growth of abnormal cells that are often widely disseminated and essentially cause damage by crowding bone marrow and other lymphatic organs to the degree that normal functioning is affected adversely. Treatment with curative intent begins with efforts to induce a remission. The specific strategy and nature of this "induction" will vary with the disease. In general, however, remission is characterized by the absence of signs and symptoms of the disease. The next phase of treatment ideally will consolidate the process begun in the induction phase. Attempts are made to be sure that any malignant cells that may remain in the body, but in locations or numbers that are not detectable, are eradicated. The final phase in the ideal paradigm is a therapeutic program aimed at maintaining the remission as long as possible with the ultimate goal of being able to discontinue treatment while the child remains in prolonged remission on the way to the elusive "cure."

The duration of treatment varies from two to five or more years. No one yet knows the optimal duration, and the decision to electively discontinue successful therapy has become one of the most emotionally charged events of the entire treatment process. It means the end of a love/hate relationship between parents, patients, and the chemotherapy. The nausea, vomiting, hair loss, painful injections, and interruptions of life-style are surrendered willingly. However, the comfort and security engendered by the successful treatments are difficult to risk, regardless of the rewards. Why, then, is treatment stopped? Because 80% of the children no longer require the drugs, but the other 20% cannot be identified until therapy is discontinued. Relapse occurs in 20% of those removed from treatment, with 10% relapsing in the first year and 10% thereafter (from two to seven or more years after stopping).

Relapses, on or off chemotherapy, are always an ominous event. From the standpoint of "treatment with curative intent," the first relapse is a significant failure. Very few malignancies (with the exception of

Wilms' tumor, discussed later) can be cured after the first relapse. Thus, treatment after relapse is conceptually quite different from initial therapy. Attempts to treat for cure necessarily become more futile and frequently are equally or even more aggressive than initial therapies. The alternatives are moderately (but less) aggressive treatment to reinduce remission and sustain it for prolonged periods, or palliative treatment directed only at providing symptomatic relief rather than focusing on the underlying cause of the illness.

Still another stage of treatment usually is instituted very late in the course of an illness. This is treatment with new and more experimental drugs. Usually, the choice for the child and/or family is "to treat or not to treat." The decision "to treat" with experimental drugs is one that is usually more sustaining of hope than life.

Acute Lymphoblastic Leukemia (ALL)   This is the most common childhood malignancy, accounting for approximately 35% of all neoplasms in children. The disease is a progressive infiltration of bone marrow and lymphatic organs by lymphoblasts. Its incidence is approximately 2.3 per 100,000 in the general population, and 1.0 per 2,880 in Caucasians under 15 years of age. Thus, there are about 2,000 new cases each year in the United States. The median age of affected children is four years with a peak incidence in the two- to five-year range, but all ages are affected and there is a slight male preponderance (1.4:1). Although the etiology is unknown and presumed to be multifactorial, predisposing factors may include genetics, radiation, viruses, and perhaps other toxic agents.

The symptomatic presentation of the disease can vary widely and may be focal or systemic, initially minor or immediately life threatening. Recent advances in therapeutics have altered the natural course of the disease dramatically. In 1950, the average survival time following the diagnosis of ALL was three months, whereas, in the late 1970s, 50% of newly diagnosed ALL patients can expect to remain free of disease for at least five years.

Treatment programs are essentially similar in most major cancer treatment centers. They are aggressive regimens, applied with curative intent, and utilize a combination of cytotoxic agents to induce and prolong disease-free periods. In addition, radiation to the brain and injections of chemotherapeutic agents into the fluid surrounding the spinal cord are usually employed as prophylactic measures against relapses in the central nervous system (Dritshila, Cassady, and Camitta, 1976). It also should be noted that newer laboratory techniques are unmasking separate disease entities, such as "T-cell leukemia," that mimic ALL but that may be much less controllable (Sen and Borell, 1975). The reader seeking more detailed information on the treatment of acute leukemia is referred to Pinkel (1976).

Acute Nonlymphoblastic Leukemia (ANLL)   This category of disease includes the rarer forms of childhood leukemia: acute myelogenous leukemia (AML), myelomonocytic, monocytic, promyelocytic, and erythroleukemia. These types constitute approximately 10–15% of childhood leukemias with no specific age peaks. The incidence of these diseases is approximately four cases per million children, or roughly 400 new cases per year in the United States. The prognosis for patients with this group of leukemias has until recently been extremely poor. Children with ANLL, like those with ALL, may present with a vast array of signs and symptoms ranging from the apparently trivial to the immediately life threatening. Although initial remissions can be achieved in 75% of the children treated, the median duration of remission has usually been little more than one year. The reader who wishes more detailed information should see Choi and Simone (1976).

Hodgkin's Disease   This illness, a malignancy of the lymph nodes, is a relatively rare disorder in childhood. Male patients outnumber females by a ratio of 1.5:1, with a marked male predominance in children under 10 years of age and an equalization of incidence between the sexes by the mid-teens.

Hodgkin's disease ordinarily presents as a gradually progressing growth of one or more lymph nodes. Less frequently, the nodal disease is accompanied by so-called "B symptoms" including fever, night sweats, and weight loss. There are four pathological subtypes of Hodgkin's disease: lymphocyte predominant, nodular sclerosing, mixed cellularity, and lymphocyte depletion. Treatment and prognosis are determined in part by the pathological subtype and also by the extent of the illness at the time of diagnosis. The latter is determined by a series of tests, often including an exploratory abdominal operation. As a result of these diagnostic tests, the disease is assigned a "stage" rating, ranging from minimal involvement (Stage I) to extensive spread (Stage IV) with or without a "B," depending on the symptoms as noted above.

Treatment of very limited disease may be only with regional radiation therapy, whereas more extensive disease is treated with chemotherapy as well. Often both of these treatment modalities are used. Expectations for successful treatment vary from over 90% for Stage I patients to about 50% for Stage IV patients. Hodgkin's disease is also somewhat unique inasmuch as chronicity, even after one or more relapses, is often the case. Thus, long-term disease-free survival suggests the possibility of cure, but relatively long-term survival followed by relapse and additional remissions is not unusual.

Patients with Hodgkin's disease, whether in remission or not, are often susceptible to unusual types of infections. These are generally mild to moderate in severity, but can be life threatening. The operation necessary for stage classification of Hodgkin's disease entails removal of the spleen. In view of that organ's role in helping the body to resist infection, the patient must cope with the lifelong risk of overwhelming bloodstream infections. Most patients will require daily doses of "prophylactic" antibiotics. This procedure, as well as the low but very real risk of instant major infection, creates chronic psychological difficulties unique to patients with Hodgkin's disease. This may be manifest in frustration and anger at frequent infections or sudden episodes of anxiety in response to what might be mild infections by usual standards. The reader wishing more detailed information should see Wiernik (1974).

Non-Hodgkin's Lymphoma   This set of diseases is quite different in children than in adults. A uniform system of classification and assessment of prognosis is lacking, and the pattern and spread of disease in children are quite different from adults as well. The incidence of these illnesses is similar to that of Hodgkin's disease and ANLL. The most common age range in childhood is four to 17 years with a median age of 11 years.

Unlike Hodgkin's disease (also known as Hodgkin's lymphoma), which usually spreads in a predictable fashion from one lymph node to another, non-Hodgkin's lymphomas are hematogenously spread. Thus, the disease is usually widespread at the time of diagnosis, much more like leukemia than Hodgkin's disease, and less readily controlled by radiation therapy. The treatment of choice, therefore, is usually chemotherapy, although occasionally radiation therapy and rarely surgery are also employed. The overall prognosis is similar to that of childhood ALL. An excellent current update on prognosis and treatment of this disease may be found in Murphy (1977).

General Issues in Treatment of Solid Tumors

Solid tumors present a set of issues different in many ways from the hematologic malignancies. To begin with, there are at least one or more sites of disease in the body. These may be visible or palpable signs of illness, which may not be present in the hematologic malignancies. Surgical intervention is almost invariably part of the therapeutic regimen, resulting in body-image change and frequent need for varying degrees of physical rehabilitation or adaptation to a surgically acquired handicap. From a therapeutic standpoint, the key issues are those of local control and systemic therapy. That is to say, one must be concerned not only about the primary tumor site, but one must also consider the potential for development of metastases or seeding of lesions at other locations in the body distant from the original tumor.

Brain Tumors   Brain tumors are the most common solid tumors of childhood, second only to leukemia in overall frequency, representing

17–20% of pediatric cancer. They are unique among solid tumors for two reasons. First, they very rarely metastasize outside of the central nervous system. Second, the prognosis is as much a function of the site as of the specific type of tumor. Treatment is complicated by the fact that surgery is frequently impossible because the tumor could only be reached by destroying vital areas of the brain. Even when the tumor is surgically approachable, total removal of the tumor is seldom feasible. Frequently, radiation therapy is employed in efforts to control brain tumors. While the role of chemotherapy has been explored over the past decade, successful drug treatment is unusual.

The presenting symptoms most commonly associated with brain tumors include morning headaches and vomiting. Both of these are signs of increased pressure within the head. Other findings may include an unsteady gait, generalized weakness, and sensory changes (especially of a visual or auditory nature). Adjunctive treatment often includes "shunting" procedures, which provide a means of removing blocked fluids within the brain. These surgical procedures can provide symptomatic relief by decreasing the pressure on the brain from fluid build-up.

With notable exceptions, such as low grade anatomically "safely located" astrocytomas and some medulablastomas, the prognosis for children with brain tumors is not good. Approximately 30–40% of these children can be expected to be alive five years after diagnosis. Detailed discussion of these tumors and their treatment in childhood may be found in papers by Wilson (1975a, 1975b) and Walker (1976).

Emotional concerns of children with brain tumors and of their families are frequently complicated by communication difficulties related to intellectual, sensory, and/or motor function losses. There is also a special subset of emotions that is evoked in response to children with impairments linked to the brain as a result of its special status as the seat of intellect and personality.

Neuroblastoma This is the most common extracranial, nonlymphomatous, solid tumor of childhood, accounting for 7–10% of childhood malignancies. The incidence of neuroblastoma is approximately one per 10,000 live births. As the name suggests, it arises from neural tissue. Usual primary sites are the abdomen (adrenal gland) and chest (sympathetic nervous system). The tumor is most common in infants and very young children, although it may occur at any age from infancy through adolescence. Neuroblastomas are also unusual in that the tumors may undergo spontaneous regression, especially in infants under six months of age.

Symptoms at the time of presentation vary with the anatomical site and extent of the disease. Adrenal tumors may present as abdominal masses, while respiratory distress may be the herald of chest tumors.

Early detection is an important factor in the prognosis for children with neuroblastoma.

The diagnosis is usually based upon a biopsy of the tumor mass, although bone marrow is often involved, making it possible to arrive at a diagnosis on the basis of a sample of marrow rather than direct biopsy of the mass itself. Urine testing can also provide diagnostic information. As in Hodgkin's disease, "staging" of the tumor at the time of diagnosis can be important in estimating prognosis.

Staging refers to the degree of dissemination or spread of the tumor. Stage I is a completely encapsulated, easily operable tumor. Stage II is a regional disease on one side of the midline. Stage III is a tumor extending across the midline with or without spread to lymph nodes. In Stage IV metastases exist at a distance from the primary site. Patients over two years of age with Stage IV neuroblastoma have less than a 7% survival rate, while children who are less than a year old at the time of diagnosis have significantly better outlook. For example, an infant less than six months old with a Stage I neuroblastoma has a better than 90% chance of long-term survival (five years or more). In general, the lower stages are treated with surgery and/or radiation therapy. Disseminated tumor is treated with chemotherapy, with or without radiation and/or surgery depending on tumor site, response to treatment, and many other variables. For an up-to-date discussion of neuroblastoma the reader should see Jaffe's (1976) paper.

When widely disseminated, neuroblastoma is a particularly unpleasant malignancy. It is often painful, resistant to treatment, and all too seldom does not permit extended periods during which the child feels well. Unlike the vast majority of pediatric malignancies, which often can be managed routinely on an outpatient basis, neuroblastoma patients must be admitted to the hospital frequently for treatment. From a psychological standpoint, the disease is more like a prolonged acute illness rather than a chronic condition. Parent-child communication is often difficult because most of the patients are too young for substantial verbal communication, and other parenting processes too often can be disrupted by nausea, pain, and irritability. When the tumor is excised easily and a continuous remission follows, the psychological prognosis is no different from that of any infant or family with an episode of acute serious illness.

Wilms' Tumor   This tumor is primarily a malignancy of the kidney, which may arise in utero. The median age at diagnosis is two years for males and three for females, with presentation in children over six years of age being quite unusual. The disease is slightly more frequent in males and is occasionally associated with other congenital abnormalities. The annual incidence is approximately 7.5 cases per million children under age 15, or roughly 450 cases per year.

Most Wilms' tumors present as asymptomatic abdominal masses, usually discovered by parents. The disease may also present with abdominal pain or blood in the urine. Initial evaluation includes a physical examination, special kidney x-rays (intravenous pyelogram or IVP), and a chest x-ray to check for possible metastases in the lungs (the most common site of spread).

As in the case of other solid tumors, the specific treatment and prognosis depend on the extent of the disease at the time of diagnosis. Except for extremely large tumors, the initial treatment is surgery. Thereafter, except for very small tumors, the tumor site and occasionally the whole abdomen are irradiated. Chemotherapy is then initiated in virtually all patients. Metastases to the lungs or other areas are treated with radiation and/or surgery. Unlike most malignancies, Wilms' tumor may be "curable" even after evidence of spread. Prognosis for a favorable outcome ranges from 85% in the case of a small localized tumor to approximately 50% in patients with extensive disease at the time of diagnosis. An update on current therapies may be found in Jenkin (1976).

Because treatment invariably involves removal of one kidney, patients are often justifiably anxious regarding urinary tract infections. A number of former patients have also expressed varying degrees of dissatisfaction with limitations placed on their activities (e.g., prohibitions against playing contact sports) as protective measures for the remaining kidney.

Bone Tumors   These consist of four tumor groups: osteogenic sarcoma, Ewing's sarcoma, bone lymphomas, and miscellaneous types. As a group, bone tumors represent less than 1% of all malignancies. They are most common in late childhood and adolescence, with a mortality rate of 1.87 per million in children under age 14 and 11.97 deaths per million in the 15 to 19 age group. Jaffe (1975) presents a detailed and up-to-date summary of these tumors.

Osteogenic sarcoma is the most common malignant tumor of bone. Characteristically the disease presents with pain at the site of the tumor, and this is often thought to be a bruise or sprain by the typical adolescent patient. Untreated, 80% of patients with osteogenic sarcoma will develop lung metastases and die. Therefore, attempts to improve upon the natural history of this tumor have focused on local control at the primary site and chemotherapy to prevent or eradicate lung metastases. The initial examination includes a physical examination, bone and chest x-rays, and a biopsy of the tumor. Additional x-ray examinations may be performed if "limb preservation" is anticipated (see below).

Local control is generally achieved by amputation, chemotherapy, and sometimes radiation. In certain cases it may be possible to attempt "limb preservation" rather than immediate amputation. When this is the treatment of choice, the section of bone with the tumor is removed and replaced with an internal prosthesis. In all cases, chemotherapy is begun early in the course of treatment based on the assumption (from the known natural history of the disease) that clinically undetectable microscopic metastases are present in the majority of patients at the time of diagnosis. Drugs are administered intermittently over one to two years. This type of approach, based on the natural history of the disease, and treatment, based on predictions of potential spread, are known as adjuvant chemotherapy. Treatment of this type in the 1970s has significantly altered the natural history of the tumor to the point that lung metastases, which predictably appear within a year or two of diagnosis, can now be eradicated in some patients and markedly delayed in appearance for most others.

New developments in the treatment of osteogenic sarcomas in the mid-1970s raise some central issues with regard to the psychological management of these patients. This tumor and its natural history were relatively unresponsive to therapeutic intervention before the early 1970s. Overall survival was poor, with 80–90% of patients developing lung metastases and dying. Then a drug called methotrexate was shown to be effective in eradicating lung metastases and shortly thereafter was in wide use for adjuvant chemotherapy. For a time the overall survival trends seemed to be reversed, with 80% of patients being disease-free and only 20% showing metastases. Slowly the apparent success of this treatment approach faded. By 1977 the disease-free survival statistics were no longer significantly different from those of 1970.

These developments, including the gradual diminution of hope and fading of the first flushes of success, extracted an enormous emotional toll from the patients, their loved ones, and the professionals caring for them. All were relatively unprepared and emotionally undefended against the shock of failure. This process aptly illustrates a new issue for cancer patients and professionals working with them: how to accept some success without really crying.

Other bone tumors (Ewing's sarcoma, lymphomas, etc.) present similarly to osteogenic sarcoma, and the principles of evaluating and treating them are also similar. First, the type of tumor and extent of involvement must be determined. Thereafter, local control (with surgery and/or radiation) and adjuvant chemotherapy for systemic treatment are the usual practices.

The specific prognosis again varies as a function of tumor type and extent of spread at the time of presentation. Ewing's sarcoma that has not spread at the time of diagnosis may be controllable for over 50% of patients, whereas it is almost universally fatal for those who present with metastases. Moreover, certain anatomical sites (e.g., ribs) may be more favorable than others (e.g., pelvic bones). Bone lymphomas in children usually are treated initially with radiation therapy and often with adjuvant chemotherapy. The overall prognosis for these patients is becoming progressively better, and long-term disease-free survival can be anticipated in over 50% of patients.

Soft Tissue Sarcomas   These tumors arise from various tissues such as muscle (rhabdomyosarcoma), blood vessels (hemangiosarcoma), and fat (liposarcoma). For all soft tissue sarcomas, presentation, treatment, and prognosis depend on the exact type of tumor, its location, and the extent of spread at the time of diagnosis. General principles of local control and adjuvant chemotherapy (as noted above) prevail in treatment. Only rhabdomyosarcomas occur frequently enough to be considered as a special subcategory.

Rhabdomyosarcomas occur primarily in Caucasians, suggesting some genetic predisposition. The age incidence distribution is bimodal with one peak in the two- to four-year range and another between ages 16 and 20. The tumors are usually classified by anatomical site of presentation: head and neck, genitourinary tract, extremities, and other. Prognosis is variable, ranging from over 80% disease-free survival in some circumstances to 40-50% in others. A detailed review on soft-tissue sarcomas in childhood may be found in Raney, Schnaufer, and Donaldson (1974).

Complications

The treatment of virtually all childhood cancer is with curative intent. This often encompasses radical ablative surgical procedures (e.g., amputation), moderately deforming radiation therapy, and aggressive recurrent courses of chemotherapy resulting in prolonged vomiting, hair loss, mouth ulcers, frequent blood tests, and occasional hospitalizations. Although very few individuals suffer all of the possible complications of treatment, and many others experience few side effects, most patients face many of these problems.

Dangerous illnesses often require treatments that can be dangerous themselves. The treatments described above often give the child and other family members more than passing doubts, and there are often times when all may wonder if they will be able to continue. Often the complaints or problems that will come to the attention of the mental health professional are of this iatrogenic nature. The thrust of most concerns relative to complications of cancer treatment relates either to the extent of body-image changes or to the side effects of chemotherapy.

"Why," a patient may ask, "did the surgeon have to cut so much when the tumor was so small?" Local control, whether by surgery or irradiation, requires that the tumor be totally encompassed. In surgery this means that the successfully removed tumor will include normal tissue around its margins. Generally some normal tissue must be removed or irradiated to ensure that all of the malignant tissue is gone. At times the full extent of disease may not even be apparent until after surgery. The goal of the cancer surgeon and radiation therapist is to eradicate the tumor while sparing as much normal tissue and function as possible.

Trying to explain to the child why chemotherapy causes problems can also be difficult. Chemotherapy is toxic for two basic reasons. First, the drugs are not tumor specific. They do not distinguish normal from abnormal cells. Second, the drugs are active only at high doses, and the maximal tolerable amounts are usually preferable for optimal killing of tumor cells. Most anticancer drug doses are limited only by normal cell tolerance. Wide individual variations exist in doses of drugs tolerated, as well as within the same individual at various times. Thus, the same dose of a drug may be subtherapeutic and toxic in one child, subtherapeutic and nontoxic in another, therapeutic and nontoxic in still another, and so forth.

The psychological components of these complications also vary between and within individual children. The set and setting of therapeutic interventions, both initially and throughout therapy, as well as the individual and collective familial strengths brought to the experience, are endlessly complex variables.

Initially, the child may be very ill and the initial therapeutic interventions may bring immediate relief, palliation of pain, and renewed energy. On the other hand, many patients feel reasonably well at the time of diagnosis, and the therapy results in their becoming "unwell." Clearly the same complications in either of these two instances will be perceived and interpreted quite differently. During the period immediately after diagnosis, the patient and family must simultaneously cope with acceptance of the serious diagnosis and acceptance of aggressive treatment. Not infrequently, coming to grips with the diagnosis is partially undone by the inability to do the same with the treatments, the former being completely out of the child's (and family's) control and the latter done only upon their agreement and with their "informed consent."

Alopecia   Hair loss, partial or total, head or whole body, secondary to chemotherapy or radiation treatment, is often an emotionally devastating occurrence. It has been well documented that children with visible physical defects, regardless of the extent of the handicap, tend to have social adjustment problems (Goldberg, 1974). Although popular opinion holds that this is particularly upsetting for adolescents, there is little empirical evidence to support that belief, and younger children are also acutely upset to find their hair coming out. Advance discussions with the child to ensure that this symptom does not come as a surprise can be helpful, as can reassurances that the hair will probably come back following cessation of treatments. Still, the emotional stress at this time in treatment will be quite high, and the child's reactions may range from defensively flippant joking to serious emotional and social withdrawal (Heffron, Bommelare, and Masters, 1973).

Other Bodily Changes   In addition to alopecia, children undergoing radical surgery or radiation therapy, as well as those on chemotherapy, will experience a number of other bodily changes. While the former are generally one-at-a-time-only events, drug treatments result in both acute and recurrent problems. These include dramatic weight gain or loss, mouth ulcers, muscle spasms, and skin rashes. Radiation treatment may leave skin discolored and lead to growth retardation of some body regions while others develop normally. The need for surgery may result in scars, organ losses, or amputations with which to cope as well. It is frightening to have one's body being altered in any fashion, but it is especially troubling to younger children who may develop magical ideas about why such things are happening to them. In a society that values beauty and normality, these changes can be devastating. Again, preparation can be helpful, but the need for adaptive coping and for easing the stress that goes with it continues unceasingly.

Chronic Vomiting   This toxic reaction to chemotherapeutic agents is virtually inescapable. Nausea and vomiting are common aspects of a treatment program that paradoxically gives the child the message that "We must make you sick to get you well." Efforts to control this symptom with available antiemetic drugs have been disappointing, but many active clinical investigations aimed at better control are underway. In some cases patients seem to develop Pavlovian-style conditioned reflex vomiting. In such instances a child may begin to vomit the day before a scheduled treatment or become nauseated simply by thinking about the hospital or clinic. Behavioral techniques, including relaxation training, and suggestion or hypnotic techniques, have occasionally been found useful with some of these children (Gardner, 1976).

Immunosuppression   Depression of a child's immune responses and the resulting increased susceptibility to all manner of bacterial, viral, and fungal infections present a constant concern. It is possible for a child whose cancer is well controlled to contract a fulminating infection and die rapidly, in a matter of hours. It is more likely, however, that the child will develop intermittent infections over the course of treatment, which may require hospitalization and be considerably more dangerous than they would be in a normal child. The frequency of these interruptions in daily living adds considerably to the whole family's stress quotient. Although the ideal treatment program is one that balances maximal effective treatment with as "normal" an existence as possible, the fine line between undertreatment and overtreatment can never be defined adequately.

Evaluating the Child's Experiences

The main point of the foregoing material is to emphasize the need for the mental health professionals who work with cancer patients to become familiar with the nature of the illnesses, treatments, and complications that are a part of each child's life experiences. This information will help put the child's and family's emotional frames of reference in perspective and will help in evaluating their emotional reactions and coping behavior. The usual situation is not one of helping emotionally troubled people overcome long-standing maladaptive patterns. Instead, basically sound families are confronting an inordinate amount of stress, which they are basically powerless to control. In such circumstances even the most well-adjusted families will be unable to escape reactive emotional difficulties linked to powerful reality events. When the family has preexisting emotional problems the onset of cancer certainly adds considerable stress.

Uncovering unconscious material and interpreting it to clients become secondary to more direct, supportive measures, including facilitating communication among family members, encouraging the expression of significant emotional concerns, assisting in the management of reactive behavior problems, and sensitizing clients to the emotional subtleties that are easily overlooked. Ironically, these tasks are not limited to the children and their families, but, as noted in the pages that follow, also apply to the mental health professional's work with the other members of the oncology team (Geist, 1977; O'Malley and Koocher, 1977).

CURRENT PSYCHOLOGICAL RESEARCH

The late 1960s and early 1970s saw the beginning of a flood of psychological studies and books on death, dying, and terminal illness. A recent, thorough review of the literature (Kastenbaum and Costa, 1977), which is both critical and selective, lists 169 important references. Unfortunately, only a small number of these papers are related to children, and those that do address childhood issues are often not directly relevant to children with life-threatening illnesses. Only recently have significant empirical studies on psychological adaptation in pediatric cancer patients begun to appear in the literature. The changing scene in cancer therapies with resulting improvements in survival statistics, and the shift in the direction of chronic life-threatening problems as opposed to conditions that were once acutely fatal, have led to many changes in the nature of psychological stress on these families.

A recent paper by Gogan, O'Malley, and Foster (1977) represents a significant effort to fill this void. The paper reviews more than 75 articles published between 1944 and 1977 and provides a background for considering psychosocial issues that bear on the treatment of the pediatric cancer patient. The review is particularly helpful because it highlights papers that seem to reflect the attitudes and trends at given time periods, that were cited frequently by other investigators, and that address issues specifically relevant to childhood cancer patients and their families.

Awareness of Death

An important paper by Vernick and Karon (1965) did much to call the attention of professionals to the pediatric cancer patient's own thinking about death. A subsequent study (Binger et al., 1969) supported Vernick and Karon's conclusion that most children above four years of age not only are aware of the seriousness of their illness but also may anticipate their own premature death. Other systematic studies have explored the development of children's conceptions of death (Koocher, 1973, 1974) and have demonstrated that young patients have a substantial awareness of death and the threat of cancer even though it may not be well articulated (Waechter, 1971). Spinetta (1974) has also carefully reviewed the literature on the dying child's awareness of death.

Anxiety Issues

Although the concept of "death anxiety" itself is a nebulous one, a number of empirical studies have documented noteworthy anxiety trends in children with cancer. Spinetta argues, "Whether or not one wishes to call this nonconceptual anxiety about the child's fatal illness 'death anxiety' seems to be a problem of semantics rather than fact" (1973, p. 844). He cautions clinicians against making general assumptions that what is true for healthy or chronically ill children will automatically be true for children with life-threatening illnesses as well. Using an innovative doll-house model, Spinetta and his colleagues (Spinetta, Rigler, and Karon, 1974) demonstrated that with each progressive hospitalization the child with leukemia tends to experience increasing personal isolation from both family and staff members as well as high levels of anxiety. He found similarly high levels of anxiety in outpatient leukemics as well (Spinetta and Maloney, 1975), in sharp contrast to children with other chronic, but not life-threatening, illnesses. In this latter study Spinetta noted that, unlike children with less dangerous chronic illnesses who become more at ease with each clinic visit, the child being treated for leukemia tends to experience heightened tension with the progression and/or increased frequency of outpatient visits. This seems to be a recognition by the child that a serious illness is worsening.

Parental Concerns

Parenting roles are particularly subject to disruption when a child develops a life-threatening illness. The parents find disciplining the sick child to be a difficult and guilt-producing task, with the net result being frequent parental manipulations by the sick child (Heffron, Bommelare, and Masters, 1973). Criticism and conflict with extended family members are not uncommon; because the child may be in treatment for several months or years, many irritating issues may remain unresolved for long periods, sometimes blocking effective parenting when the child needs it most (Hamovitch, 1964). There is a real danger of one or both parents abdicating their parental responsibility.

Few studies have looked beyond the parents to the patient's siblings, although there is growing recognition that they must not be overlooked. Heffron et al. (1973) noted that sibs tend to be caught in a cycle of jealousy (as a consequence of special attention given the patient), which leads to teasing, which leads in turn to intense feelings of guilt if the patient's condition worsens. A variety of behavior problems including enuresis, headaches, poor school performance, school phobia, depression, severe separation anxiety, and persistent abdominal pains have been reported as sibling reactions (Binger et al., 1969).

Many families are able to cope effectively with the stresses of having a child with cancer. Although there are some particularly well-written reports on family coping and stress reactions (Chordoff, Friedman, and Hamburg, 1964; Hamburg, 1974), writers often seem to have discrepant findings, probably because of differing definitions of "coping." Despite much attention in recent years, a clear, behaviorally oriented, testable definition has not yet been developed.

Anticipatory Grief The process of coping by preparing for the child's death before it occurs is known as "anticipatory grief," a term first coined by Lindemann (1944). More recent studies have demonstrated the impact of this process (Friedman et al., 1963; Binger et al., 1969) by which family members gradually separate themselves from the patient, mourning not only the illness but also the impending death. When first describing this phenomenon of anticipatory grief, Lindemann observed that, while it may serve the family well as a coping process, it may not be in the patient's best interests. Many recent studies (Waechter, 1971; Spinetta, Rigler, and Karon, 1973, 1974; Spinetta and Maloney, 1975) have actually demonstrated the fact that the child senses an increasing emotional distance and accompanying sense of loneliness as the illness progresses.

The Child's Death   If death occurs, it is important that the family not be abruptly abandoned. A number of studies have suggested that at least one family member (more often several) can be expected to react strongly enough to need psychotherapeutic help no matter how "well prepared" they may seem (Binger et al., 1969; Kaplan et al., 1973). Kaplan and his associates also have noted that families that are able to employ a shared coping pattern fare better than those in which individual family members guard their fears and concerns privately. The institution where the child was treated and a familiar caregiver can provide invaluable transitional help during the period of mourning and even intermittently thereafter. One must be mindful of those who survive, even though a family member has died.

The Caregivers

In the days when children with cancer generally lived only a short time, the caregivers had only two substantial tasks: to minimize the child's distress and to prepare the family for a death. As the foregoing material has made clear, today's situation is far more complex. Now there are usually much longer periods of survival and, in some cases, even an elusive "cure." All of this occurs in the context of oft traumatic treatments that are in the child's best medical interests. The notion of preparing the family for a death is replaced at the onset with hope for survival, shared by both the family and caregivers. To counsel a patient with widespread disease or many relapses about the life-threatening aspects of the disease is a difficult challenge to the caregiver's self-esteem, not to mention a sad and emotionally draining experience.

The notion of a caregiver who is enjoined to "know thyself" in the emotional sense is not new to psychotherapists, but it may require considerable effort on the part of many members of the treatment team. Two papers full of poignant anecdotes are truly obligatory reading for the professional who plans to work with these children and their families. One is a fairly recent paper on the makings of a good psychological consultant on a pediatric surgery ward (Geist, 1977). The other ranks as a classic comment on children with cancer and their caregivers and is aptly titled "Who's Afraid of Death on a Leukemia Ward?" (Vernick and Karon, 1965).

CURRENT PRACTICES OF PSYCHOLOGICAL CARE

Communications and Honesty

Clinicians have long debated the question "to tell or not to tell," as well as the issues of deciding when "to tell" and then "how much." In the 1950s and 60s, a "protective" approach of "benign lying" was widely advocated. Proponents considered the life-threatening aspects of the child's disease to be an unneeded burden and advised parents to shield the child from any realization of the severity of the illness. The goal was to maintain a sense of normalcy in the family, and children were often assured cheerfully they would soon be well and out of the hospital (Evans, 1968; Toch, 1964).

Our view is that this sort of deception helps no one and simply weaves a web of white lies that ultimately captures the child, parents, and caregivers alike while creating unnecessary emotional distances and stress when they are needed least. We do not, on the other hand, advocate "truth" as an absolute good because, in the final analysis, truth per se is meaningless. We advocate an approach of humane honesty that recognizes that the giving of specific information often serves the patient and family well, but sometimes does not.

A child with a life-threatening illness should be told the name of the condition, given an accurate explanation of the nature of the illness (up to the limit of his ability to comprehend), and told that it is a serious illness of which people sometimes die. At the same time, however, the child and family can be told about treatment options and enlisted as allies to fight the disease. An atmosphere must be established in which all concerned have the opportunity to ask questions, relate fantasies, and express concerns, no matter how scary or far fetched they may seem.

When a patient is feeling sick, weak, and dying, there is no need to remind him of the prognosis. If a family and patient know a prognosis is poor but persist in clinging to hope, one has no right to wrest that from them. The truth, humanely tempered, is important, but we must be mindful of the patient and how his needs are served. To tell the "whole truth" or a "white lie" for the benefit of the teller serves no one in the end.

Availability of Psychotherapeutic Services

The availability of psychological consultation services in pediatric oncology treatment centers can no longer be considered a luxury. As outlined earlier in this chapter, the ever increasing complexity and variables of the treatment programs demand a relatively sophisticated consultant who can function smoothly as a member of an oncology treatment team.

Issues about side effects of treatment, troublesome symptoms, relations with staff members, and a hundred other potential concerns cannot be met efficiently by a therapist at the local mental health center, a school counselor, or a private practitioner away from the clinic. The other members of the oncology treatment team must have consultants they know, whose judgment they trust, and with whom they can relate on a regular basis (see Geist, 1977).

The frequency and nature of services offered to these patients and their families also will necessarily be quite different from those that a psychotherapist generally provides. Most of the children and families will be people without significant psychopathology, but who are experiencing a number of emotional stresses of a reactive reality-based nature. The needs of most will not fall into the once-a-week insight-oriented psychotherapeutic paradigm. To begin with, the frequency of needed interventions will vary widely. There may be some weeks when a family or specific child may need several hours of intensive assistance from a mental health professional. This may be followed by a period of weeks or months when only intermittent consultations are needed. In general, the child and family can be expected to most need assistance during peak stress episodes, and these episodes come and go as a function of the course of the child's illness.

The critical periods in the natural history of the child's illness can be taken as emotional stress markers as well. The initial diagnosis probably is the first key stress event, even if the child has been ill for a period before that, because it is then that the life-threatening aspects of the condition first become clearly known in most cases. This may be followed by a period of reduced tension while treatment is begun, only to again reach critical levels with the onset of chemotherapy side effects, serious infections, surgical procedures, hospitalizations, relapses, and so on. The result is a series of stress peaks interspersed with relative periods of normalcy. In most cases the periods of normalcy are of long duration with only rare stress peaks, the greatest of which are reached at the time of initial diagnosis and at the time of death. Still another major stress point occurs with the elective cessation of chemotherapy and the "it's finally over" celebration. Here is a time when it might seem that universal elation ought to be the rule, but the psychologist with a knowledge of the diseases involved will see the need to avoid overemphasizing the event to protect those destined to relapse later. The point to be made here is that psychological services to these children and their families cannot be effective if made available only through traditional service models. Availability of psychotherapeutic assistance must be a well-integrated segment of the overall treatment of the whole child.

Skills and Techniques

It is evident that the psychologist or other mental health professional working as a member of the pediatric oncology team will need to have some specialized knowledge about childhood cancer and current cancer treatments, but there are other specific skills and techniques that will be particularly useful. Consultant skills are very important. This is the ability to flexibly respond to highly specific problem situations in a task-oriented fashion. A good consultant must also be "a team player," that is to say, a person who is able to communicate well with parents and staff as well as with the sick children and who can help in reducing confusion by having many caregivers in many different roles.

The ability to be in touch with many families and to monitor their progress without necessarily intervening is also a helpful talent. This requires a degree of flexibility and a special sensitivity to signs of anxiety or deviation from normal family patterns, often correlated with events in the treatment of the disease itself. Recognition that each family has a different baseline and coping pattern, and knowing when there is a significant deviation demanding intervention, are a subtle talent but a necessary one because time invariably will be at a premium.

Crisis intervention skills are a must for the effective consultant. Acute anxiety and assorted crises will strike each child or family sometime during the course of the illness, not to mention crises other members of the treatment team may experience in doing their jobs. A talent for sharing techniques and knowing when to enlist the aid of another team member or family member as a surrogate therapist is also important. The good consultant knows the limitations of his time, energy, and skill, and will not hesitate to use effective others for the benefit of the child or family.

Psychological Issues in Patient Care

A number of specific issues of a psychological nature can be anticipated in work with childhood cancer patients. Some of these have been alluded to earlier in this chapter, but a specific listing of recurrent psychological issues deserves particular attention. The categories of issues include general considerations, individual patient concerns, and family issues.

General Considerations Frequent themes in therapeutic intervention with child clients and their families involve educative issues, patient advocacy, roadblocks to effective treatment, and general emotional support. Both parents and children will often misunderstand or misinterpret various tests, procedures, or treatment events related to the disease, despite the best efforts of the staff at offering information. The psychologist can often be in the position of recognizing the nature of the misconceptions and being able to provide additional input of an educative nature. There are times when patients or families have special gripes or concerns that they are unwilling or unable to voice to relevant members of the treatment team. In cases such as these the psychologist can act as the advocate of the patient and raise the issues with the appropriate team member. At other times in the course of treatment, various roadblocks of an emotional nature (e.g., lack of cooperation in taking medication or acting-out behavior on the hospital ward) may pose significant management problems. This is another situation when the psychologist's ability to size up the nature of the emotional concerns and suggest appropriate strategies to the staff or parents could be of major benefit. Basic supportive psychotherapy is also a major source of strength in facilitating the ongoing emotional care of both children and their parents.

Individual Patient Concerns One significant problem is that of forced dependence on others as a function of various transient or more enduring incapacities. Older children and adolescents who have just begun to appreciate independence that comes with maturation suddenly find themselves becoming dependent on others as caregivers, with the attendant embarrassing losses of privacy. Younger children too can be expected to react with frustration at times in the face of painful procedures to which they must submit willingly. This problem is illustrated with some specific case examples and intervention strategies in O'Malley and Koocher (1977).

Another frequent concern involves the loss of bodily control. This may be manifest in painful muscle spasms, nausea, or cognitive disorientation as a function of chemotherapy and analgesic medications. Neurological deficits also accompany the progressive course of some diseases and cause additional concern. Typical examples of the child's reactions include one youngster whose disorientation while on morphine made her fearful that she was ". . . going crazy." Another youngster in the hospital for initial chemotherapy was terrified of his vomiting in response to chemotherapy and became panic stricken fearing that he was about to choke and die. In instances such as these, the availability of a psychologist or other mental health professional who can recognize the emotional issues, provide support, and offer reassuring educational information can be very important.

There are many other concerns of a much more specific or individual nature, and these will vary as a function of the child's developmental level and the specific point in the course of the illness. The consultant must be especially mindful of the magical thinking and real-life events that might combine at any point to place considerable stress on the child with cancer.

Family Issues Among the most common of family concerns, broadly defined, is the protection of the child. Sometimes it is the intent of the family to protect the child from anticipated anxiety, sometimes from pain and suffering. Sometimes one may wonder if the protection is not for the benefit of family members other than the child. The psychological consultant is in a unique position of being able to independently assess the concerns of the individuals involved and to facilitate family communication in the most advantageous fashion. For example, a 14-year-old amputee who was hospitalized for chemotherapy seemed unusually depressed and shared her concern that her illness was breaking up the marriage of her parents. In fact, the parents had been quarreling over the issue of whether or not to discuss the illness in front of the girl. In an extended family session it was possible to draw out the individual concerns of each family member and to leave an emotional climate in which "protectionism" was not a roadblock.

There are many cases when family members (including the patient) adopt defense mechanisms that seem unrealistic or that do not permit full realization of the facts of the patient's condition. This is not invariably a bad thing but rather illustrates the differences in coping styles. Unless a particular coping style is seriously endangering the patient's care, it should be respected as legitimate. When it is necessary to confront a family member on some aspect of coping that is harmful to the patient, the professional must be ready to supply support and alternative suggestions to help take the place of the defense mechanism he is asked to abandon.

Another common family issue that is closely tied to the behavior of other team members has to do with the direct care of the child. Some parents are immobilized or unable to care for their child during periods of relapse in the course of the illness. Others want very much to care for their child but are preempted by a thorough and efficient treatment staff. There will be times when the psychological consultant may have to take an active role in helping the parents to participate actively in the care of their children. It is terribly frustrating for a parent to sit with a child for long hours in a clinic or hospital room with "nothing to do" for the child when they desperately want to be expressing their concern in some way. There are many ways in which families can become involved directly in the care of the pediatric cancer patient, and, when this is a key concern, the psychologist is often in a position to facilitate matters.

Emotional Costs to the Caregivers

Although some papers have sensitively touched on the feelings of those who care for children with life-threatening illnesses (Geist, 1977; Vernick and Karon, 1965), it is difficult to categorize these people or to summarize succinctly why they work in this field. One generality that seems to hold is that people either leave the field after a few years or make it a permanent career. The reasons behind this and the coping styles of caregivers or oncology team members never have been fully studied. The emotional costs to oncology team members are most evident when there is a group of deaths over a short period of time or when a number of patients who have been in remission all relapse in close temporal proximity. As the caregivers go about helping people to cope, inducing remissions, and watching many patients go home well, it is easy to feel as though "We win some and lose some." It is when a victory suddenly turns into defeat, a series of losses come in rapid succession, or a particularly close relationship ends in death that a contagious depression characterized by short tempers and black humor seems to hang in the air.

Why then would anyone want to work with these patients and families? The answer may be that, although the emotional costs are high, the rewards are higher. For the medical staff there is the knowledge that life is being sustained and the quality of it kept at a higher level than was ever possible for these patients in the past. For the mental health professional there is the opportunity to work with highly motivated patients and families and to see significant beneficial progress in relatively short periods of time. For all members of the treatment team there is the continuous reward of playing an important helping role at a crucial time in the life of a family.

There is no good way to tell a family that their child has cancer, or to tell the child either, for that matter. Our research with childen who survive cancer, however, underscores the importance of openness, honesty, and consistent support from the primary caregivers. Often the parents or children will not be able to ask questions that are important to them at the outset, but this should not be taken as a sign that they do not want to "know." To function effectively in this regard, the caregiver must know his own feelings and be comfortable with them. Some patients die. There are many depressing days. These are real facts and legitimate feelings for the caregiver to have, and the most well-adjusted people are those who realize this and can reasonably accept them.

SUMMARY

This chapter is a relatively brief attempt to convey some basic information and principles to the mental health practitioner. The key points that it is hoped the reader will carry away include the following: First, pediatric cancer is a complex set of chronic life-threatening illnesses with many highly individual factors bearing on the treatment and prognosis for any given patient. Second, psychological problems that these children and their families experience usually are linked directly to the stress of the illness and related therapies. It is therefore of crucial importance that the mental health treatment staff be knowledgeable regarding the nature of the illnesses, types of treatment employed, and nature of variability to be expected. Third, it is highly desirable that psychological support services be available as one arm of the overall treatment team whenever possible. That is to say, the mental health practitioners should be working closely with the physicians, nurses, and other team members to deliver the most efficient and effective care to the patients and their families. Finally, because of the strong motivation for closeness and sharing that is often generated during such illnesses, a strong potential for significant facilitation of family relationships is frequently present. In such circumstances the timely and sensitive intervention of the mental health staff can meet a critical family need and simultaneously offer many highly rewarding moments to the professionals involved.

REFERENCES

Binger, C. H., Balin, A. R., Feverstein, R. C., Kushner, J. H., Zoger, S., and Mikkelsen, C. 1969. Childhood leukemia: Emotional impact on patient and family. N. Engl. J. Med. 280(8):414–418.

Choi, S. I., and Simone, J. V. 1976. Acute nonlymphatic leukemia in 171 children. Med. Pediatr. Oncol. 2:119–149.

Chordoff, P., Friedman, S. B., and Hamburg, D. 1964. Stress, defenses and coping behavior: Observations in parents of children with malignant disease. Am. J. Psychiatry 120:743–749.

Dritshila, A., Cassady, J. R., and Camitta, B. 1976. The role of irradiation in central nervous system treatment and prophylaxis for acute lymphoblastic leukemia. Cancer 37:2729–2735.

Evans, A. E. 1968. If a child must die . . . N. Engl. J. Med. 278(3):138–142.

Friedman, S. B., Chordoff, P., Mason, J. W., and Hamburg, D. A. 1963. Behavioral observations on parents anticipating the death of a child. Pediatrics 32(4):610–625.

Gardner, G. G. 1976. Childhood, death and human dignity: Hypnotherapy for David. Int. J. Clin. Exp. Hypnosis 24:122–139.

Geist, R. A. 1977. Consultation on a pediatric surgical ward: creating an empathic climate. Am. J. Orthopsychiatry 47:432–444.

Gogan, J. L., O'Malley, J. E., and Foster, D. J. 1977. Treating the pediatric cancer patient: A review. J. Pediatr. Psychol. 2:42–49.

Goldberg. R. T. 1974. Adjustment of children with invisible and visible handicaps: Congenital heart disease and facial burns. J. Counsel. Psychol. 21(5):428–432.

Hamburg, D. A. 1974. Coping behavior in life-threatening circumstances. Psychother. Psychosom. 23:13–25.

Hamovitch, M. B. 1964. The Parent and the Fatally Ill Child. Delmar Publishing Co., Los Angeles.

Heffron, W. A., Bommelare, K., and Masters, R. 1973. Group discussions with parents of leukemic children. Pediatrics 52(6):831–840.

Jaffe, N. 1975. Malignant bone tumors. Pediatr. Ann. February.

Jaffe, N. 1976. Neuroblastoma: Review of the literature and an examination of factors contributing to its enigmatic character. Cancer Treatment Rev. 3:61–82.

Jenkin, R. D. T. 1976. The treatment of Wilms' Tumor. Pediatr. Clin. North Am. 23:147–160.

Kaplan, D. M., Smith, A., Brobstein, R., and Fischman, S. E. 1973. Family mediation of stress. Soc. Work 18(4):60–69.

Kastenbaum, R., and Costa, P. T. 1977. Psychological perspectives on death. Ann. Rev. Psychol. 28:225–249.

Koocher, G. P. 1973. Childhood, death, and cognitive development. Dev. Psychol. 9:369–374.

Koocher, G. P. 1974. Talking with children about death. Am. J. Orthopsychiatry 44:404–411.

Lindemann, E. 1944. Symptomatology and management of acute grief. Am. J. Psychiatry 101:141–148.

Murphy, S. B. 1977. Prognostic features and obstacles to cure in childhood non-Hodgkin's lymphoma. Sem. Oncol. 4:265–272.

O'Malley, J. E., and Koocher, G. P. 1977. Psychological consultations to a pediatric oncology ward. J. Pediatr. Psychol. 2:54–58.

Pinkel, D. 1976. Treatment of acute leukemia. Pediatr. Clin. North Am. 23(1):117–130.

Raney, R. B., Schnaufer, L., and Donaldson, M. H. 1974. Soft-tissue sarcomas in childhood. Sem. Oncol. 1:57–64.

Sen, L., and Borell, L. 1975. Clinical importance of lymphoblasts with T markers in childhood acute leukemia. N. Engl. J. Med. 292:828–832.

Spinetta, J. J. 1974. The dying child's awareness of death: a review. Psychol. Bull. 81(4):256–260.

Spinetta, J. J., and Maloney, L. J. 1975. Death anxiety in the outpatient leukemic child. Pediatrics 65(6):1034–1037.

Spinetta, J. J., Rigler, D., and Karon, M. 1973. Anxiety in the dying child. Pediatrics 52(6):841, 845.

Spinetta, J. J., Rigler, D., and Karon, M. 1974. Personal space as a measure of a dying child's sense of isolation. J. Consult. Clin. Psychol. 42(6):751–756.

Toch, R. 1964. Management of the child with a fatal disease. Clin. Pediatr. 3(7):418–427.

Vernick, J., and Karon, M. 1965. Who's afraid of death on a leukemia ward? Am. J. Dis. Child. 109:393–397.

Waechter, E. H. 1971. The child's awareness of fatal illness. Am. J. Nurs. 7:1168–1172.

Walker, M. D. 1976. Diagnosis and treatment of brain tumors. Pediatr. Clin. North Am. 23:131–146.

Wiernik, P. H. 1974. Hodgkin's Disease 1974. Johns Hopkins Med. J. 135:25–32.

Wilson, C. B. (ed.). 1975a. Brain tumors. Sem. Oncol. 3:1.

Wilson, C. B. 1975b. Surgical treatment of childhood brain tumors. Cancer 35:950.

Young, J. L., and Miller, R. W. 1975. Incidence of malignant tumors in U.S. children. J. Pediatr. 86:254–258.

11
Pulmonary Disorders
Asthma and Cystic Fibrosis

Suzanne Pochter Bronheim

Life and breath are linked so strongly in human existence that any condition that threatens breath is experienced as terrifying and dangerous. Before she even counts the toes of her newly born offspring, the mother wants to hear the cry that proves her baby is breathing well. The young infant instinctively fights anything that might impede his breathing. Death is portrayed in drama as a futile gasping for air. Only recently has the concept of death become sufficiently sophisticated to allow for the idea of life without breath and to provide resuscitation to those who to a layman are "obviously dead." An acute episode of pulmonary disease (such as acute bronchiolitis or pneumonia) is, therefore, frightening. The presence of chronic pulmonary disease and the accompanying feeling of always being in danger of dying have long-range psychological impact. These psychological complications of chronic pulmonary disease are illustrated here by the discussion of two diseases with different types of psychological involvement: 1) asthma, which has a strong psychological component in both its symptoms and treatment, and 2) cystic fibrosis, which cannot be ameliorated by psychological intervention, but which has a devastating effect on the psychosocial development of its victims and their families.

Many diseases involve the lungs in infancy and childhood and, if numerous, take their psychological toll. Most of these diseases, however, are caused by external pathogens and with proper treatment can be cured. Cystic fibrosis and asthma are, however, conditions or states of the organism. The symptoms can be managed and their life-threatening nature negated, but the underlying problem cannot presently be cured. Patients grow up having to incorporate in their self-image the fact that they are always in danger of losing breath and life. These two diseases have been chosen for discussion because of this intractable psychological quality and its impact on the child and his relationships with significant others.

ASTHMA

Medical Aspects of Asthma

The Committee on Diagnostic Standards for Nontuberculous Respiratory Diseases proposed the following definition of asthma: an illness that is manifest clinically by intermittent episodes of wheezing and dyspnea (shortness of breath), generally associated with a hyperresponsive state of the bronchi, which may be antigen mediated. It is differentiated from other obstructive airway diseases by its usual reversibility (Aaronson, 1972). In short, asthmatics are likely to respond with attacks of wheezing and shortness of breath because their bronchi respond more readily to stimuli (including allergens) than do normal bronchi. This wheezing and shortness of breath are generally only episodic, and the asthmatic child has symptom-free intervals.

The prevalence of asthma and its sociological impact are considerable. It is estimated that 2–4% of the population have asthma. In 1964, 1.2 million school children were known to have asthma. These children accounted for 6.5 million days of school absence or 25% of school days lost for all chronic diseases combined. This disruption alone suggests that the disease is going to involve a major social-psychological factor, no matter what its etiology (Aaronson, 1972).

The onset of asthmatic symptoms may be during infancy, but the most common period of onset is between three and eight years of age. Often the asthma has been preceded by a chronic allergic rhinitis (runny nose) or, in infancy, by repeated respiratory infections. A positive family history for atopic diseases (asthma, allergic rhinitis, or eczema) is often present, and genetics are strongly implicated in the cause of this condition (Cohen, 1971; Aaronson, 1972; Kempe, Silver, and O'Brien, 1974).

The life-threatening aspect of asthma is associated with the severe attack that will not clear with usual drug treatment—*status asthmaticus*. The child is usually considered in status asthmaticus only after wheezing has become severe over hours and cannot be reversed after several doses of both oral and intramuscular medications. When the child has reached this point, fatigue and diminished pulmonary function can lead to a dangerously high level of CO_2 in the blood and, with other changes, cause respiratory failure. At this point a series of emergency medical measures are needed to prevent tissue damage from anoxia (Ellis, 1975). All measures used to treat asthma—daily medication to prevent wheezing, environmental control to decrease irritants, hyposensitization, home and emergency room treatment to stop wheezing that develops despite preventive measures—are directed against the child's going into status asthmaticus. However, it cannot always be prevented, and many families with asthmatic children experience this scare at some point. Some severely asthmatic patients do die from status asthmaticus, although with proper treatment and compliance to treatment death is not a necessary nor a common part of the picture.

The prognosis for asthma is generally better than that of many chronic diseases, because, if adequately treated, it tends to get better rather than worse with age. People often talk of "outgrowing" asthma. Long-term studies indicate that 50% of patients will be completely symptom-free 20 years after the onset of the symptoms with proper treatment. Only 10% will still have severe symptoms at that time. The fatality rate from asthma over that 20-year period is less than 1% (Ellis, 1975).

Etiology   The question of etiology has created a great deal of friction between medical personnel and mental health professionals (Mattson, 1975). The major thrust of the literature on the psychological aspects of asthma has been to establish a psychogenesis of this disease. Medical caregivers have focused on allergies and infections as the etiology of asthma. Both approaches have mistaken conditions correlated with exacerbation of symptoms with causative factors. Psychological stress, allergens, and infections are all external agents. More recent findings and theories place the etiology within the individual. There seem to be physiological differences in asthmatics that cause them to react to a variety of stimuli with bronchoconstriction. The various agents that trigger attacks in the asthmatic do not affect nonasthmatics. The difference seems to be in the fact that asthmatics have a chronic increase in bronchial lability, even when symptom-free (Jones, Buston, and Wharton, 1962). Even young adults who have "outgrown" their childhood asthma and have been symptom-free for four or more years have been found to have abnormally high bronchial lability, no matter what agent supposedly triggered the attacks (Jones and Jones, 1966).

The exact mechanism that is defective in asthmatics has not been firmly established. Current thinking suggests that asthmatics have a deficient or inadequate adenylate cyclase system so β-adrenergic stimulation by catecholamines does not take place (Criep, 1976). Adenylate cyclase is a receptor enzyme in the cells that responds to stimulation of the sympathetic nervous system. When stimulated by chemical mediators of the sympathetic nervous system this receptor substance produces those changes in organ functioning associated with sympathetic stimulation. In the case of the bronchi, sympathetic stimulation causes dilatation. Thus, if there is an insufficiency in the receptor system the sympathetic nervous system will not be able to effectively counteract the constriction caused by parasympathetic stimulation (Guyton, 1977). Parasympathetic stimulation is increased by such nonspecific factors as cold, infection, and emotions. Chemicals can inhibit β-adrenergic stimulation specifically, and changes in cell chemistry caused by immunological factors produced by the body in reaction to allergens can also increase constriction (Criep, 1976).

What were once viewed as possible causes of asthma can now be identified as triggering agents. Respiratory infection can set off an attack. Allergies can trigger wheezing. The child may be allergic to inhaled substances such as the dust and molds in his house, the dander of a pet, or the pollens of grasses, weeds, and trees. Ingestants such as milk, eggs, wheat, chocolate, and peanut butter can trigger asthma via allergic response (Ellis, 1975). Many other nonimmunological or infective factors can also contribute to wheezing: cold, pungent odors, exercise and rapid respiration, emotional upset, tobacco smoke, acetic acid (Criep, 1976), and psychological stimuli. A combination of factors can trigger any one child's wheezing. Only a small percentage of cases can be traced to only one agent (Rees, 1956).

Treatment   Treatment of asthma is aimed at relaxing the bronchi through use of medication to prevent attacks or to prevent their becoming severe and by using measures to minimize the impact of triggering agents. Asthmatics at home may be given medication to ingest or to inhale. Sympathomimetic drugs, phosphodiesterase inhibitors (such as theophylline), and, in severe cases, corticosteroids are the most frequently prescribed drugs given to asthmatics to enhance dilatation of the bronchi. If home treatment fails, emergency room treatment may be required. Some medications given to children in treating asthma may cause them to be restless and irritable, particularly if the dose is excessive. This factor is of course important in assessing behavioral functioning of these children. Skin testing is often done to determine which inhalent allergens might exacerbate the asthma. Based on the results of this testing, a course of injections to desensitize the child to these allergens is common. Food allergies are investigated through blood tests and changes in the diet. If particular ingestants are found to exacerbate symptoms, they must be eliminated totally from the diet. (Because milk, wheat, and eggs are common offenders, this restriction of diet is often difficult to enforce.) The child's physical environment may need changes: measures to reduce dust and mold, separation from pets, air filtration, and air conditioning. Finally, emotionally stressful situations may need to be resolved as part of the treatment (Kempe, Silver, and O'Brien, 1974; Ellis, 1975). All of these measures are aimed at preventing the asthma attack.

Psychological Aspects of Asthma

Much of the literature on the psychological aspects of asthma has viewed the disease as one with a psychogenesis. The types of phenomena observed by mental health professionals working with asthmatic children certainly reinforce this view, particularly without current models of the disease to explain them at a physiological level. The psychological component of asthma is so striking that even the earliest reports note it. Hypocrites reminded asthmatics that they must guard against their anger (Cohen, 1971). In more recent times, Dutch asthmatic children were often sent to boarding school in Switzerland. These children showed marked improvement in the mountain air, but curiously the local asthmatic children accrued no such benefit. After World War II when money was scarce, a boarding school was built by the Dutch in their own country. They found that this removal from the home had equally positive results. In both cases children were more symptomatic on visiting day (Bastiaans and Groen, 1955. Luparello et al. (1968) found that when a group of asthmatic patients were told that the nebulized saline solution they were inhaling was an allergen or irritant they developed increased airway resistance and in some cases full-blown attacks. When they were treated with a saline placebo, symptoms subsided. One of these subjects went so far as to have hay fever symptoms when told the inhalent was pollen and asthma alone when told it was dust. Dekker and Groen (1956) were able to evoke asthma attacks in the laboratory by exposing subjects to anxiety-arousing stimuli. (In one case riding in an elevator produced an asthma attack.) The evidence that lends most credence to the idea of psychogeneses is the numerous case reports in which the asthma cleared with the resolution of intrapsychic or intrafamilial conflicts. However, all of these data and the rest of the massive literature can only be put in proper perspective with an understanding of the present formulation of the physiology of asthma.

Very little, if any, literature on the psychological aspects of asthma takes into account an understanding of the disease based on the adenylate cyclase insufficiency model. Aside from ignoring the physiology of this disease studied, most studies involving asthmatic children have been embarrassingly inadequate in terms of design. Freeman et al. (1964), reviewing 195 articles on psychological variables of allergic disorders (most involving asthma), leveled a variety of criticisms at the literature. First, much of the research and all of the case studies involving psychological aspects of asthma used as subjects asthmatic children referred for psychiatric treatment, often because the medical management of their asthma was ineffective. Numerous conclusions about the dynamics of asthma or the personality of the asthmatic child or his mother were based on this skewed population. Medical diagnosis was often questionable. In one study mentioned by Freeman et al. (1964), the diagnosis of allergy was based on self-report by acutely psychotic patients. Many studies took no pains to ensure blindness of raters. Often the doctor who treated the child rated both the child's personality and his medical improvement. Almost all studies were post hoc. Mothers were described as rejecting or overprotective after the onset of asthma with no regard for the fact that the child's illness has an obvious impact on the mother's reactions to the child. With these criticisms in mind, a review of the literature is almost reduced to a presentation of the psychological folklore about asthma. The theories and information advanced in the literature are not totally discountable, but they must be viewed within the framework of the physical causation suggested earlier. There is useful information in case studies about approaches to the patient and the dynamics of family interaction. Attributions of causal nature must, however, be suspect. If nothing else, the literature (except for more recent, controlled studies about interventions) is of historical interest and raises some tantalizing questions that might be reinvestigated with more stringent controls.

The Folklore of Asthma   Since the mental health field has taken such an interest (based on the number of articles) in asthma, it is no surprise that asthmatics have been assumed to have a higher index of psychopathology than nonasthmatics. Various attempts were made to demonstrate this difference using personality inventories, projective tests, or evaluative interviews. Many studies did not establish the medical diagnosis. Several studies using inventories found asthmatics to be more like nonasthmatic neurotics than like normals (Leigh and Marley, 1956; Dekker, Barendregt, and deVries, 1961). Using projective techniques, Neuhaus (1958) compared 84 asthmatic children and their 25 siblings with 84 chronic cardiac patients and their siblings and a matched group of normal controls. The Rorschach, the Dispert Fables, and the Brown Personality Inventory were used. This study added the key factor of comparing asthmatic children with other chronically ill children. Chronic illness has an impact on the families and on the child's development. It is important to determine whether psychopathology measured is the cause or result of asthma. Neuhaus' (1958) results indicated the latter. Asthmatic children were more neurotic, insecure, and dependent than normal children, but they were not different from children with cardiac disease or their own siblings (who also would feel the effects of a chronically ill child in the family).

Williams and McNicol (1975), in a controlled, prospective study of 400 asthmatics and 100 controls drawn from a population of 23,000 school children, compared the groups at ages seven, 10, and 14 years. Asthmatics as a whole did not have more behavioral disturbances; in fact they had few. More interestingly, those disturbances noted were in the group of children with most severe asthma—those who had remissions of less than one month or had 10 attacks in the previous three months. Of this group 79% were boys. (Males tend to be more susceptible to asthma, and in this study they were more highly concentrated in the groups with severe asthma.) These children were less socially mature, more demanding for material possessions or maternal attention, and more likely to exhibit displaced aggression. Again, the question remains as to cause or effect, with psychological disturbances as the result of serious illness being strongly implied.

This failure to solidly demonstrate higher levels of psychopathology in asthmatics does not destroy the premise of a psychogenesis of the disease for many theorists. If anything, it may support some of the more popular theories, which hold that the asthma itself is the psychopathology, thus no other symptoms would necessarily be present. It has been called both an abnormal defense against ego disintegration (Freeman et al., 1964) and an abnormal way of discharging anxiety (Mattson, 1975). The first premise has led to a series of studies attempting to demonstrate that psychosis and asthma are incompatible. The second arises from the best known, most elaborate dynamic formulation of asthma.

The attempts at showing that asthma is not present in psychotics have centered on comparisons of incidence in hospitalized versus normal populations. Ross, Hay, and McDowell (1950) and Swartz and Semrad (1951) found a lower incidence of asthma in psychotic populations. Freeman et al. (1964) point out, however, that incidence statistics gathered in 1928 were being used as the basis of comparison. Other studies report no consistent findings to support this supposition.

The observations of children separated from their families for the treatment of asthma (mentioned earlier) led workers to investigate the parent-child relationship as the source of disturbance in asthma. It was hypothesized that asthmatic children had an excessive, unresolved dependence on mother. Any threat of separation could bring on an attack. The wheezing and dyspnea were equated with the child's suppressed cry for his mother. Crying is a way to reestablish the dependent bond and the asthma may develop when the crying—the longings it represents—is not tolerable to the mother (French, 1950; Weiss, 1950; Saul and Lyons, 1951).

Support for this theory has come from three sources: individual case studies, studies of groups of cases, and research reports. Anecdotal reports are of interest to the clinician, in that they suggest ways of formulating the dynamics of a problem child with asthma. These reports cannot, however, support French's theory because most clinicians use it to explain and label the phenomenon observed. The other two types of evidence usually employ some set of rating tools to classify the type of mother or type of parent-child relationship in the asthmatic group. A typical study by Miller and Baruch (1948) compared 63 allergic children with 37 nonallergics in an attempt to demonstrate the importance of maternal rejection as the etiology of allergy. Twenty-four (64.8%) of the nonallergic children had rejecting mothers, while 98% of the mothers of allergic children were rejecting. In most of these studies, as with much of the literature in this field, design problems raise serious questions about the results. There is no description of criteria for ratings and no mention as to whether raters were blind to the subject's classification. Numerous other studies suffer from the same defects and those that do not, as Freeman et al. (1964) point out, do not show such favorable results. In fact Dubo et al. (1961) and McLean and Ching (1973) did a well-controlled study and found no relationship between maternal-child interaction factors and severity of asthma or its failure to respond to medical treatment. These factors relate only to the child's social-psychological adjustment, his adaptation to the illness, and the level of limitation the asthma imposes. The last two factors are present as part of the picture with any chronic disease, whether psychogenic or not. Both Cutter (1955) and Fitzelle (1959) compared large groups of mothers of asthmatics with mothers of children who came for treatment of other medical problems and found no differences.

Similar attempts have been made to delineate the personality of the asthmatic child himself. Most such studies have taken groups or subgroups of asthmatic children and delineated an "asthmatic personality," which usually involved a number of negative traits such as impatience, impulsivity, "pseudo-independent behavior," depression, or immaturity (Little and Cohen, 1951; Bastiaans and Groen, 1955). Because these investigations were looking for pathology and specific conflicts, it is no surprise that they were found. The evidence, gained in this way, is difficult to interpret. A few studies (Ring, 1957; Graham et al., 1962) have asked the question the other way. Raters were asked to predict what disease the patient had based on psychological characteristics. Raters in these studies were able to identify the disease from personality assessment data. The exact nature of the "asthmatic personality" varies to such an extent from study to study that the clinical mental health worker seems best advised to approach each child individually, without preconceived ideas of what conflicts or characteristics he will have beyond those problems that often plague children with chronic disease.

A final area of exploration in the psychological literature about asthma has been the family system of the asthmatic child. It is based on the same sort of case reports and experiences that prompted psychoanalytical formulations, but, instead of focusing on the maternal-child bond, the emphasis is on the process within the entire family. Minuchin et al. (1975) are some of the more articulate proponents of this viewpoint. Their model for explaining psychosomatic illness in children is based on a triad of factors within the family: 1) a family organization that encourages somaticization (members constantly ask one another, "Do you feel all right?" "Are you tired?" etc.), 2) involvement of the children in parental conflict, and 3) physiological vulnerability. Pathological family interactions may trigger the onset or hamper the subsistence of the psychophysiological processes of the disease. The symptom serves to keep a homeostasis; it keeps conflict within tolerable bounds. Thus, a child may have an attack when parental conflict reaches a level not tolerated within the system and thus divert attention and lower anxiety. This model makes good sense (to some extent) in view of the physical basis in asthma. Because wheezing is a response easily brought on by stress and is also conditionable (Miller, 1969), it is not surprising that attacks would become more frequent during family stress, particularly if they were reinforced by a reduction in anxiety following their appearance. The specificity of family conflict mentioned by Minuchin et al. (1975) may reflect more about the manageability of the stress placed on a youngster and the patterns of reinforcement within the families studied, than it suggests specific familial conflicts as the cause of symptoms. Again, these formulations come from therapy cases and probably apply to children whose asthma does not respond well to medical management, but they do not explain the *cause* of all asthma.

Psychological Intervention in Childhood Asthma

Although the literature on the psychological aspects of asthma has established little, if anything, about the psychogenesis of the disease, it has identified numerous factors that can be related to its exacerbation. Some individuals can be affected by anxiety (induced by imaginary or real stimuli). A poor family situation or psychopathology in the parents or child can interfere with the successful medical management of the child. Finally, those changes noted in parent-child relations should not go unheeded, because the presence of chronic, potentially life-threatening disease can easily color this relationship in such a way that the child's social and emotional development is negatively affected by the physical disease.

A variety of interventions has been delineated in the literature, with widely different goals. Basically, these interventions have one of two foci: 1) to give the patient greater control over his symptoms, increase his ability to follow treatment, and lessen inadvertently conditioned internal cues that trigger attacks; or 2) to change the environmental response to the child and his symptoms so as not to reinforce them by providing the family system (and child) with more adaptable means of dealing with conflict to lessen stress in the environment and increase the system's (and child's) ability to tolerate anxiety. Not every patient needs psychological intervention. Some may need only minimal intervention to help them gain more control over symptoms caused by suggestibility in order to reduce the need for medication. Others require intensive psychotherapy and at times temporary removal from the family to get symptoms under control. Finally, there are those children who may need help, not because their asthmatic symptoms are negatively affected by emotional factors, but because their development of self seems negatively affected by their own and/or parent reactions to the disease. Each case requires a different approach and, fortunately, many methods have been reported to be successful with asthmatic children.

Biofeedback and Relaxation Therapy   There are ways in which the mental health worker (either alone or with the respiratory therapist) can provide an important service to most asthmatic children. These treatments are indicative of the changing role of psychological input into the treatment of asthma, since there is no supposition of pathology. There is, instead, an emphasis on increasing coping skills. In some settings in which asthmatic children are treated, relaxation therapy, a form of "psychological intervention," is offered to all asthmatic children. Respiratory therapists teach children a set of exercises, incorporating Jacobson's progressive relaxation techniques, to help them develop more control over their symptoms without the need for added medication. The goal of these exercises is to learn to relax the bronchi at the first sign of constriction and thus prevent a full-blown attack.

By combining relaxation therapy with biofeedback, Feldman (1976) and Vachon and Rich (1976) both report positive results with asthmatics in decreasing airway resistance. Biofeedback was provided by a light that came on when the subjects breathed into a machine in a way that indicated better expiratory flow and/or volume (decreased airway resistance). The subjects in one study were not aware of its intent; thus, suggestion is an unlikely cause of the results. Reportedly, severe asthmatics are not helped as much by this technique, perhaps because they suffer from more permanent, nonreversible damage.

Desensitization   Moore (1965) reports success in helping the asthmatic child free himself from internal cues and suggestion as sources of wheezing. Some asthmatics become so sensitized that the mere thought of wheezing or having an attack will set them off. Moore (1965) used pulmonary function testing, as well as subjective report, as the index of improvement. Three treatments were used: 1) relaxation (Jacobson method) for five minutes twice daily at home, 2) relaxation plus the suggestion to be a more relaxed person, and 3) relaxation plus desensitization to three hierarchies based on imagined situations involving allergens or infectious substances, psychologically stressful situations from the patient's own life, and psychodynamically formulated situations thought to trigger asthma. All subjects improved, but those who were specifically desensitized to internal triggering cues did best. This form of treatment can be useful for the child in whom suggestion plays a large role or who has trouble tolerating the family stress in a situation that is not particularly pathological or of sufficient difficulty to warrant family psychotherapy. It can be added to breathing exercises and biofeedback when the child seems unable to use those techniques in actual triggering situations because of overwhelming anxiety. The imaginal practice of the desensitization approach can first provide experience in using these techniques in the face of less potent stimuli.

Hypnosis   Because suggestibility has been implicated in the exacerbation of asthma, hypnosis has been used to introduce suggestions against wheezing and anxious responses. Smith and Burns (1960) hypnotized 24 subjects with a mean age of 11 who had suffered from asthma for many years. A variety of subjective and objective measures were used. A control group showed no changes, and the hypnotized children (four sessions of hypnosis) showed only subjective improvement. Hypnosis, in this study, did not decrease the number of wheezing attacks nor the amount of medication used. It seems more fruitful to teach the asthmatic child techniques such as relaxation and breathing exercises (boosted, if necessary, by initial desensitization) that give him *active* control over his symptoms, rather than using a technique of "being cured" passively.

Other Behavior Modification Techniques   Behavior modification techniques can be used in another way to enhance the child's active role in controlling his symptoms and reducing the need for emergency-room visits and hospitalizations. Most asthmatic children are on some regimen of medication. Many may also have dietary restrictions. Parents can provide the control and guidance needed to follow these treatment regimens when the child is very small. As the asthmatic child gets older, it is necessary (because of his frequent separations from home) and desirable for him to monitor his own diet and medications. It is extremely difficult for the child to take medicine and watch his diet *every* day, particularly when he is feeling healthy. The psychologist, either directly or in consultation with a physician or visiting nurse, can help set up a schedule of reinforcements using stars or points to help the child perform these behaviors regularly. Both parents and physicians can be enlisted to praise the child or to give a tangible reinforcer for proper adherence to the medical regimen.

Family Therapy and Group Therapy   All of the treatments mentioned above can be of help to many asthmatic children because they aim at enhancing positive, active control of symptoms and are not predicated on the presence of psychopathology. For some asthmatic children, however, this type of intervention is not enough. Their asthmatic symptoms have become enmeshed in the conflict of the family or have come to serve a maladaptive psychological purpose for the child himself. In these cases, medical regimens are often ignored or are ineffective. Attempts to increase the child's control over symptoms seem to have little or no effect. A more intensive or individualized form of treatment is needed in these cases. Again, the severity of the problem and its resistance to less invasive or drastic interventions will dictate what form of treatment is appropriate. The exact modality (family therapy, group therapy, etc.) may be dictated by the nature of the problem and the resources available. Any of these modes also is appropriate for the child with emotional problems who also has asthma. Therapy, however, may help with the maladaptive behaviors but may have no effect on the asthma (Sclare and Crochet, 1952). Assessment of the role the disease plays in the child's functioning is essential in determining how to intervene. The observation of patterns—what precipitates attacks, what follows them that could reinforce them, what function they might serve—will be the clue to the intervention needed.

When a maladaptive family process is the source of difficulty in managing the child's asthmatic symptoms, it is likely that attempts at changing medication or providing the child with greater self-control over the psychological stimuli that trigger his attacks will be of little help. Environmental response to the child and his symptoms becomes the controlling variable. If the parents respond to wheezing with overprotective, solicitous behavior, which may include keeping him home from school for unnecessary amounts of time, allowing him to shirk household duties, or allowing him to be pampered and get extra attention (beyond what is medically indicated), then the wheezing is reinforced and may increase in frequency. When the child begins to wheeze during a family conflict or confrontation that the family is unable to resolve, the family's attention is diverted to caring for the "sick child" and the resulting decrease in tension also may reinforce the appearance of symptoms during family conflicts. When the family system perpetuates this symptom by reinforcing it, then intervention must focus on changing the system. Again the specific nature of the intervention depends on the severity of the problem.

If there are only one or two isolated areas (such as going to school or doing chores) during which symptoms appear, then a circumscribed approach is useful. The mental health worker can help parents find out what, if any, problems exist that cause the child to avoid school, etc. After these difficulties are resolved, the parent needs help in using behavior modification approaches to change the child's responses. For example, the child must finish the chore, go to school, etc. as soon as the symptoms are cleared. He may even be reinforced for appropriate behavior and absence of symptoms in the problematic settings.

When parents are unable to identify the areas of difficulty or are unable to easily change their responses to the wheezing, family therapy is indicated. Liebman, Minuchin, and Baker (1976) suggest five specific goals in their approach to the asthmatic child's family. Their form of therapy is directive as well as exploratory, and, by focusing on the specific issues involved with the asthmatic symptoms, it is relatively short term. They suggest that the family therapist help the family to: 1) delineate the dysfunctional patterns that produce stress and the attacks, and change them to functional patterns, 2) change maladaptive relationships that are maintained by the presence of symptoms, e.g., the overly protective mother, 3) work on the concrete problems of the siblings such as poor school performance or needing braces, 4) give no special treatment to the patient regarding discipline or responsibility, and 5) get away from home more and encourage the child to become involved with peers.

Psychotherapy   In some instances the asthmatic child or a member of his family may be so severely emotionally disturbed that the asthmatic symptoms become part of an extremely complicated, symbolic attempt to resolve neurotic or psychotic conflicts. In these cases, even changes in the family environment may have insufficient effect because the symptoms have taken on a personalized meaning. Traditional psychotherapies for the child and/or parent may be the answer here. This type of problem is the one often described in case histories of the psychological treatment of asthmatics, and many conclusions about asthmatics have been drawn from this extreme population.

Residential Placement   At times the child's health is endangered to such a point or the family's resistance to change is so great that more drastic measures are needed to eliminate psychological environmental control of symptoms. In these cases the treatment needed may be one of the oldest: residential placement or what has been termed the parentectomy (Peshkin, 1968). When the home situation cannot be changed, the child may need to be in a setting that frees him from the factors that aggravate his symptoms while providing medical care as well as psychological support services. After a year or two in such a setting, the child hopefully will have developed new response patterns and enough ego strength to re-enter the home situation without the return of severe asthmatic symptoms. Optimally, the parents and/or family would continue in treatment to change the environment to which the child returns. Unfortunately, when residential treatment is needed, the family often has great difficulty making substantial changes.

Role of the Mental Health Worker

The spectrum of psychological treatments that can be useful in working with asthmatic children is great. In many ways the approaches to protecting the child from the "psychological allergens" that aggravate his symptoms parallel those used to control medical aspects of the disease. The child can learn to control his response to stress by relaxation just as he can take antihistamines or other drugs that will block his response when faced with physical causes of symptoms. Changes in, or a move to a new, environment help medically (dust-free, pollen-free arrangements) as well as psychologically (family and residential treatment). Finally, desensitization to irritants, both physical and psychological, has been helpful to asthmatics.

All of the types of intervention and the ongoing assessment needed to determine when it is needed and what approach is appropriate necessitate a very active role for the mental health worker in relation to the asthmatic child. While all the disciplines within the mental health field can provide any of these services, traditionally there have been areas of expertise designated to each. Psychologists generally have had the most experience and training in behavior modification and biofeedback approaches. Social workers often have the knowledge needed to make a good residential placement. Psychiatrists have traditionally had greater experience with severely disturbed patients. Beyond these traditional skills, family, group, or individual psychotherapy to treat asthmatic children should be offered by whoever is best trained within a given setting. A variety of people who could consult with physicians, nurses, and physical therapists treating the asthmatic child would be optimal, since the professional who possesses all the skills mentioned here is rare, indeed.

The mental health professional who interacts with asthmatic children has another responsibility as well. Because so much of the psychological literature on asthma in the past has asserted the view of psychogenesis, many physicians have become disenchanted with the mental health profession as a source of help in managing their asthmatic patients. Most of the children they treat are not disturbed or severely neurotic; thus, the services of the mental health professional are not considered. Education of physicians about approaches such as relaxation therapy, biofeedback, and behavior modification, which may benefit many patients, is a part of the mental health professional's role. Information about environmental approaches to change as well as about intrapsychic modes of therapy needs to be provided. Service and education, then, are the roles to be filled by the mental health professional involved with asthmatic children.

CYSTIC FIBROSIS

Dealing with the cystic fibrosis patient is, for the mental health professional, light years removed from the uncertainties and ambiguities of involvement with the asthmatic child. There is no question here of psychogenesis, no real debate about the role of the psychologist or other mental health professionals. Cystic fibrosis is a genetically transmitted, mendelian recessive trait affecting the exocrine glands. It leads an ever lengthening, but relentless, path to early death that is marked by physical discomfort and psychological pain. There is little the psychologist or other mental health professionals can do but stand by and help pick up the pieces of shattered lives and families. As will become evident, there is a prolonged process of coping necessary, and few individuals or families are equipped to sustain this process alone. To understand the role of psychological intervention in the treatment of the cystic fibrosis patient and his family, it is first necessary to know about the disease itself. In many ways, just the description of the symptoms and course of this disease point to the need for and direction of intervention. Although limited, the literature on the psychosocial aspects of cystic fibrosis and effective interventions points to a framework for approaching the crises of this disease.

Medical Aspects of Cystic Fibrosis

As mentioned, cystic fibrosis is a genetically transmitted, mendelian recessive trait affecting the exocrine glands. Most of the serious consequences are caused by the chemical change in and increased viscosity of mucous secretions. Sweat and salivary glands are also affected negatively. These changes lead to clogging of the pancreatic and bile ducts (and thus pancreatic insufficiency), clogging of air passages and chronic pulmonary disease, excessively high sweat electrolytes, and sometimes cirrhosis of the liver.

When this disease was first identified as a separate clinical entity in 1938, the mortality rate was 75% in the first year, and over 95% of the patients died by their third year of life. At present, when cystic fibrosis patients benefit from early diagnosis (preferably within the first three months of life), aggressive medical therapy, and psychosocial support, they can expect a greatly increased longevity (Kulczycki, Regal, and Tantisunthorn, 1973). Children followed in one of the cystic fibrosis centers that provides care by a multidisciplinary team survive to an average age of 15 (90% diagnosed by three months), and more and more patients are surviving into adulthood. Although careful management can extend the lifespan for cystic fibrosis patients, there is no cure for this ultimately fatal disease. At some point pulmonary symptoms cannot be contained, and death caused by the complications of pulmonary insufficiency follows. Often this final process is a long, drawn out series of nearly fatal episodes, with the family and patient repeatedly having to face imminent death. Because of the lethal nature of the pulmonary symptoms and the presence of these symptoms in almost all patients, cystic fibrosis care traditionally has fallen primarily upon the pulmonary specialists.

There are, however, a multitude of symptoms affecting the life-style, self-image, and development of the cystic fibrosis patient.

Pulmonary symptoms begin with partial bronchial obstruction, because the abnormal secretions interfere with the normal cleaning process to remove dust and bacteria from the lungs and bronchi. As a result, repeated infections cause further bronchial and bronchiolar obstruction, which again increases chance of infection. At first, patients have a dry, hacking cough and some difficulty breathing. This process progresses until breathing becomes more labored and the cough becomes productive and sometimes paroxysmal, followed by vomiting. The child becomes more and more listless, has reduced muscle tone, and is likely to develop a barrel-chest deformity and clubbing of fingers and toes caused by cyanosis. Nasal polyps and paranasal sinus abnormalities are common with cystic fibrosis.

The abnormal secretions that block the flow of pancreatic digestive enzymes into the duodenum (in approximately 80–85% of cases) cause malabsorption of fats and proteins. As a result of this malabsorption, the child has frequent, foul-smelling stools, which are often preceded by severe abdominal pains. The patients may also have a voracious appetite but fail to grow and to gain weight. Many cystic fibrosis patients look much smaller and younger than their age and show signs of malnutrition such as protuberant abdomens and wasted buttocks.

Diabetes mellitus is more prevalent in cystic fibrosis children than normal children. These children are prone to rectal prolapse, fecal masses, and, because of excessive sweat salinity, are vulnerable to severe salt loss, heat prostration, circulatory collapse, and death during hot weather or when febrile. Some patients also show liver involvement, often portal hypertension and its complications. In addition, male cystic fibrosis patients who survive to adulthood are sterile (some females have been known to conceive and bear children) (Holsclaw et al., 1973).

The genetic nature of this disease adds a further, insidious aspect to its impact. It is a recessive trait, thought to be carried by 5% of the population. (There is presently no test for the heterozygote.) Thus, when both parents carry the gene, the probability is that one child in four will have the disease, two will be carriers, and one will be normal. This means that a positive diagnosis of cystic fibrosis in a family arouses anxiety for future generations and also for the presence of cystic fibrosis in siblings. It is not uncommon for families to lose more than one child to cystic fibrosis.

The disease is diagnosed by testing the sweat (these children taste "salty" when kissed) and pancreatic functions. Chest x-rays are used to assess pulmonary status. This step is crucial because early intervention is the key (Kulczycki et al., 1973) to increasing longevity if it is followed by aggressive treatment.

Understanding the medical treatment is essential to an understanding of the overwhelming burden it places on the family. Treatment directed against bronchial obstruction includes postural drainage. The patient is positioned to achieve maximal drainage of mucus from each pulmonary lobe. While the patient or parent pounds on the chest or uses vibrators to loosen the mucus, the child tries to cough up as much sputum as possible. This procedure is usually done two times a day.

In addition to these procedures, the patient is often on some regular regimen of antibiotics to fight the rash of chronic infections.

The pancreatic symptoms are treated by giving replacement enzymes to improve digestion and thus reduce the number and bulk of stools, improve weight gain, and decrease excessive appetite. Diet should be high in protein, low in fat, and include extra salt.

In short, the patient with cystic fibrosis and his family face the tragedy of early death at an unknown point in the future. The wait for this death is made even more difficult by symptoms that are not only physically dangerous but socially embarrassing (e.g., coughing, foul-smelling stools and flatus, distorted appearance), by the diversion of family energies to the demanding treatment, by loss of time in school (or job) and with peers as a result of frequent illness and hospitalizations, and by the financial strain caused by this prolonged involvement with the medical community.

It takes very little imagination to picture the effects of this process on a child or adolescent trying to develop a sense of self, to grow more independent, and to feel that his life, which may be cut short at any time, is worth living. Only the slightest amount of empathy is needed to understand the anguish of parents, the resentment of the overwhelming task, and the effects on siblings and the marriage relationship of such a disease (Holsclaw et al., 1970, 1973).

Psychological Aspects of Cystic Fibrosis

The literature relating to the psychological effects of cystic fibrosis and the means most effective in ameliorating these is mostly descriptive in nature. There are numerous renditions of the devastating effects of this illness on the child, the parents, and siblings. Each article has a slightly different focus (different age group, different type of family, different theoretical model) and a variation on the basic theme of multidisciplinary support for the cystic fibrosis patient and family. Some articles (Tropauer, Franz, and Dilgard, 1970; Meyerowitz and Kaplan, 1973; Boyle et al., 1976) list the results of questionnaires or scientific evaluations: numbers of parents able to cope, types of reactions, amount of psychopathology in this population. Others describe touchingly, in subjective, human terms, the experience of the patients, families, and staff during the crisis points in the disease process (Bushman, 1973; Dooley, 1973; Lorin, 1973). In general, much of what is known about the chronically ill and dying child has been applied to the specifics of cystic fibrosis. It is these specifics that are presented here, set in a framework that can help the pediatric psychologist and other mental health professionals assess what sorts of intervention would be most helpful to the cystic fibrosis patient and his family at any point in time.

The Three Crises of Cystic Fibrosis

A disease, such as cystic fibrosis, which runs a course over many years, can be thought of as having a development much like that of its human victim. There is a successive pattern of events and a series of crises which must be resolved if subsequent events and crises are to be handled adequately. If an earlier crisis is not resolved adequately, the unfinished issues it arouses will reappear later to make resolution more difficult, if not impossible. In the development of the child, it is understandable that a child who has not fully resolved questions of autonomy will have difficulty with the later developmental crisis of establishing his identity. In a chronic disease, it is similarly a problem for parents and patients who have not resolved issues around accepting the diagnosis to cope adequately (or with *manageable trauma*) with the later crisis of imminent death. Cystic fibrosis is a disease that typically presents at least three such crises: the diagnosis, the adolescence of the patient, and death. Understanding of these crises, the issues they arouse and interventions to facilitate maximal resolution appears to be the most appropriate role for the pediatric psychologist on a cystic fibrosis team. Both of these tasks cannot be carried out in a vacuum—cooperation with the primary physician, nurses, physical therapists, and social workers is essential to the successful handling of the psychological aspects of the disease.

The First Crisis: Diagnosis and the Beginning of Treatment Parents often reach the first crisis after a period of tests, hospitalizations involving a series of doctors, and tentative diagnoses and prognoses. The diagnosis sends shock waves through the family and is confusing: on the one hand the parents are given a death sentence for their child, while at the same time they are told that there is hope for prolonging that life if they actively involve themselves in elaborate treatment procedures.

Initial reactions to the diagnosis of cystic fibrosis have been observed to parallel those seen to other lethal diagnoses and to death itself. Sabinga, Friedman, and Huang (1973) suggest the following pattern: 1) shock, 2) disbelief or denial, 3) distortion or blocking, 4) eventual acceptance and depression, and 5) either resigned, realistic coping or extreme defensive maneuvers. This process follows its own pace in each family and can be facilitated but not hurried. The problems arise when families and patients get stuck at the points of denial and distortion and cannot get on with the business of treatment. Fathers seem to have particular difficulty at this point, often reacting angrily toward the diagnosing physician (Patterson, 1973) and refusing any involvement in psychological treatment for the family (Belmonte and St. Germain, 1973). Often the denial melts in the face of the child's first relapse (Meyerowitz and Kaplan, 1973), but, while facts can overwhelm the defense of denial, they cannot help resolve the underlying issues of the family, parents, and patient that made them unable to resolve this initial crisis on their own.

Giving up one's denial of the diagnosis of cystic fibrosis means more than accepting the fact of an early death for the child. There are other common issues aroused by the specific nature of cystic fibrosis. The one that often hits first is the guilt usually aroused by a damaged child, which is particularly a factor when the damage is genetically determined. Mothers often experience conflicting feelings about the birth of a child. When the child is born with a defect, the mother feels guilt for having "hurt" her child (Patterson, 1973). The "bad seed" complex hits hardest those couples who have no other "normal" children (Sabinga et al., 1973). Because of the genetic aspects of cystic fibrosis, the extended family becomes involved and can add to the stress. Often the husband's mother suggests that there is "nothing like that in our family," particularly because women tend to "marry up" (socioeconomically) and are seen as coming from inferior stock (Patterson, 1973). Whether this attitude is expressed or not, many parents see their children as a way to please their own parents, and the production of a damaged child dashes these hopes and confirms negative self-feelings. Parents' guilt can be further fueled by intimations by medical staff that the child should have been brought sooner for diagnosis.

The treatment required for a cystic fibrosis child causes a monumental interruption of a family life-style. Meyerowitz and Kaplan (1973) found that 54% of the mothers they surveyed were employed before the diagnosis of cystic fibrosis, but only 26% remained working outside the home postdiagnosis. One in three fathers gave up job mobility and thus career advancement so that his cystic fibrosis child could remain near one of the special centers offering optimal care. These losses are in addition to the financial strain of medical care (McKey, 1973). The family's social life can be affected negatively by the amount of time given to treatments and by the embarrassment over socially unacceptable symptoms (foul-smelling stools, paroxysmal cough, etc.) (Doctor, 1973; Patterson, 1973). Mother spends so much time with the sick child that father is shut out, siblings feel neglected (Belmonte and St. Germain, 1973), and family communication patterns are disrupted.

All these disruptions are ultimately resented, and the resulting angry feelings are often difficult and uncomfortable for the parents of the cystic fibrosis patient to resolve in a useful way. Parents who have always had difficulty with anger are most susceptible because they repress the hostility and end up missing treatment regimens or displacing the anger onto other family members. Even when treatment regimens are followed obsessively (perhaps in reaction formation), there is little loving care given, and the children do worse than in families where treatment is more lackadaisical but given more freely. When the parents are able to overtly express this anger and resentment they are better caregivers, not only for the sick child, but for the entire family (Tropauer, Franz, and Dilgard, 1970). Free expression of these feelings is a major step, however, because these feelings usually re-arouse the parents' guilt about having "damaged" their child. This trap can hold families back in their attempts to resolve the crisis of accepting the diagnosis.

Even when guilt and anger are within bounds, the parents of the cystic fibrosis patient must strike a viable balance between the work of anticipatory mourning that comes with full acceptance of the diagnosis and the job of being totally and actively involved in the long-term treatment of their child. They must be letting go at the same time that they are totally involved. They cannot let go so much that they do not provide the daily treatment; yet, they must yield to the reality of assured death to make a successful resolution of this first crisis as a basis for meeting later crises in the disease (Farkas and Schnell, 1973).

Finally, there are practical problems that must be resolved, which revolve around the issues of denial, guilt, and anger. What to tell the child is a major concern. All three alternatives—hiding the truth, telling all, and telling part of the information—have been recommended. The physician must certainly bear part of the burden, but, for a young child, parents are still the ultimate authority. This task is extremely stressful for most parents; there is an increased incidence of stress-related illnesses such as ulcers in parents whose children ask questions about cystic fibrosis (Meyerowitz and Kaplan, 1973). Parents who cannot accept the diagnosis will mislead the child about his condition, to the point of suggesting that the cough is "from a cold." The child himself will pick up on this denial, leaving both himself and his parents poorly equipped to deal with the realizations during adolescence of the true nature of cystic fibrosis. Others, often out of guilt, will "protect" the patient with a "web of silence" (Lawler, Nakielny, and Wright, 1966). Even in the best of circumstances parents need guidance on how to explain cystic fibrosis to their child.

The other "practical" question for parents is whether or not to have more children. Parents need both genetic counseling, to understand the risks, and psychological support, to explore the underpinnings, of their decision. Again, resentments over growing up, the dream of the ideal family, can be aroused and must be addressed.

This first crisis for most cystic fibrosis patients mostly involves the family, because the child is usually young. When the diagnosis is made in an older child or adolescent, the family's input is important, but the patient also may manifest feelings of anger, denial, or depression. In these cases, the reactions of the patient are much like those of long-diagnosed cystic fibrosis patients as they enter adolescence, and the focus of intervention will be the individual as well as the family.

All the issues mentioned above occur to some degree for all families during the initial crisis of accepting the diagnosis and beginning treatment. Given the extreme nature of the situation, it is impossible to say what "normal" behavior will be. Parents of cystic fibrosis patients have repeated bouts of depression (Tropauer, Franz, and Dilgard, 1970); yet, this is not an inappropriate reaction. The task for the family of a cystic fibrosis patient is to carry through responsibly on treatment with minimal disruption of family functioning and without causing development of psychological symptoms by other family members. For each family, the behaviors involved will differ, and the nature of the family's communication patterns, ability to support one another emotionally, and stability will affect the impact of the diagnosis. "Healthier" families tend to cope better (Tropauer et al., 1970), but, even in these families, father is often shut out and the patient may play one parent against the other (Findlay et al., 1969; Belmonte and St. Germain, 1973). A typical pattern is an overprotective mother and a withdrawn father (Boyle et al., 1976). The other side of this picture is the overtly rejecting mother. Neither approach represents an adequate resolution of guilt and resentment. Somehow in the midst of the emotional stress and treatments families can regain normal activity—as one mother put it, "You've got to work in enough time for fun" (Kulczyski, Regal, and Tantisunthorn, 1973, p. 123).

All families may need some help counteracting the forces that tend to diminish communications within the family of a cystic fibrosis child and create the maladaptive patterns mentioned. (The thrust of this help is discussed later.) When there is psychopathology in family members and/or very disrupted family functioning, the impact of the diagnosis of cystic fibrosis becomes a further stress that cannot be processed in a helpful way. This pathology can manifest itself in a variety of ways. Refusal to participate in treatment is one extreme. The other extreme is probably equally as common: the disease and the routine of treatment become organizational points for the disturbed mother or family. The mother finds ego-organization in the routine required and gratification in the forced dependency of her child. She may now have an ego-syntonic way to inhibit separation and growth by her child. Disorganized families can find this same sort of focus in the crises of the sick child. Davies and Addington (1973) describe the case of such a disrupted family. Father was often absent for long periods of time, mother abused alcohol, and the younger sibling manifested pathological behavior. When the cystic fibrosis patient was acutely ill and hospitalized, this family was able to function and draw together. The patient herself was thus often sick and depressed. This example stresses the point that the actual ability to provide treatment for the child is not a sufficient criterion for judging the adequacy of a family's psychological adjustment to the diagnosis and the treatment. One must be alert to the process and the toll it takes on family members, in particular the cystic fibrosis patient. The subtleties of this process may not be initially apparent in the interactions with medical staff if the medical results are positive. Extra assessment of families during the initial phase is crucial and may need to be initiated by treatment staff because families often wish to avoid voicing the issues involved.

Two other specific types of families are mentioned in the literature as having particular difficulty accepting the diagnosis and/or initiating treatment. One is the family that has already suffered death or deaths of other siblings because of cystic fibrosis. There is, at times, a sense by these families of wanting to abandon the sick members and devoting energies to those who will survive. The other type of family is one in which the death wish for the cystic fibrosis child is particularly intense. The families of chronically ill patients all entertain a death wish to some degree in that it affords relief from the suspense, pain, loss of freedom, and disruption of family caused by the patient's illness. The death of the cystic fibrosis child also removes the albatross of "bad genes" from the parents' necks. Finally, it can be a way of proving to the doctors that the hope they offer is false. In some families this subconscious wish grows to such proportions that the child's treatment and life are endangered. In an area where organized help is readily available, these families find reasons *not* to take advantage of these facilities: it is too far, too expensive, not useful to *their* child, etc. (Warwick and Shapero, 1973).

This sort of pattern should be a "red flag" to medical staff or other team members, since intervention has been shown to be helpful in lessening the impact of this death wish on the conscious behavior of parents (Warwick and Shapero, 1973).

What difference does the resolution of denial, anger, guilt, resentment, and death wishes in the family of newly diagnosed cystic fibrosis patients make in the patient's development, the family's functioning, and the success of medical treatment? When mothers have not fully resolved their feelings of guilt, when they do not accept the inevitability of their child's worsening condition, they often suffer guilt over inevitable setbacks (Tropauer, Franz, and Dilgard, 1970), such as infections, and redouble their efforts at the cost of family functioning. Fathers are shut out and offer less support, leaving the mother isolated and resentful (Belmonte and St. Germain, 1973). Other siblings often act sick to get attention (Tropauer et al., 1970) and harbor a growing resentment toward the cystic fibrosis patient, which interferes with the gains of normal sibling interactions and can diminish their ability to deal with the cystic fibrosis patient's ultimate death without lasting emotional scars (Farkas and Schnell, 1973). The patient himself is more limited than necessary in the development of independence and competency needed for a positive self-image and a base for adolescence if mother is overly involved. He will be depressed and see himself as even more deficient than most children with his disease if mother is rejecting because she cannot face her guilt or resentment. In either case he will often not become more involved in his own care as his age and competencies increase, leaving him vulnerable to the next crisis in the course of cystic fibrosis—adolescence.

Medical prognosis is also affected by the way a family deals with this initial crisis. The family that denies the illness and eschews help greatly diminishes the patient's hope for extended life. The overly protective mother, however, also seems to have a negative effect on treatment. Boyle et al. (1976) found that patients who were infantilized did worse. Those who were competent and had a more typical psychological development did better. The factor affecting this variable appeared to be mother's ability to maintain an active life outside the home. This ability was *not* related to severity of the child's illness but to mother's ability to maintain perspective and her determination to keep family life as "normal" as possible.

Aside from enhancing the family's ability to provide treatment and continue to function in a way that meets major needs of all members, the other crucial reason for ensuring an adequate resolution of this first crisis is the need to lay the groundwork needed to weather the crisis almost always precipitated by the onset of adolescence in the cystic fibrosis patient himself. During the years between these crises the patient is gleaning information about who he is (how frail is he? how loveable? how damaged?), what he is like compared to other children, what his disease is about, and the importance of his medical treatments. He learns whether or not to be ashamed of his symptoms. He picks up on whether or not he is a burden or a disruptive force in his family. He senses his parents' death wish for him if it is intense. At the same time his family may have worked out a tense equilibrium in which their guilts, resentments, and distortions can be submerged, unquestioned. They are not prepared to face the re-arousal of these issues when the patient himself reaches adolescence and begins to grapple with the same conflicts.

The Second Psychological Crisis: Adolescence   Pairing the words adolescence and crises seems almost embarrassingly easy and even glib. New issues face the cystic fibrosis patient as he becomes a teen and young adult. What appears to precipitate the crisis for these patients is not the hormonal changes (onset of puberty is often delayed) but the increased cognitive powers of hypothetical abstract reasoning. The younger child may fear separation from parents as a result of hospitalization or may not like the inconvenience of his treatments (Tropauer et al., 1970), but he does not have the ability to understand the concepts of chronicity, fatality, or even future in an abstract sense. When the cystic fibrosis patient develops this greater understanding, the awareness of his disease changes radically. It is as if he has heard the diagnosis for the first time (Liggens, 1975), and his reactions will run the same course as those of his parents when the diagnosis was first made. If the family members have not resolved their issues around the diagnosis—if they have not provided proper treatment, have hidden the reality of the disease, etc.—the adolescent will feel betrayed or else supported in maintaining his denial. Even if the family has worked through the issues of guilt, anger, denial, overprotection or rejection, and resentment, the adolescent cystic fibrosis patient has a particularly difficult task in dealing with the age-typical concerns of independence, identity, and heterosexual intimacy, because his symptoms and prognosis interfere with normal resolutions. Just as his parents had to learn to juggle their anticipatory mourning and their total involvement with his treatment, so now the adolescent must learn to deny death (live "as if") but not deny the disease (Helman, 1973). With today's medical care the adolescent may live another 15 years, but he may not. He may be able to be active and may enjoy relatively good health, or he may be in the end stages of chronic pulmonary disease. In either case he is now an independently thinking person, who must make his own adjustment to his disease—a process that is often painful for his caregivers to watch.

Cystic fibrosis interferes with almost every aspect of life that is crucial to an adolescent. He is working toward greater independence psychologically at a time when his disease may be making him physically more dependent. Even if his condition is stable, he must rely on parents and medical staff in a way that chafes, where the anxiety about individuation can be dealt with by regression that is sanctioned because of the illness. Parents can make the process more complicated if overprotection has been their way of dealing with their guilts and anxieties about their child. They cannot bear to relinquish control over treatments or the child's life-style because they cannot tolerate any setbacks. For more pathological parents, too, the illness gives an excuse for limiting their child's separation. If there has been good resolution of the crisis of diagnosis, then by the time the cystic fibrosis patient reaches adolescence he has already assumed responsibility for much of his care and he can achieve independence relative to his own previous state.

For the adolescent part of his search for identity leads him to find out who he is relative to his peers. Parental approval becomes relatively unimportant compared to peer acceptance. Having any chronic disease makes a child different, and, if he has not developed a comfortable self-view including his disease, he will expect peer rejection as well. For the cystic fibrosis patient his altered appearance (small stature, extreme thinness, barrel chest, etc.) puts a particular strain on his interpersonal relations (Liggens, 1975). Most cystic fibrosis patients view their bodies as distorted, a fact reflected in their human figure drawings (Boyle et al., 1976). Wanting desperately to be like everyone else, adolescent patients will try to hide their disease (Kulczycki, Regal, and Tantisunthorn, 1973) and forego treatment that would mark them as different. Sexual development is also delayed in many cystic fibrosis patients, adding further anxieties to those around the heterosexual relationships and intimacy experienced by most teenagers. Males are sterile, and this fact must be incorporated into a sense of self at a time when any difference is painful and a true deficit is devastating.

Another path of the search for identity includes projecting oneself into the future: "What will I be?" is as much a question as "Who am I?" For the cystic fibrosis patient with an uncertain life-span this is a question that makes him anxious and depressed (Boyle et al., 1976). He doesn't know how much future there is. To function he must deny death but not his disease. Career goals are uncertain or limited because the cystic fibrosis patient may be too sick or weak for many jobs. Like many who have been cared for, cystic fibrosis patients want to be helpers, but few have the stamina to complete rigorous professional training (Boat and Helman, n.d.). Careers must also be limited to areas in which the patient is not exposed to infection, dust, fumes, or other irritants that could exacerbate pulmonary symptoms. Future marriage and children are also questionable because of the disease. Spouses must be willing to deal with frequent illness, special treatments (like sleeping with the mist tent), and possible financial difficulties because of high medical bills. Helman (1973) suggests that much of the depression for adolescent boys at present comes from the realization that they will not attain career goals. Girls are mostly depressed about their poor appearance and thus lowered desirability as dating and marriage partners.

The typical adolescent response to any limitation is rebellion. When a chronically ill child rebels against the rules adults impose on him, he may also ignore those restrictions essential to his health. In cystic fibrosis patients, "death through rebellion" is a concern because failure to follow imposed treatment can easily be fatal. Patients defy warnings against smoking and drinking and refuse treatments that interfere with their independence (Helman, 1973; Kulczycki et al., 1973). Adolescents generally explore the limits of their own mortality as part of their experimentation with hypothetical thinking. Death is considered tentatively. But as the cystic fibrosis patient considers it, he cannot then push it away as "not me." Depression and hopelessness then take over and the patient may refuse treatment. This tendency is more marked when the patient's condition is worsening, which is often the case during adolescence (Helman, 1973).

Parents and staff become increasingly upset as an adolescent repeatedly fails to come home for postural drainage and eats improperly. When these actions result in his condition worsening and his ultimate death, the adolescent's passive suicide triggers particularly intense feelings in those who have been unable to reverse the process. If the family members have never resolved their guilt and resentment, they will respond to this gesture with tremendous anger that cannot be resolved. Even when they have worked it through, they can be overwhelmed with a sense of helplessness, and both the patient and his family may need help to come through this second crisis. Again resolution here will affect the family's ability to·deal with the death of the patient. If the patient actually dies because of rebellion-suicide, the guilt and anger of the family can be a tremendous obstacle to adequate mourning. There is a close interplay between psychological and physical factors, even when overt rebellion is not involved.

It has been noted that more males than female cystic fibrosis patients survive into young adulthood. A variety of explanations has been offered, but one raises interesting questions about the necessity for counseling even when there is not overt rejection of treatment or failure to cope with adolescent issues. An essential part of the cystic fibrosis patient's treatment for pulmonary symptoms is physical exercise. Adolescent males, as part of their peer relations and sense of self, remain as active or become more active than when younger. Girls, on the other hand, begin to take on the more passive, nonphysical role traditionally considered feminine and reduce their activity to conform to peer expectations.

A special case of the adolescent crisis in cystic fibrosis is when the disease is first diagnosed in the teens or early twenties. These patients have no chance to adapt to their prognosis and the treatments before the crisis of establishing one's identity. Getting the diagnosis at this point is like finding out that one is not who one always thought one was. All hopes, plans, and ideals are thrown into question. This patient can be high-risk both emotionally and medically and deserves routine psychological intervention (Boat and Helman, n.d.).

Aside from the psychological difficulties that the cystic fibrosis adolescent must face, reality factors interfere and require outside management help. There is at present a lack of financial assistance for cystic fibrosis patients over 21 years old. Crippled children societies provide services to younger patients, vocational rehabilitation gives only interim help while the patient is being trained, and welfare is available only if the patient is willing to be labeled "permanently and totally disabled." Some health insurance programs cover treatment, but at least 30% of young adult cystic fibrosis patients have none. Many (80–85%) are capable of at least part-time work, but employers are reluctant to hire them because they are too weak or miss too much work. In addition, a job must include time for postural drainage, which many young adults need to perform several hours a day.

These problems in the real world in many ways verify the adolescent's feelings of hopelessness and anger. As he tests himself in the adult world he finds his strengths, but he also finds himself and the world lacking in many essential ways.

The Final Crisis   The psychological process of dying and the death of a cystic fibrosis patient are not basically different from other diseases. The anticipatory mourning and the stages of grief are the same. The description of that process is complex and well documented elsewhere (Kubler-Ross, 1969). Those aspects of this process specific to cystic fibrosis include uncertainty about life expectancy and, thus, difficulty with anticipatory mourning, as well as the strains of multiple brushes with death.

Uncertainty is always the added factor of psychological stress in dealing with cystic fibrosis. Some patients die very young, but more and more survive into adulthood. Death, when it comes, is rarely sudden. It is often a lingering process with many episodes of critical illness during which the family is told there is no hope. Each time the patient faces death and deals with his fears; each time the family members go through anticipatory mourning and begin withdrawing their emotional investment in the patient. When the patient suddenly rallies and often even returns home to normal functioning, there can be anger, confusion, and guilt on both sides. Bushman (1973) describes a case in which an adolescent girl improved after two weeks of a seemingly downhill course. When her mother was told of the recovery, her response was, "This is so difficult. Already I have said my farewell." The girl, however, again became critically ill and died shortly thereafter. This see-saw is particularly difficult for families who have not learned to be comfortable with their resentments and death wishes for the patients. They have felt the relief and release as well as the pain of the imminently anticipated death. When their child does not die, the guilt can be overwhelming.

If the family has to go through the process of deinvestment too many times, the patient is likely to find himself isolated. He may feel abandoned by his family at a time when he is fearful and dealing with the sadness of leaving them through death (Bushman, 1973; Helman, 1973), compounding the isolation that frequently occurs when family, friends, and medical staff are reluctant to talk to the dying patient about death.

The resolution of this crisis—both the false alarms and the patient's ultimate death—depends greatly on the patient's and family's abilities to resolve the earlier crises. Again the family is the focus, because they survive. Parents who have not resolved their initial guilt or who cannot bear to imagine that the fate of their children is beyond their control, suffer the guilt of the omnipotent—if only mother had performed the treatments better, if only they hadn't let the patient go where he was exposed to infection. All parents may have these thoughts, but those who have never resolved the basic issues cannot let go of this guilt, cannot finish the mourning process, and cannot move on. In families where there was discomfort about telling siblings or denial of the prognosis, surviving children have no reality to counteract their fantasies that their rivalrous wishes and resentment of the time given the sick sibling have caused the death. This guilt, if it is not addressed, can be the seed for future psychopathology. These surviving children are at risk (Farkas and Schnell, 1973). When the patient has died through an adolescent suicide equivalent, the guilt and anger will also inhibit the natural course of mourning and lock families into a permanent state of depression. If the parents have not been able to accept the appropriate strivings for independence in an adolescent or young-adult cystic fibrosis patient, they may blame the child for dying, because he did not care for himself as well as they could have.

All these examples illustrate the necessity for resolution of critical issues at each stage in the psychosocial course of cystic fibrosis. Each family will have its own content, but the process is virtually universal. The framework presented here is suggested as a way to judge the need for intervention and to suggest the points at which support could prevent a long course of psychological maladjustment for cystic fibrosis patients and their families.

Intervention: What Kinds and When

The literature on cystic fibrosis unanimously recommends that patients be followed in one of the special multidisciplinary centers established in conjuction with the Cystic Fibrosis Foundation. (A complete list of the centers is available from the national headquarters of the Cystic Fibrosis Foundation in Atlanta, Georgia.) Aside from the medical benefits of such a center, the patient's psychosocial progress can be monitored and promoted through a close relationship between physician and mental health personnel. If the mental health professional is part of a team (at such a center or in other settings) and knows and is known by the patient and family throughout the illness, he is more likely to be able to have impact at points of crisis. It can be very difficult for these families to tolerate another new, intrusive face during particularly stressful times.

A variety of interventions can be used to help families and patients adjust during the initial diagnosis phase. Meeting other parents and patients to share experiences and pain and to find realistic hope is recommended (Kulczyski, Regal, and Tantisunthorn, 1973). This can be done both informally (the waiting room can be a very therapeutic place for parents, if they can be helped to make contact with healthier families) and through organized parent groups. Meyerowitz and Kaplan (1973) point out that there is the danger in parent groups that unrealistic hopes of a "cure" can be reinforced. When there is a professional consulting with the group this trend can be noted and hopefully overcome. There may also be a time limit to the usefulness of such groups. Families who have worked through the pain of initial diagnosis may not benefit by an endless reliving of it by ongoing group participation (Meyerowitz and Kaplan, 1973).

Contact with other parents is helpful in providing support through a sense of universality, but parents may need to work separately with a mental health professional to deal with idiosyncratic issues attributable to personal history and maladaptive family interaction patterns. Part of this process can be educational—sharing with families the kinds of difficulties that often arise (shame, overprotection, resentment, lessening of the marital bond, etc.). Most families can then benefit from short-term work, which has a double focus: 1) understanding family communication and interaction patterns and changing them to maximize support for all members, and 2) working on the gradual process of accepting the diagnosis and exploring the reasons for difficulty at any point in this process. An approach like Minuchin et al.'s (1975), which is short-term, focused, and in which the therapist is active and at times directive, is an effective way to encompass both issues (Liebman, Minuchin, and Baker, 1976). Parents need special sessions for themselves, but it is essential that siblings and the patient be included (when age allows) in such sessions. Meyerowitz and Kaplan (1973) also suggest groups for the siblings of cystic fibrosis patients, because they, too, share issues that peers at school or in the neighborhood do not. The relationship built during this initial phase can be called into play at stress points throughout the course of illness. It is for this reason that a stable team member who has continuous contact with patients and staff can be most helpful.

The medical staff can aid in other ways to help promote adjustment and prevent crises. Patterson (1973) recommends that patients and families be told early that once patients reach the age of 15 they will be seen medically without their parents. This announcement can aid in having the child take over increasing responsibility for his care and can avert some of the problems in adolescence. Winder and Medalle (1973) also recommend therapy groups for adolescent patients. At this point patients may need the kind of support that their families needed at the time of initial diagnosis, and group treatment is often felt to be effective with adolescents because it minimizes the resistance to treatment as a sign of resistance to adult intervention. For older adolescents and young adults self-help groups have been useful. These can focus on shared solutions of common problems with schooling, jobs, social life, etc. (Boyle et al., 1976; McCoy, 1976). The group can even plan outings to provide recreation and medically advised exercise in a protective group with medical personnel available. Experiences that show the cystic fibrosis patient that he can do "normal" things are of great help in developing a more positive, potent self-image and in instilling the hope for an enjoyable life needed to continue to fight the disease.

Finally, families should be afforded the same opportunity to meet with a professional when the cystic fibrosis patient is dying as that that they were given initially. Help should be available informally (visits to the patient's room or to the patient's waiting area by staff) and in traditional therapy sessions. The patient should also have some person with whom he can discuss his feelings about dying. (This person may be the psychologist or social worker, but can be a favorite nurse, doctor, medical student—whoever is able to be there and listen.) After a patient's death, follow-up with the family is critical. First, they may need help on the process of mourning. (Siblings are, as mentioned, at particular risk and need evaluation during this time.) Second, the staff of the center and/or hospital have become an integral part of the family's support system, and it would greatly compound the loss of the child if all these people were "lost" at the same time.

The total approach to psychological intervention should emphasize parsimony. The less intervention the better. The goal can best be accomplished by using observations by other staff members and knowledge of the disease to take preventive steps that are geared specifically to the particular crisis or issue facing the cystic fibrosis patient and his family at any given time. More global, traditional psychotherapeutic approaches should be reserved for those times when psychological problems based on *internal* conflict necessitate a basic personality change. Otherwise, the approach can be most helpful and acceptable if it is issue specific. For example, talking to other cystic fibrosis parents may help the parents with feelings about the initial diagnosis but be of little use in dealing with a rebellious, suicidal adolescent. If help in an appropriate form is offered during the crises before a maladaptive solution is developed by the child and family, then the amount of psychological intervention will be minimal.

Role of the Pediatric Psychologist and Mental Health Professionals

A multidisciplinary team consisting of medical, nursing, social work, physical therapy, and psychology or psychiatry staff is the optimal approach to providing services to the cystic fibrosis child and his parents. Medical problems can certainly impinge on social and emotional well-being and vice versa. The patient will need the help of all these professionals at some point, and a group that meets regularly and is aware of all input can provide effective, well-coordinated sharing of information with and about the patient and can protect the child from conflicting approaches.

The mental health professional who is affiliated with a multidisciplinary team treating cystic fibrosis patients can perform a variety of services. He can, of course, provide direct service via psychotherapy and counseling to patients and their families. Education of medical staff is also crucial. Sensitizing staff to the psychological pitfalls of the disease and helping staff to listen for the signs of emotional difficulty, as well as physical distress, is a task for the mental health worker. The psychologist or psychiatrist (who traditionally have had a consultation role) should also consult with the staff on ways they can deal with problems such as parental resistance to treatment, adolescent rebellion, etc. Sensitized physicians, nurses, and physical therapists can (and must) provide important psychological support to the cystic fibrosis patient and his family through their more frequent and continuous contacts. Finally, the mental health professional can serve as a support person and sounding board to the staff. The psychological stress of dealing with these patients is great, and, in a center where staff deal almost exclusively with cystic fibrosis patients, they, at times, will need help in dealing with their feelings toward a difficult parent, a rebellious adolescent, or the loss of a long-time patient.

In addition to these duties, the mental health professional involved with cystic fibrosis patients has a responsibility to keep abreast of new developments in the diagnosis and treatment of the disease. The exact causes of the disease are unknown and the variety of ways it is manifest are poorly understood. (Recently a 44-year-old man was diagnosed as having cystic fibrosis. There is a report of a 63-year-old with the disease (Scully, Galdabini, and McNeely, 1977).) Some patients and their families are usually aware of new information and may use it or distort it to fit their own psychological needs. The psychologist or social worker cannot hide behind his nonmedical position if families are to be helped in the assimilation of such information realistically. The physician can provide factual material to the parents, but the mental health professional may be more aware of the emotional issues involved and can be instrumental in helping the family assimilate the physician's facts.

SUMMARY

Any disease that affects breath is terrifying, but those chronic conditions affecting the lungs have a particularly strong psychological effect. Asthma and cystic fibrosis demonstrate two aspects of the psychological aspects of chronic pediatric pulmonary disease.

Asthma, which is a physiologically based disease, can be exacerbated by emotional stress, psychological suggestion, and conditioning of wheezing through social reinforcers. It is a disease in which psychological intervention can be helpful in decreasing the frequency and severity of attacks. This intervention can have one of two foci: 1) control of symptoms, or 2) change of environmental response to symptoms. Most children can benefit from such techniques as biofeedback, disensitization to psychological stimuli, and behavior modification methods to increase compliance to treatment, which enhance their active control over their disease. In addition, children whose family situation is such, or whose own personal conflicts are such, that compliance to treatment or reduction of stress is difficult may need more traditional forms of psychotherapy or residential treatment to eliminate emotion-triggering agents. Mental health professionals can aid asthmatic children by providing these services and by educating medical personnel about the variety of interventions available.

Cystic fibrosis is a genetically transmitted disease involving the exocrine glands. While many organs are affected, pulmonary symptoms are the aspect of the disease that proves fatal. Parents must be actively involved in time-consuming treatments, which can postpone death to adolescence or early adulthood at best. Psychological intervention cannot change the course of this disease. It is crucial in helping patients and families deal with the devastating effects of the disease. The time of initial diagnosis, the adolescence of the patient, and the patient's death comprise three critical points or crises in the psychological course of the disease. Resolution of the issues at each point may be facilitated by appropriate psychological intervention and is important to the emotional well-being of the patient and of the family members who will survive him.

Chronic disease requires involvement over time by the mental health professional. This, however, does not mean continuous involvement. It is important in dealing with the psychological aspects of chronic pulmonary disease to assess the parameters of a crisis at any point in time and to provide services directed specifically toward those issues.

ACKNOWLEDGMENTS

I would like to thank Robert T. Scanlon, M.D., and members of the interdisciplinary team of the Pediatric Pulmonary Center of the Georgetown University Medical Center for their advice in preparing this chapter.

REFERENCES

Aaronson, D. 1972. Asthma: General concepts. In R. Patterson (ed.), Allergic Disease: Diagnosis and Management, pp. 197–239. J. B. Lippincott Co., Philadelphia.

Alexander, F. 1950. Psychosomatic Medicine, Its Principles and Application. W. W. Norton & Co., New York.

Bastiaans, J., and Groen, J. 1955. Psychogenesis and psychotherapy of bronchial asthma. In D. O'Neill (ed.), Modern Trends in Psychosomatic Medicine, pp. 242–268. Butterworth & Co., London.

Belmonte, M., and St. Germain, Y., 1973. Psychosocial aspects of the cystic fibrosis family. In P. R. Patterson, C. R. Denning, and A. H. Kutscher (eds.), Psychosocial Aspects of Cystic Fibrosis, pp. 84–92. Columbia University Press, New York.

Boat, T., and Helman, B. n.d. Educational and Vocational Counseling for Young Adults with Cystic Fibrosis. Cystic Fibrosis Foundation, Atlanta, Ga.

Boyle, I. R., diSant'Agnese, P. A., Sack, S., Millican, F., and Kulczycki, L. 1976. Emotional adjustment of adolescents and young adults with cystic fibrosis. J. Pediatr. 88:318–326.

Bushman, P., 1973. Care of the dying adolescent: A case history. In P. R. Patterson, C. R. Denning, and A. H. Kutscher (eds.), Psychosocial Aspects of Cystic Fibrosis, pp. 98–102. Columbia University Press, New York.

Cohen, S. I. 1971. Psychological factors in asthma: A review of their aetiological and therapeutic significance. Postgrad. Med. J. 47:533–540.

Criep, L. 1976. Pharmacologic modulation of antigen antibody release of chemical mediators. In L. Criep (ed.), Allergy and Clinical Immunology, pp. 109–118. Grune & Stratton, New York.

Cutter, F. 1955. Maternal Behavior and Childhood Allergy. Catholic University of America Press, Washington, D.C.

Davies, M., and Addington, W., 1973. Psychosocial aspects of cystic fibrosis family life as they affect medical management. In P. R. Patterson, C. R. Denning, and A. H. Kutscher (eds.), Psychosocial Aspects of Cystic Fibrosis, pp. 59–70. Columbia University Press, New York.

Dekker, B., Barendregt, J., and deVries, K. 1961. Allergy and neurosis in asthma. J. Psychosom. Res. 5:83–89.

Dekker, E., and Groen, J. 1956. Reproducible psychogenic attacks of asthma. J. Psychosom. Res. 1:58–67.

Doctor, J. 1973. The chronically ill child: Soma and Psyche. In P. R. Patterson, C. R. Denning, and A. H. Kutscher (eds.), Psychosocial Aspects of Cystic Fibrosis, pp. 19–26. Columbia University Press, New York.

Dooley, R., 1973. Management of the terminal adolescent. In P. R. Patterson, C. R. Denning, and A. H. Kutscher (eds.), Psychosocial Aspects of Cystic Fibrosis, pp. 202–212. Columbia University Press, New York.

Dubo, S., McLean, J. A., Ching, A. Y. T., Wright, H. L., Kauffman, P. E., and Sheldon, J. M. 1961. A study of relationships between family situation, bronchial asthma and personal adjustment in children. J. Pediatr. 59:402–414.

Ellis, E. F., 1975. Allergic disorders. In V. Vaugh and R. J. McKay (eds.), Nelson Textbook of Pediatrics, pp. 492–521. W. B. Saunders Co., Philadelphia.

Farkas, A. and Schnell, R., 1973. A psychological study of family adjustment to cystic fibrosis. In P. R. Patterson, C. R. Denning, and A. H. Kutscher (eds.), Psychosocial Aspects of Cystic Fibrosis, pp. 202–212. Columbia University Press, New York.

Feldman, G. 1976. The effect of biofeedback training on respiratory resistance of asthmatic children. Psychosom. Med. 38:27–34.

Findlay, I. I., Smith, P., Graves, P. J., and Linton, M. L. 1969. Chronic disease in childhood: a study of family reactions. Br. J. Med. Educ. 3:66–69.

Fitzelle, G. 1959. Personality factors and certain attitudes toward child rearing among parents of asthmatic children. Psychosom. Med. 21:208–217.

Freeman, E. H., Feingold, B. F., Schlesinger, K., and Gorman, F. J. 1964. Psychological variables in allergic disorders: a review. Psychosom. Med. 26:543–575.

French, T. M. 1950. Emotional conflict and allergy. Int. Arch. Allergy Appl. Immunol. 1:28–40.

Graham, D. T., Lundy, R. M., Benjamin, L. S., Kabler, J. D., Lewis, W. C., Kunish, N. O., and Graham, F. K. 1962. Specific attitudes in initial interviews with patients having different "psychosomatic" diseases. Psychosom. Med. 24:257–266.

Guyton, A. 1977. Basic Human Physiology. Normal functions and mechanisms of disease. 2nd Ed. W. B. Saunders Co., Philadelphia.

Helman, B., 1973. Death and bereavement in chronic lung disease. In P. R. Patterson, C. R. Denning, and A. H. Kutscher (eds.), Psychosocial Aspects of Cystic Fibrosis, pp. 95–97. Columbia University Press, New York.

Holsclaw, D., Dooley, R., Gibson, L., Grand, R., Hilman, B., Huang, N., Selden, R., Jr., Schwachman, H., and Talamo, R. 1973. Cystic Fibrosis Medical Information: A summary of symptoms, diagnosis and treatment. Cystic Fibrosis Foundation, Atlanta, Ga.

Jones, R. H. T., and Jones, R. S. 1966. Ventilatory capacity in young adults with a history of asthma in childhood. Br. Med. J. 2:976–978.

Jones, R. S., Buston, M. H., and Wharton, M. J. 1962. The effect of exercise on ventilatory function in the child with asthma. Br. J. Dis. Chest 56:78–86.

Kempe, C., Silver, H., and O'Brien, D. 1974. Current Pediatric Diagnosis and Treatment. 3rd Ed. Lange Medical Publications, Los Altos, Cal.

Kubler-Ross, E. 1969. On Death and Dying. The Macmillan Co., London.

Kulczycki, L. L., Regal, D., and Tantisunthorn, C. 1973. The impact of cystic fibrosis on the parents and patients. In P. R. Patterson, C. R. Denning, and A. H. Kutscher (eds.), Psychosocial Aspects of Cystic Fibrosis, pp. 117–133. Columbia University Press, New York.

Lawler, R., Nakielny, W., and Wright, N. A. 1966. Psychological implications of cystic fibrosis. Can. Med. Assoc. J. 94:1043–1046.

Leigh, D., and Marley, E. 1956. A psychiatric assessment of adult asthmatics: A statistical study. J. Psychosom. Res. 1:128–136.

Liebman, R., Minuchin, S., and Baker, L. 1976. The use of structural family therapy in the treatment of intractable asthma. Am. J. Psychiatry 131:535–540.

Liggens, M., 1975. Cystic fibrosis into the teens and beyond. Patient Care 120–144.

Little, S. W., and Cohen, L. D. 1951. Goal-setting behavior of asthmatic children and of their mothers for them. J. Pers. 19:376–389.

Lorin, M., 1973. The twilight hours. In P. R. Patterson, C. R. Denning, and A. H. Kutscher (eds.), Psychosocial Aspects of Cystic Fibrosis, pp. 27–33. Columbia University Press, New York.

Luparello, T., Lyons, H. A., Bleecher, E. R., and McFadden, E. R., Jr. 1968. Influences of suggestion on airway reactivity in asthmatic subjects. Psychosom. Med. 30:819–825.

McCoy, J. 1976. Psychosocial aspects of cystic fibrosis in young adults. Presented at Cystic Fibrosis in Young Adults. A Clinical Symposium, December 17, Washington, D.C.

McKey, R. Jr., 1973. Coping with a family-shattering disease. In P. R. Patterson, C. R. Denning, and A. H. Kutscher (eds.), Psychosocial Aspects of Cystic Fibrosis, pp. 93–94. Columbia University Press, New York.

McLean, J., and Ching, A. 1973. Follow-up study of relationships between family situation and bronchial asthma in children. J. Am. Acad. Child. Psychiatry 12:142–161.

Mattson, A. 1975. Psychologic aspects of childhood asthma. Pediatr. Clin. North Am. 22:77–88.

Meyerowitz, J., and Kaplan, H., 1973. Cystic fibrosis and family functioning. In P. R. Patterson, C. R. Denning, and A. H. Kutscher (eds.), Psychological Aspects of Cystic Fibrosis, pp. 34–58. Columbia University Press, New York.

Miller, H., and Baruch, D. W. 1948. Psychosomatic studies of children with allergic manifestations. I. Maternal rejection: A study of 63 cases. Psychosom. Med. 10:275–278.

Miller, N. E. 1969. Learning of visceral and glandular responses. Science 163:434–445.

Minuchin, S., Baker, L., Rasman, B. L., Liebman, R., Melman, L., and Todd, T. C. 1975. A conceptual model of psychosomatic illness in children. Family organization and family therapy. Arch. Gen. Psychiatry 32:1031–1038.

Moore, N. 1965. Behavior therapy in bronchial asthma: A controlled study. J. Psychosom. Res. 9:257–276.

Neuhaus, E. C. 1958. A personality study of asthmatic and cardiac children. Psychosom. Med. 20:181–186.

Patterson, P., 1973. Psychosocial aspects of cystic fibrosis. In P. R. Patterson, C. R. Denning, and A. H. Kutscher (eds.), Psychosocial Aspects of Cystic Fibrosis, pp. 3–12. Columbia University Press, New York.

Peshkin, M. 1968. Analysis of the role of residential asthma centers for children with intractable asthma. J. Asthma Res. 6:59–92.

Rees, L. 1956. Physical and emotional factors in bronchial asthma. J. Psychosom. Res. 1:98–114.

Ring, F. O. 1957. Testing the validity of personality profiles in psychosomatic illnesses. Am J. Psychiatry 113:1075–1080.

Ross, W. D., Hay, J., and McDowell, M. F. 1950. The association of certain vegetative disturbances with various psychoses. Psychosom. Med. 12:170–178.

Sabinga, M., Friedman, C., and Huang, N., 1973. The family of the cystic fibrosis patient. In P. R. Patterson, C. R. Denning, and A. H. Kutscher (eds.), Psychosocial Aspects of Cystic Fibrosis, pp. 13–18. Columbia University Press, New York.

Sadler, J. E. 1975. The long term hospitalization of asthmatic children. Pediatr. Clin. North Am. 22(1):173–183.

Saul, L. J., and Lyons, J. W. 1951. The psychodynamics of respiration. In H. A. Abramson (ed.), Somatic and Psychiatric Treatment of Asthma, pp. 93–103. The Williams & Wilkins Co., Baltimore.

Sclare, A. B., and Crochet, J. A. 1952. Group psychotherapy in bronchial asthma. J. Psychosom. Res. 2:157–171.

Scully, R. E., Galdabini, J., and McNeely, B. U. 1977. Case records of the Massachusetts General Hospital: Case 26-1977. New Engl. J. Med. 296:1519–1526.

Smith, J. M., and Burns, C. L. C. 1960. The treatment of asthmatic children by hypnotic suggestion. Br. J. Dis. Chest 54:78–81.

Swartz, J., and Semrad, E. V. 1951. Psychosomatic disorders in psychoses. Psychosom. Med. 13:314–321.

Taussig, L. M., Lobeck, C. C., diSant'Agnese, P. A., Ackerman, D. R., and Kattwinkel, J. 1972. Fertility in males with cystic fibrosis. New Engl. J. Med. 287:586–589.

Tropauer, A., Franz, M. N., and Dilgard, V. W. 1970. Psychological aspects of the care of children with cystic fibrosis. Am. J. Dis. Child 119:424–432.

Vachon, L., and Rich, E. S. 1976. Visceral learning in asthma. Psychosom. Med. 38:122–130.

Warwick, W., and Shapero, B., 1973. The parental death wish. In P. R. Patterson, C. R. Denning, and A. H. Kutscher (eds.), Psychological Aspects of Cystic Fibrosis, pp. 193–196. Columbia University Press, New York.

Weiss, E. 1950. Psychosomatic aspects of certain allergic disorders. Int. Arch. Allergy 1:4–28.

Williams, H. E., and McNicol, K. N. 1975. The spectrum of asthma in children. Pediatr. Clin. North Am. 22:43–52.

Winder, A., and Medalle, M. 1973. Support for growth in cystic fibrosis teenagers. In P. R. Patterson, C. R. Denning, and A. H. Kutscher (eds.), Psychosocial Aspects of Cystic Fibrosis, pp. 103–114. Columbia University Press, New York.

Index